NEW, UPDATED EDITION

Dr. Pitcairn's Complete Guide to

NATURAL HEALTH
FOR
DOGS & CATS

Dr. Pitcairn's Complete Guide to

NATURAL HEALTH
FOR DOGS & CATS

Richard H. Pitcairn, D.V.M., Ph.D. & Susan Hubble Pitcairn, M.S.

Rodale Press, Inc.
Emmaus, Pennsylvania

NOTICE

This book is meant to supplement the advice and guidance of your veterinarian. No two medical conditions are the same. Moreover, we cannot be responsible for unsupervised treatments administered at home. Therefore, we urge you to seek out the best medical resources available to help you make informed decisions on pet care.

Printed in the United States of America on acid-free ∞ , recycled paper ♻

Cover Designer: Lynn N. Gano
Cover Illustrator: Deborah Chabrian
Illustrator: Frank Fretz

Library of Congress Cataloging-in-Publication Data

Pitcairn, Richard H.
    Dr. Pitcairn's complete guide to natural health for dogs and cats/
  by Richard H. Pitcairn and Susan Hubble Pitcairn. — Rev. ed.
     p. cm.
    Includes index.
    ISBN 0–87596–243–2 paperback
    1. Dogs. 2. Cats. 3. Dogs—Health. 4. Cats—Health. 5. Dogs—Diseases.
6. Cats—Diseases. I. Pitcairn, Susan Hubble. II. Title. III. Title: Complete
guide to natural health for dogs and cats.
SF427.P63 1995
636.7'083—dc20   94–44229

Distributed in the book trade by St. Martin's Press

8   10 9   paperback

— OUR PURPOSE —

*"We inspire and enable people to improve
their lives and the world around them."*

CONTENTS

Foreword viii
Preface xi
Acknowledgments xiii

PART 1 NATURAL HEALTH FOR PETS

CHAPTER 1   We Need a New Approach to Pet Health Care 2
CHAPTER 2   What Do They Really Put in Pet Food? 7
CHAPTER 3   Try a Basic Natural Diet—With Supplements 22
CHAPTER 4   Easy-to-Make Recipes for Pet Food 43
CHAPTER 5   Special Diets for Special Pets 60
CHAPTER 6   Helping Your Pet Make the Switch 80
CHAPTER 7   Exercise, Rest and Natural Grooming 89
CHAPTER 8   Creating a Healthier Environment 104
CHAPTER 9   Choosing a Healthy Animal 114
CHAPTER 10   Emotional Connections and Your Pet's Health 144
CHAPTER 11   Neighborly Relations: Responsible Pet Ownership 149
CHAPTER 12   Lifestyles: Tips for Special Situations 174
CHAPTER 13   Saying Good-Bye: Coping with a Pet's Death 183
CHAPTER 14   Holistic and Alternative Therapies 189
CHAPTER 15   How to Care For a Sick Animal 207

PART 2 QUICK REFERENCE

How to Use the Quick Reference Section 222
Abscesses 227
Allergies 229
Anal Gland Problems 232
Anemia 233
Appetite Problems 234
Arthritis 235
Behavior Problems 237
Bladder Problems 239
Breast Tumors 244
Cancer 245

Constipation 248
Dental Problems 250
Diabetes 253
Diarrhea and Dysentery 255
Distemper, Chorea and Feline Panleukopenia 257
Ear Problems 261
Epilepsy 265
Eye Problems 267
Feline Immunodeficiency Virus 269
Feline Infectious Peritonitis 270
Feline Leukemia 272
Foxtails 274
Hair Loss 275
Heart Problems 275
Heartworms 277
Hip Dysplasia 280
Jaundice 281
Kidney Failure 282
Liver Problems 286
Lyme Disease 288
Pancreatitis 290
Paralysis 291
Pregnancy, Birth and Care of Newborns 293
Rabies 296
Radiation Toxicity 296
Reproductive Organ Problems 297
Skin Parasites 299
Skin Problems 303
Spaying and Neutering 308
Stomach Problems 309
Toxoplasmosis 315
Upper Respiratory Infections 317
Vaccinations 321
Vomiting 326
Warts 327
Weight Problems 327
Worms 330

SPECIAL GUIDES

Handling Emergencies and Giving First Aid 337
Schedule for Herbal Treatment 346
Schedule for Homeopathic Treatment 348
Additional Recipes 350
Sources of Natural Pet Products 352
Recommended Reading and Tapes 357
Normal Values of Vital Signs 360
Index 363

TABLES

Recommended Grains 28
Recommended Legumes 30
Best Ingredient Choices for Feeding Your Pet 32
Nutritional Composition of Recipes for Dogs 54
Nutritional Composition of Recipes for Cats 56
Average Caloric Needs for Adult Dogs 59
Average Caloric Needs for Adult Cats 59
Feeding Dogs with Extra Needs 64
Feeding Cats with Extra Needs 66
Kitten Feeding Schedule 69
Nutritional Composition of Growth Recipes and Vegetarian Recipes for Dogs 72
Nutritional Composition of Growth Recipes and Vegetarian Recipes for Cats 74
Common Ingredients in Flea-Control Products 98
Behavioral Patterns and Congenital Defects in Dogs 124
Behavioral Patterns and Congenital Defects in Cats 138

FOREWORD

It is a refreshing change to write a foreword for a book such as this, written by a kindred spirit who, in grasping the holistic principles of health and disease and with courage and conviction, dares to go against the narrow mainstream and consensus of veterinary medicine to open up new frontiers.

As a recent graduate in veterinary medicine in 1962, I wrote a clinical treatise on "sympathy-lameness" in dogs, describing how emotionally disturbed dogs and those soliciting the attentions of their owners will actually feign injury to one of their legs. Some veterinarians publicly ridiculed this study, since it was inconceivable that animals could be afflicted with emotional and psychosomatic disorders.

Today there is more widespread recognition of such phenomena: Humans are not the only intelligent, sensitive beings on Earth. Our animal kin can also suffer from a wide variety of emotional problems, as Dr. Pitcairn describes in this book. Yet the suggestion that animals have emotions that can affect their health will still be met with strong resistance, because many "experts" believe that such interpretations are anthropomorphic.

Similarly, most people never even consider that animals should be accorded rights and become part of the community of moral concern. The usual view is that animals are inferior to us, so we can exploit them as we choose without a twinge of conscience.

Above and beyond the ethical consideration of our dealings with animals is the pervading view that mind and body are separate. Nature is thus demystified or desanctified into a mere resource to be conquered and exploited for our exclusive use. Animals are "mechanomorphized"—seen as unfeeling machines, and treated as commodities. And humanity is likewise dehumanized, the body being considered just a survival machine for our genes or a biomechanical container holding the mind. Furthermore, with this fragmented world view, humanity becomes increasingly separated and alienated from nature, animals and from the totality of our own being and becoming.

Such erroneous beliefs and values are being challenged today, since they lie at the roots of our contemporary social and environmental ills. Modern physics, ecology and various Eastern philosophies all have shown that we live in a unified field. It is imperative for our own health and our future survival that we think and act *eco*centrically rather than *ego*centrically. Our values, beliefs and wants must become attuned to the totality of life, so that enlightened self-interest is in concord with the greater good. This new, world-embracing ethic includes a universal reverence for all life, including animal life. It is urgently needed.

Such is the philosophy behind the holistic medicine that Dr. Pitcairn and a handful of other veterinarians are applying to animals. As is often the case, Dr. Pitcairn's introduction to holistic medicine began with personal experience, first with experiencing the effect of changing his dietary habits and then of treating his own child with herbal medicine. This led him to the realization "that many chronic and degenerative diseases we see today are caused or complicated by inadequate diets." Since the immune system is especially vulnerable to dietary imbalances, Dr. Pitcairn did graduate research, obtaining a Ph.D. in advanced studies in immunology. Yet such specialization had limited practical application and seemed to confuse rather than clarify the nature of health and disease. So, after his graduate studies were completed, he reassessed the modern approach to animal health problems and realized the narrowness and ineffectuality of such an approach, especially in chronic, degenerative and psychosomatic disorders.

He knew intuitively that it is bad medicine not to see health problems "in relation to the whole and to become lost in the division of our artificial labels and definitions." Furthermore, he learned through personal experience that healing (and health maintenance) entails not only specific therapies, but also major lifestyle changes.

As an animal doctor with such insight and knowledge, he has made the obvious and most intelligent decision: to develop a holistic health care and maintenance program for pets, together with a valuable encyclopedia of treatments for veterinarians and pet owners (ideally under the supervision of their pets' doctors) to use. Certainly, much more research is needed, especially in veterinary chiropractic, herbology and homeopathy. Veterinary acupuncture is being practiced by an increasing number of veterinarians, and my own book on pet massage, *The Healing Touch: The Proven Massage Program for Cats and Dogs*, opens up new vistas for pet owners and veterinarians to help pets through sickness and also maintain their overall physical and psychological well-being.

Holistic medicine respects and is attuned to the "wisdom of the body." This body wisdom—the connection between body-sensitivity and mind awareness—has almost been lost to modern civilization, which separates mind from body, man from animal and humanity from nature. We have to relearn the fact that our bodies are not machines, nor are animals'.

Albert Schweitzer, the great humanitarian and healer, said that the good doctor simply awakes "the physician within" the patient. Similarly, as Dr. Pitcairn so ably shows in this book, both the good veterinarian and the pet owner can help awaken and support the natural processes within the animal to help prevent illness and combat stress and disease.

The presence of the healer is part of the healing process. Talking to a person or animal in a quiet, gentle voice has a very similar effect to comforting (petting) or gentle, rhythmic massage. Researchers have shown that the effect is quite profound, the cardinal signs being a dramatic decrease in heart rate and a general relaxation in muscle tension. The change in heart rate is an indication that the parasympathetic nervous system is being stimulated. This is, I believe, part of the healing or tonic effect of gentle vocal or physical contact. When the parasympathetic nervous system is stimulated, the digestive system is stimulated; this is why the tender loving care of a mother rocking her baby and singing it a lullaby, or a cat or dog licking its offspring or companion, facilitates the digestive process.

Being emotionally deprived of the essential energy of another's affection is as bad as being deprived of some essential dietary nutrient. In fact, there are many physical, social and emotional "nutrients," such as exercise, play and recreation, affection, touch and companionship, that are vital components of total health care for human and beast alike.

The healer, by influencing the mind of the patient, together with directly affecting the body (via drugs, massage and so on), activates the physician within, restoring balance. Therefore, an animal is more likely to benefit if it is emotionally attached to the healer than if it were not attached or were being treated by a stranger. This is why the therapies suggested by Dr. Pitcairn for home use hold such great potential for pets and pet owners. Their effectiveness is enhanced by the close emotional bond between pet and owner.

Holistic living is living in harmony with ourselves, each other and with nature as a whole; it is knowing that the quality of relationships influences our state of health as much as our temperament, perceptions, genetic constitution and such. The same holds true for the health of our pets. And the more removed we and they are from nature, the more disharmony and privation, the more sickness and suffering there are in the world.

This book will help pet owners make a better life for their pets and for themselves as well. Dr. Pitcairn provides the essential enlightenment for a fully responsible, fulfilling and healthful relationship between humans and animals.

With this book, pets have never had it so good!

MICHAEL W. FOX, D.SC., PH.D.,
   B. VET. MED., M.R.C.V.S.
Vice President of the
Humane Society of the United States

PREFACE

I am a very lucky man.

There are few of us that have the good fortune to have their dreams come true. One of my dreams, from an early age, was to be able to relieve the suffering of disease and even cure (in the true sense of the word) the terrible diseases that afflict our animal friends. Sixteen years ago, I "discovered" homeopathic medicine. Along with nutrition, this wonderful method of treatment became the tool that I needed to bring this dream to fruition.

Since converting my practice to the use of homeopathy and nutrition, my experience of being a veterinarian has been transformed. I am really, truly seeing animals get well from conditions that are simply considered incurable and hopeless from the conventional perspective.

Not all patients can be helped, of course. It depends on how much damage has been done. However, a much larger percentage of chronically ill animals can be brought to health than one would ever expect from our experience with the dominant school of medicine.

To me, this has been a most illuminating experience. I never thought that there was a system of medicine that could do a better job than what I was taught in veterinary school. How could I have gone through all those years of training and not have heard of it? I now realize that this is the situation for many veterinarians who are looking for a better answer. Responding to this need, in the last few years, I have turned my attention to the training of other veterinarians in this system of healing. As Susan and I put the second edition of this book "to bed," we are in the middle of the second Professional Course in Veterinary Homeopathy with close to 40 participating veterinarians. We are also establishing the Academy of Veterinary Homeopathy, which will serve as the guiding organization for training and research.

These are very exciting developments for those of us in alternative medicine. I am very grateful for my good fortune in seeing these things come to fruition. I am also very thankful for the wonderful acceptance our book has had among both the public and the veterinary profession, so my final thanks is to you, the reader, for your interest and for your support.

RICHARD H. PITCAIRN

Everything connects to everything, which connects to everything else. You can't understand life in fragments. That has been a guiding principle behind this book and, I believe, the key to its success and endurance.

From a wider perspective, the topic of natural care for dogs and cats offers an enormous opportunity to show the value of taking a holistic approach to any aspect of life.

That has been the real joy in creating it, as a kind of tribute to the sacred wholeness of creation.

Now, even more than the first time around, I see this book as our admission that, despite our specialized scientific knowledge, we simply cannot grasp the wholeness of life from the details of its workings. So, ultimately, the best we can do in caring for a living creature is to approximate the natural conditions under which it thrived for millions of years, and, where we can, to gently stimulate the natural vital force to right itself when it has become unbalanced. From this perspective, one can meaningfully look anew at every detail of how we care for animals: their diet, their living quarters, their social interactions with other animals and with us, the ways they are affected by the environment, and the use of natural remedies.

From this larger perspective, we are also freed, indeed impelled, to explore past the limits of old assumptions: Perhaps "pet food" is not the only thing that pets can eat; perhaps animals are affected by our thoughts and feelings; perhaps there is a system of healing that trusts and goes with the body's intelligence rather than tinkering with its expression; perhaps we have come to the point that, for our mutual survival, we must consider the ecological impact of our choices.

If this book serves to communicate a healthy respect for the intelligence behind creation and a sense that we would do well to interfere with natural processes as little as possible, then I would know that its deeper purpose, and mine, has been fulfilled.

SUSAN HUBBLE PITCAIRN

ACKNOWLEDGMENTS

Producing a book is a lot like making a film. It's a team effort. Yet the authors' or actors' names and faces appear so prominently that we can easily overlook the tremendous contributions made by those working behind the scenes.

Though this is the second edition of this book, we want to repeat our thanks to the editor of the first edition, who helped make it accessible and helpful to so many pet owners. Carol Keough lovingly coached us through the original edition. She carved away the excess, sanded the rough spots and polished the surface until the whole thing began to shine. To her we owe tremendous thanks for the success that this book has become. For this updated, revised and much expanded edition, Charlie Gerras offered patient, encouraging support and helped us stay at least somewhat on schedule as we struggled to meet the deadlines. (Busyness usually goes hand in hand with success and no one understood better than Charlie.)

Our appreciation extends no less to the many dedicated people at Rodale Press who worked on both editions, particularly to John Feltman and Mark Bricklin, whose faith and encouragement originally convinced us that we should put our earlier understanding to pen and typewriter, and to Sharon Faelten and Rob Sayre, who urged us to put our increased experience to scanner and keyboard (a lot has changed in 14 years, personal computers being just one of them).

Just as essential were the tireless teams of fact-checkers, whose job it was to verify every calculation and every reference. We especially owe a debt of thanks to Susan Rosenkrantz, Holly Clemson, Carol Baldwin, Carol Matthews, Martha Capwell, Sue Ann Gursky, Christy Kohler, Susan Nastasee and Joann Williams. Credit to Roberta Mulliner for seeing to the translation of the disks we sent. And a salute to Mary Lou Stephen for patiently incorporating editorial changes as the manuscript made its way to the final version. We could go on naming the contributors at Rodale—from the copy editors, typesetters, designers and illustrators, to those who handled the mysteries of marketing, finance and sales. We thank each and every one.

For the development of our ideas and experience, we are very grateful to the many wonderful clients, readers and colleagues whose shared commitment to natural healing for animals has made all the difference. Special thanks for the first edition go to those who tested our original recipes and to my ever-supportive co-workers, Tootie Truesdell and Dottie Warner. For the second edition, special thanks go to my associate Jana Rygas, D.V.M., for her detailed contributions to behavioral issues in chapter 11 and for her unflagging enthusiasm. To Deborah Kearns and Sheya Rondeau, my dedicated assistants, goes great appreciation for years of positive, intelligent service on behalf of natural medicine. Without them it would have been impossible to find the time this last year to write and revise.

In the wider circle of our lives, we are very blessed to have some of the finest clients and colleagues that any veterinarian could ever hope for. You are too many to name, but we treasure the difference you have made in our lives and in this work. To our former neighbor, author and editor Al Strickland goes a special thank you for guiding us through the intricacies of book contracts. To Anitra Frazier, author of *The New Natural Cat*, heartfelt thanks for years of support, encouragement and bringing many clients our way.

When it comes to the heart of this book, the ideas behind it—the unseen crew is graced by hundreds of pioneers whose commitment to healing and understanding has inspired, informed, challenged, taught and healed us and many others. To name just a few: Samuel Hahnemann, the father of homeopathy; James Tyler Kent, after Hahnemann the most gifted homeopathic physician; George Vithoulkas and Bill Gray, who together wrote *The Science of Homeopathy*, the book that started Richard on his life-work in homeopathy; Constantine Hering, T. F. Allen and H. C. Allen, John Henry Clarke, J. Compton Burnett, C. M. Boger and countless other physicians who refined homeopathy and gave it to the world; Paavolo Airola, who taught us to trust nature's ways; Juliette de Bairacli-Levy, who shared the wisdom of ages of folk medicine; J. Allen Boone, who showed us that animals are far more than we imagine them to be; and John Robbins and Debra Dadd, who made us more acutely aware that individual health is inseparable from the choices we make about the health of our environment.

Lastly, to all the animals of the world—both domestic and wild—who feel, who suffer, who delight, who share in the fate of this increasingly fragile planet—we offer our appreciation and the hope that this work will be of benefit.

To them, and to all the human members of the "crew," we dedicate this book.

RICHARD H. PITCAIRN, D.V.M., PH.D.
SUSAN HUBBLE PITCAIRN, M.S.

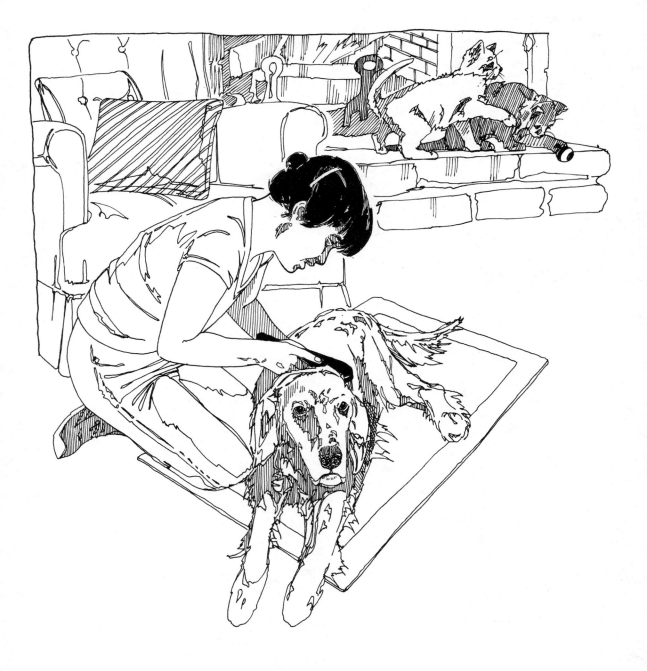

Part One
Natural Health for Pets

CHAPTER ONE

WE NEED A NEW APPROACH TO PET HEALTH CARE

Why don't you take care of this one?" my colleague asked me, with the look of someone about to unload an unwelcome problem. He pointed through the door to a little middle-aged dog sitting forlornly on the examining table. If his coat had ever been sleek, soft and healthy, it was no more. Obviously, his hair had been falling out for some time, revealing large greasy patches that had an unpleasant odor. Even his spirits were low. Unfortunately, I'd seen cases like his all too often.

Waiting nearby were the dog's equally dejected guardians, an aging couple who had "tried it all," and still cared enough about their little companion to try once more. The dog's hospital record showed a long history of treatments—cortisone shots, medicated soaps, ointments, more shots, more salves—none of which brought any noticeable improvement.

"The poor little guy is just *so miserable*, doctor," began Mrs. Wilson anxiously. "We would do anything if we thought it would help."

It didn't take me long to decide that it was finally time to step off the beaten path and try out a new nutritional approach to this kind of case, an idea that had been brewing in my mind for some time. We were at a medical dead end and there was nothing to lose. But more important, I knew there was a good chance that what I had in mind might work. As I examined Tiny, I explained to the Wilsons why I thought an improved diet was their animal's best chance for recovery.

"Skin problems like his are probably the most common and frustrating of the conditions we try to deal with," I told them. "Because the skin is such a visible area of the body, it can show the first signs of underlying problems, particularly those caused by inadequate diet. The skin grows very rapidly, making a whole new crop of cells about every three weeks. It needs a lot of nourishment, so when the diet lacks what's really needed, the skin is one of the first tissues to break down and show abnormalities like the kind we see here in Tiny."

As we went on talking about the effects of diet and the shortcomings of highly processed pet foods based on low-quality food by-products, the Wilsons saw that a change could make a big difference. So we worked out a suitable feeding program for Tiny, emphasizing fresh natural foods.

Starting now, Tiny would eat meat, whole grains and fresh vegetables. In addition, the Wilsons would give him several supplements rich in nutrients important to the health of the skin as well as to the rest of the body—brewer's yeast, vegetable oil, cod-liver oil, kelp, bonemeal, vitamin E and zinc. I also recommended that they bathe Tiny occasionally with a mild nonmedicated shampoo to help remove irritating, toxic secretions from his skin without burdening his body with harsh chemicals.

During the next few weeks, my mind often went to Tiny, wondering how he was doing on this new treatment. A month after their first visit, the Wilsons returned to show the results of the treatment. Tiny was like a new dog.

"You wouldn't believe the difference!" Mrs. Wilson exclaimed. "He runs around and plays like he's a puppy again." Tiny was indeed full of life, jumping around excitedly on the examining table. His coat was much healthier, and hair was rapidly filling in the previously bare spots.

It was very rewarding to all of us, but most of all to Tiny. For the Wilsons, there was the added benefit of realizing that their dog's health was now in their control and that keeping him well did not require monthly injections of cortisone or other medications.

A NEW SENSE OF PURPOSE TAKES HOLD

Tiny's case was one of my first clinical attempts to apply the results of a long learning process concerning the vital role of nutrition in health. Now, after 17 years of seeing successes such as this with improved diet, the essential importance of nutrition in restoring health is obvious to me.

However, I did not always approach cases in such a manner. My veterinary school training in nutrition had included little more than the admonition: "Tell your clients to feed their animals a good commercial pet food and to avoid table scraps." Beyond that, nutrition just wasn't considered an important part of our education. I accepted this attitude at face value, and after graduation I set out to conquer disease armed with the usual arsenal of drugs and surgical techniques gleaned from my years of schooling.

Faced with the day-to-day challenges of my first job in a busy mixed practice (small and large animals), I soon learned that many diseases simply did not respond to treatments as I had been told they would. In fact, it often seemed that what I did to help mattered very little. I was like a bystander at the battle for recovery—doing a lot of cheering and occasionally making a contribution of sorts, but often feeling ineffectual.

So I tried to make sense of what I saw and gradually several basic questions arose: Why do some animals recover easily, while others never seem to do well, regardless of which drugs are used? Why do some animals in a group seem to have all the fleas and catch all the diseases going around, while others are never affected? I knew there must be some basic understanding that I just didn't grasp about the ability of an animal's body to defend and to heal itself.

When you ask a question long enough and deeply enough, life seems to provide the opportunity to find an answer. Soon a job offer as an instructor at a veterinary school was dropped in my lap. Always eager to be in a climate of learning, I immediately accepted.

Once I was back in academia, I decided to take a course or two myself, and the next thing I knew, I was a full-time graduate student in veterinary immunology, virology and biochemistry. Surely here, I thought, I can learn the real secrets of the body's defense systems. And so I set about studying and researching various problems, particularly the body's immune response to cancer.

Some five years and a Ph.D. degree later, I found that the answers to my questions still eluded me. Though I had acquired an even greater wealth of factual information about the mechanisms of immunology and metabolism, I still did not feel a sense of real insight about the issues that concerned me.

THE BIG PICTURE: THE HOLISTIC APPROACH

I had begun to realize what was causing me to feel baffled by conventional veterinary medicine. Knowledge was fragmented, and specialists clung to narrow academic disciplines. For example, one group of immunologists would hold a particular viewpoint on disease mechanisms and a second group, a different view. It seemed that no effort was being made to reconcile the opposing positions. And then there were the microbiologists, the virologists, the biochemists, the pathologists and a host of others, all of whom tended to see things through different sets of filters! Our research aims had become so narrowly defined and carried out that we were missing the whole picture. I didn't fully realize it at the time, but I felt, somehow, that what we really needed was a holistic approach to the problem of disease.

As a result, I started doing two things that were decisive and that have continued to be my style of operation ever since. One was to read broadly in many fields and from many sources to get a larger scope of concepts and ideas. The other was to experiment with new ideas that made sense to me by trying them out on myself.

I made it first priority to learn more about nutrition. After some self-directed study, I was convinced that nutrition was a very significant factor in maintaining health and treating disease. Therefore, it amazed me to find that the indifference to nutrition that prevailed when I was a student in veterinary school was still in place. There was a wealth of research, for example, showing that a number of specific vitamins are essential to the normal functioning of the immune system—though they were never mentioned throughout my years of graduate study. Most surprising to me was the fact that proper nutrition could boost the body's natural resistance to disease. Here was an incredible truth—unique in that it meant the body need not rely on drugs for better health. With this information, people could take charge of their own health. At last I was beginning to find some answers to my questions.

PERSONAL DIVIDENDS FROM A DIET CHANGE

I decided to change my own diet. I began to use whole grains, to cut out sugars and other junk foods, to eat less meat and to take supplements like nutritional yeast, wheat germ and various vitamins. Before long I was feeling better than I had in years.

I also started exercising regularly, using herbs and exploring my inner life. All these measures eventually played a part in removing some things from my life that I didn't need—like a potbelly I was developing, plus colitis, ear infections, excess tension, susceptibility to colds and flu, and a number of negative psychological habits.

Though these personal experiments didn't constitute so-called statistically significant studies, they were tremendously valuable to me. There is nothing more convincing about the value of a treatment than feeling better after using it. You don't need the interpretation or opinion of any authority to acknowledge positive changes in your own body and mind.

After helping myself, I began to apply my newfound knowledge to animals—first my own pets and then, as I returned to clinical practice, some "hopeless" cases like Tiny's. At one point, I adopted a stray kitten half-starved and ragged from life in the woods. We named her Sparrow because she looked like a small bird made up mostly of feathers and fluff. At first, I fed her a conventional kibble and she did all right. But when she became pregnant a year or two later, I decided to boost her strength. I faithfully added fresh raw beef liver, raw eggs, bonemeal, fresh chicken, brewer's yeast and other nutritious foods to her daily fare.

Unlike many cats I've seen, she never lost any weight or hair during pregnancy, and her delivery was exceptionally fast, easy and calm. She always had plenty of milk to nurse her three large, thriving kittens, and all of them grew up to be much larger than their mother. I kept one of these kittens and continued adding supplements to the diets of both mother and offspring. I was always amazed at how remarkably healthy they were. I never needed to use any flea control on them. And if one of these cats got scratched or bitten in a fight, the injury healed quickly and never developed into an infection or abscess. Sparrow lived to the ripe age of 18 years and never needed veterinary care for any of the common cat problems.

One thing led to another and soon I became deeply interested in using herbs as a treatment. A particular occasion convinced me that these natural remedies could bring about almost miraculous cures. It was late one Sunday night and my son, Clark, (then about six) was besieged by a high fever, flushed face, swollen throat glands and incipient bronchitis (to which he was prone). He was very restless and cried with extreme discomfort and pain. I had nothing in the house to give him except some aspirin, which neither reduced his fever nor enabled him to get to sleep.

I felt stuck, and I threshed about in my mind, desperately searching for some way to help Clark. Then all at once I remembered I had some goldenseal (*Hydrastis canadensis*) capsules in the house. Goldenseal has been found very useful for reducing inflammation of the lining of the bronchial tubes, the nose and the eustachian tubes (which drain the ears to the throat), especially when the inflammation is accompanied by a harsh, dry cough and fever. I gave him one capsule with a little water. Five to ten minutes later, Clark suddenly got up and, for the first time in hours, went to the bathroom and voided a large quantity of urine. Afterward, he lay down, relaxed and fell asleep. Clark's fever dropped rapidly and by the next morning, he was normal.

As you can imagine, this experience was very encouraging to me. Looking back, I realize how fortunate I was to have hit it so perfectly. Goldenseal was quite appropriate for the symptoms my son showed. This remarkable experience inspired me to pursue many fruitful directions later on, such as herbology, naturopathy and, especially, homeopathy. This last has completely changed my understanding of the nature of disease and its cure.

Though I eventually branched out in other directions, I have found over the years that proper nutrition is the essential foundation of a holistic approach to health and healing. Without it there is little to work with in helping an animal to recover. And I feel certain that many of the chronic and degenerative diseases we see today are caused by or complicated by inadequate diet.

After all, the physical body requires certain substances it cannot make internally. As with any complicated and delicate machinery, one missing element in the fuel that powers the body can bring the whole mechanism to a standstill. For example, it appears that the immune system with its production of specialized white blood cells and antibodies is particularly susceptible to nutritional imbalance. Perhaps, because of the fast growth of these specialized cells and their complex function, deficiencies show up sooner here than in, say, the skeletal system.

That said, let's take a closer look at what your animal friend is actually eating. What is and *isn't* provided by the diet can make a big difference in your pet's health.

CHAPTER TWO

WHAT DO THEY REALLY PUT IN PET FOOD?

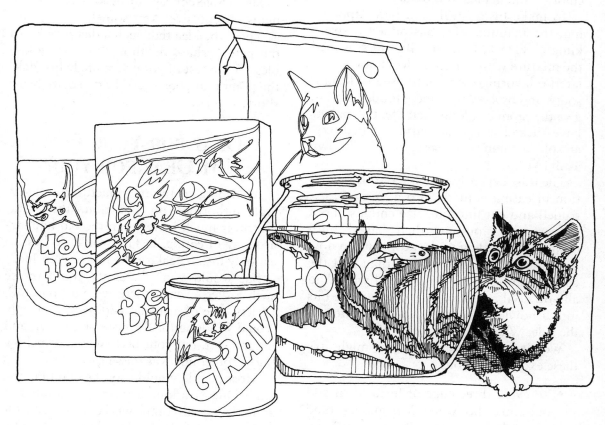

Sensitive assays have detected residues of over 100 different foreign chemicals and metals in our tissues—compounds and substances that were virtually absent from the environments of our predecessors.
—*Marc Lappé*

Imagine that somebody has just developed and marketed a "complete" packaged diet for human beings called Insta-Meal. At last, science and business have combined their know-how to provide you with a simpler, cheaper way to handle the daily chore of planning and preparing meals. According to the label, this product contains all the daily requirements for fats, carbohydrates, protein, vitamins and minerals needed to keep you ticking. To compensate for any loss of nutrients in processing, the manufacturer has added an array of synthetic vitamin and mineral compounds bearing such impressive names as pyridoxine hydrochloride, calcium pantothenate, iron carbonate, potassium chloride and manganous oxide.

To make Insta-Meal look more appetizing, the manufacturer has added a sprinkling of FD&C Red No. 40 and seasoned the mixture with a dash of disodium guanylate (a flavoring commonly used in instant soups and processed Chinese foods). And to give the product a long shelf life, the makers have tucked in a little butylated hydroxyanisole (a common preservative also known as BHA).

The least expensive version of this revolution in eating is made into a mixture, extruded and cut into bite-size chunks about the size of croutons, then baked until crunchy. According to the ads, you can now have a complete diet for less than half the cost of eating the old-fashioned way. And all you need to do is shake some of the bits into a bowl and serve a little tap water on the side. What could be simpler?

Worried about variety? You might try these exciting versions.

◆ To every three cups of Insta-Meal add one cup of hot water. Mix and let stand a couple of minutes. New Insta-Meal makes its own tasty sauce.

◆ Mix two cups of Insta-Meal with two cups of milk, broth or water in your blender. Pour into a greased loaf pan and bake at 350°F for 20 minutes. Presto— "Insta-Casserole"!

◆ Prefer a hearty, meaty style? Try our five canned flavors—Tuna Twist, Chunky Chicken, Mulligan Stew, Turkey Dressing or, for vegetarians, Savory Soylinks.

◆ For that occasional sweet tooth, try new soft, moist "Insta-Patties," preserved with sugar. This item comes in four fruity flavors.

The whole concept of Insta-Meal for humans is repulsive. Yet, somehow we have accepted the idea that such a diet is right for our pets. Perhaps the thought of eating kibbles for the rest of your own life helps make the point that pets forced to do so are being shortchanged.

OKAY FOR YOUR PET, NOT OKAY FOR YOU?

According to the manufacturer and several authorities on nutrition, the insta-system is much better than the old haphazard way of eating. In fact, you'd do best to eat only Insta-Meal for the rest of your life.

But would you? Certainly you'd refuse such a diet, even if there were a "natural" variety, free of artificial additives. Not only would you long for the taste of a varied and natural diet, but your body would somehow know something was missing.

Most people would soon be climbing the walls in frustration, desperate for a salad or some fruit—anything whole and fresh. Or just different! And while lying awake at night, you might wonder about the true meaning of some common Insta-Meal label ingredient terms: bakery by-products, poultry meal and (shudder) sterilized restaurant by-products.

I have nothing personal against the makers of processed foods for pets, nor do I seek to put them out of business. They're probably doing their best to provide nutritionally balanced products at reasonable prices, making use of materials that might otherwise go to waste or just be used as fertilizer. It's just that I don't think *any* kind of completely cooked, dried, canned or frozen prepared food constitutes an optimal diet for the good health of either human or beast. I believe all of us—humans and animals—should have a variety of fresh, wholesome, unprocessed food included in our daily diets.

At first many are surprised at the thought of feeding pets what they call people food. It doesn't seem proper. Feeding animals (and often ourselves) highly processed convenience foods may be accepted as the normal and correct thing to do, but I believe it is wrong. It's simply a practice our culture has adopted over a few short decades, true merit aside.

Europeans feed their dogs much more naturally, minimizing the use of commercial foods. Many breeders have commented to me that these European dogs are far healthier than American dogs. No diet we can formulate from least-cost products and process for convenience and long storage will ever rival those mysteriously complex fresh-food diets offered for aeons by Nature herself.

The many objections we can make about the nutritional quality of animal convenience foods boil down to two sorts. First, they *don't* contain some things we wish they *did* (adequate quantities and/or qualities of proteins, fats, vitamins and minerals as well as the more intangible qualities unique to live, fresh foods). Second, they *do* contain other things we wish they *didn't* (including various slaughterhouse wastes, toxic products from spoiled foodstuffs, non-nutritive fillers, heavy-metal contaminants, sugar, pesticides, herbicides, drug residues and artificial colors, flavors and preservatives).

When you feed your pet convenience foods, you help create another problem: The presence of various toxins and pollutants actually *increases* the body's need for high-quality nutrients necessary to combat or eliminate these same contaminants. When overall nutrition is already lower than it should be, we are inviting trouble.

WHAT'S MISSING IN PET FOODS?

Pet food manufacturers make a big effort to produce competitive, consistent products whose ingredients are drawn from a fluctuating market of least-cost raw materials. Using computerized analyses, they select the constituents they need to make a product that meets or exceeds the recognized minimal nutritional standards for dogs and cats.

Along with a list of ingredients that usually includes categorical terms like *meat meal* or *dried animal digest*, the product label tells you what percentage of the food is protein, fat, fiber, moisture and sometimes ash, carbohydrates and calcium. These label analyses not only provide a way to compare various products, they also assure the public that a given feed meets minimum standards.

So let's say you want to purchase a high-protein food for your dog. All you have to do is look for the label that promises the highest percentage of protein in the product, right? Unfortunately, no. Two factors make such easy evaluations more difficult:

First, not all proteins are created equal; some are much more useful to animals than others. Second, you can't really compare the "percentage of crude protein" in two products, for example, unless you also consider the moisture content of each. This is especially important when comparing a dry food with a canned one. Let's consider each factor in turn.

LABELS CAN BE MISLEADING

To examine protein content (one of the most important nutrients for an animal) you must first understand a few terms.

A protein's *biological value* (also called the nitrogen balance index) depends on each food's unique composition of amino acids, which are the building blocks the body uses to construct its own tissues. In this context, eggs are given an ideal value of 100, which means they are the most useful form of protein known. On this relative scale, fish meal is ranked 92, beef and milk, 78, rice, 75, soybeans, 68, yeast, 63 and wheat gluten, 40.

The *digestibility* of a protein (or any food) is simply the extent to which the gastrointestinal tract can actually absorb it. For example, one source might be 70 percent digestible, another 90 percent. Some proteins—like those in hair—are less digestible because they are difficult or impossible for the body to break down.

Also, the prolonged high temperatures used to sterilize some pet foods can destroy much of the usefulness of even those proteins that have high biological value. That's because the heat causes some proteins to combine with certain sugars, forming compounds that can't be broken down by the body's digestive enzymes.

Since manufacturers need list only the amount of *crude protein* contained in the product, rather than the amount your pet can actually digest and use, producers can and do include inexpensive sources that may supply your pet with much less usable protein than you are led to expect. Most people don't realize that the general pet food label terms that refer to various meat industry by-products can actually mean poultry feather meal, connective tissues, leather meal, fecal waste from poultry and other animals and horse and cattle hair. All these have reputedly been used in pet foods. Such ingredients would certainly boost the *crude* protein content, but provide relatively little nourishment. (It's surely not *my* idea of a good meal for an animal.)

To understand how deceptive this crude protein figure can be, imagine two cans of dog food, each claiming a content of 10 percent protein. Product A protein comes from a good-quality beef with a biological value of 78, carefully processed so that it will be about 95 percent digestible. This means it actually contains about 7.4 percent *net usable protein* (10 percent protein content × 78 biological value (0.78) × 0.95 digestibility). The protein in Product B, on the other hand, comes mostly from chicken feather meal with a biological value of 40 and a digestibility of 75 percent. This means it has less than half the net usable protein of the first can, or 3 percent (0.10 × 0.40 × 0.75). Obviously, a pet will fare much better on Product A. But remember, both labels correctly state the same crude protein content.

Because of the use of such tough, fibrous ingredients, dogs are typically able to utilize only about 75 percent of the protein in meat meal. And all meat meal is made even less digestible by the high cooking temperatures needed to sterilize it. Dried blood meal, another cheap ingredient, contains even less usable protein.

Other basic ingredients in pet food can vary widely in both quality and digestibility, just as the protein does.

Carbohydrates in soft-moist dog foods usually come from such empty-calorie sources as sugar (sucrose), propylene glycol and corn syrup. I have also been told that leftover doughnuts from the fast-food industry have been used as carbohydrates in pet food, as have moldy and rancid grains deemed unacceptable for human consumption. Higher-quality products, on the other hand, may contain complex carbohydrates from whole grains, which are much more nutritious. Except for the sugars, it is difficult to tell by reading the label exactly what you are getting in your pet food.

Fats most often come from animal fats rejected for human consumption. Such fats may be rancid, a state that makes the fats very toxic to the body. Rancid fats also rob the body of essential vitamins.

Fiber may simply come from whole grains and vegetables or it can mean extra filler fiber has been added from sources like peanut hulls, hair or even newspapers.

So by itself, the chemical analysis on the label does not mean a whole lot. To underscore this point, one veterinarian reputedly concocted a mixture containing the same proportions of protein, fats and carbohydrates found in a common brand of dog food, by using old leather shoes, crankcase oil and wood shavings. While things are not that bad, the point is that labels don't always tell us enough. Be especially wary of a pet food that lists its ingredients in categorical terms like these:

- Meal and bonemeal
- Meat by-products
- Dried animal digest
- Poultry by-product meal
- Poultry by-products
- Digest of poultry by-products
- Liver glandular meal
- Chicken by-products
- Dried liver digest
- Fish meal
- Fish by-products

The Pet Food Institute, which represents the industry, has repeatedly sought permission from the Food and Drug Administration (FDA) to use more of these collective ingredient terms. The industry members argue that it allows them to choose a "least-cost mix" from each class of ingredients. Some of the sought-after collective ingredient terms have included "processed animal and marine protein products," "vegetable products" and "plant fiber products." What if some of these terms were interpreted by disreputable manufacturers to allow inclusion of such garbage ingredients as feathers, hair and sawdust in your pet's dinner? The idea isn't far-fetched. I remember reading a news story some years back about a large commercial bakery that was using wood pulp as a fiber source in one of its bread products for *humans*.

THE MATHEMATICS OF MOISTURE VARIATIONS

The second factor that complicates comparisons among pet food labels is varying moisture content. To compensate for its effect on the nutritional analysis, you'll have to do a little math. For instance, the label on a can of dog food may say that the protein content is 6 percent. Yet the label on a box of inexpensive kibble may say the protein content of the product is 20 percent. Sounds like a lot more, doesn't it? However, that is probably incorrect.

To compare percentages of any nutrient in pet foods accurately, you must first level the playing field by refiguring each number as a percentage of the total dry weight. To understand what this figure represents, imagine squeezing every drop of water out of the canned food or the kibble and then measuring the proportion of protein in the solids that remain. That figure is the percentage of protein by dry weight. And, usually, canned foods with water removed actually have a higher proportion of protein than dry foods.

So, for a true comparison of nutrients in different brands, you must, in theory, omit the moisture content. Here's how: Find out what percentage of the food is actually solid (dry weight). Do that by subtracting the listed moisture content of the food from 100 percent. The difference is the dry weight. Using our example, let's say the moisture is 75 percent for the canned food and 10 percent for the kibble. That means our canned food is 25 percent solid and our kibble is 90 percent solid. This is where the nutrients are (the water part simply passes from the body as urine).

Once you know what percentage of the food is dry weight, then you can simply divide the percentage of protein (or any other listed nutrient you wish to determine) by the dry weight. Our examples come out like this.

Canned food example

$$\frac{6\% \text{ protein (label)}}{25\% \text{ dry solids}} = \begin{array}{l} 24.0\% \text{ protein} \\ \text{(dry weight basis)} \end{array}$$

Kibble example

$$\frac{20\% \text{ protein (label)}}{90\% \text{ dry solids}} = \begin{array}{l} 22.2\% \text{ protein} \\ \text{(dry weight basis)} \end{array}$$

It's easy once you get the hang of it. When calculated on this basis, most dog foods contain at least 22 percent crude protein, while cat foods contain at least 32 percent. But remember the significance of the term *crude protein*; there's no easy way to determine what percentage of it is really usable by the animal.

WHAT ABOUT VITAMINS AND MINERALS?

While various vitamins, minerals and amino acids are usually added to pet foods, the exact amount is seldom stated. Additionally, some of the vitamins present in the original ingredients or added by the manufacturer may be lost before your animal ever eats the food. The nutrients can be destroyed by heat processing, particularly in the presence of oxygen, as well as by interactions with other ingredients, like chemical contaminants, during the shelf storage of the product.

Vitamins A, E and B_1, all important in fighting disease, are particularly susceptible to such loss. For example, researchers report that a number of cat foods are so low in vitamin B_1 that they produce deficiencies after only a few weeks of feeding. Another study shows that the processing method used in a certain cat food altered its vitamin B_6 in a way that made it useless to cats' bodies, and deficiency symptoms followed. Furthermore, cats fed low-fat diets absorb vitamin A rather poorly. This problem is of most concern when cats are fed dry food, which is, by necessity, fairly low in fat.

Minerals added to a product may be chemically complete in their basic form, but can lack the complex organic structures found in natural foods. These natural structures in which minerals are held in the body are often referred to as chelates. Sometimes this association is created artificially and sold as "chelated minerals" in natural food stores, but, of course, the best form is that found in whole foods.

Undoubtedly, there is a great deal we still don't understand about the way nutrients act and interact within the body. As a result, manufacturers might add a number of synthetic or isolated vitamins and minerals and still not fully replace those natural forms lost in processing or insufficiently supplied in the first place. As I see it, this also means that we are safer in trying to provide a natural diet that is as nutritious as possible than in using denatured or low-quality food and trying to compensate by adding a few isolated nutrients. Through ignorance, we might omit one or more crucial but little-understood ingredients.

ANOTHER MISSING INGREDIENT: LIFE

All processed pet foods—whether sold in cans, bags or frozen packages, at huge supermarkets or local health food stores—are missing something that seems to me the most important "nutrient" of all. This key ingredient is practically ignored by nutritional scientists, but we can occasionally sense its presence. It is a quality found only in freshly grown, uncooked whole foods: *Life energy!*

Those accustomed to mechanistic explanations of the universe might consider this viewpoint a bit extreme. Yet researchers have used laboratory tests to confirm the presence of something described by people around the world for centuries—a subtle force field that permeates and surrounds all living things. Exactly what this field is and how it operates is still mostly a mystery. However, a number of successful therapies (such as acupuncture and homeopathy) address healing at this level.

Through a special medium of photography developed in Russia by the Kirlians, a husband and wife team, a number of investigators are discovering a whole new world of colorful and complex emissions and "auras" of energies given off by living organisms. They seem to vary according to the individual's emotional state, health and drug use, among other factors.

The Kirlians were the first to discover that the field around "a withered leaf (shows) almost no flares. . . . As the leaf gradually dies, its self-emissions also decrease correspondingly until there is no emission from the dead leaf." What are the implications of this finding for animals (or people) who never or rarely eat anything still fresh or raw enough to retain this mysterious energy?

PROVING THE POTENCY OF RAW FOODS

Almost everyone knows that raw food contains more vitamins and minerals than cooked food, because cooking destroys and depletes many nutrients. When nutritional standards were originally determined for dogs and cats, it was presumed that raw foods, not cooked, would be used. Yet all the pet foods available commercially are very thoroughly cooked and none are nutritionally equal to what was established by these original standards.

The living testimony exemplified in the many people and animals who thrive on diets that include plenty of fresh raw vegetables, fruits, dairy products and other foods is enough to convince me that a diet of cooked foods alone will not keep a pet in top-notch condition. Moreover, my clinical experience over the last 20 years confirms this. The positive change in many animals given a home-prepared, raw-food diet after eating processed foods is nothing short of amazing.

One illustration of this point concerns a remarkable experiment run by Sir Robert McCarrison, a doctor stationed in India some years ago. Impressed by the enviable degree of health enjoyed by the Hunza, Pathan and Sikh peoples, he wondered if a diet similar to theirs could produce comparable physiques and health in experimental rats.

For 27 months Dr. McCarrison fed over 1,000 laboratory rats a variety of live foods, including sprouted beans, fresh raw carrots and cabbage and raw whole milk, along with whole-wheat flatbread and a bit of meat and bones (once a week). He also provided the rats with good air, sunlight and clean living quarters. At the close of the experiment, when the rats had reached an age equivalent to about 55 years in human terms, he sacrificed them and autopsied them thoroughly for signs of disease. To his amazement, he could find none. The only deaths that *had* occurred among those rats were from accidents.

Later Dr. McCarrison fed two other diets—one that was typical of poor people from England and the other typical of poor people in parts of India—to groups of laboratory rats. Rats on the poor Indian diet had disease in every organ they possessed. Those that lived on the boiled, sweetened and canned foods commonly eaten by the English poor grew so high-strung that they ate each other, the weaker rats succumbing first.

One of the most fascinating sources of information about the importance of raw foods comes from what is now known as the Pottenger Cat Studies. Dr. Pottenger did not set out to study cat nutrition, but he became intrigued by differences in the health of a number of cats he was using in experimental studies. Turning his attention to this topic, he did a series of nutritional comparisons. For several generations one group of cats was fed completely raw food (meat, bones, milk and cod-liver oil). Another group of cats was fed the same foods either partially or completely cooked. What he found is of definite importance to those of us who want to raise really healthy pets.

- Cats on the entirely raw-food diet were completely healthy, never needing veterinary attention.
- The more the food was cooked, the less healthy were the cats that ate it.
- The health problems seen in the experimental cats on the cooked diet were remarkably like those commonly seen in cats today—mouth and gum problems, thyroid disorders, bladder inflammation and the like.
- Over a period of three generations, the

cats on the cooked-food diet continued to deteriorate until they could no longer reproduce.

♦ When the cats were put back on a raw-food diet, it was not until four generations later that the animals totally recovered from the physical effects of the cooked diet.

Why is this? Foods are so complex that there is still much we don't understand about them. Researchers have discovered, for example, that cats require a dietary source of taurine, an amino acid that many mammals, including humans, can synthesize. Taurine, found only in animal tissues, is largely destroyed by cooking. One study shows that an average of 52 percent of the taurine in raw meats is lost through baking and an average of 79 percent through boiling. As a result of processing, many commercial cat foods once had low levels of taurine. Now it is added to cat foods and supplements.

In caring for our own cats, my wife and I came to the conclusion that we would rather not wait for more such discoveries. Instead, we would rather be cautious, choosing to feed our cats a diet that most closely resembles that of their evolutionary history. (When the meat is fed raw as recommended, by the way, calculations show that our recipes for cats contain taurine in amounts comparable to taurine in the wild diet.)

THE PERILOUS INGREDIENTS PUT IN PET FOODS

Now that I've discussed what's missing in commercial pet food, let's look at the unsavory ingredients that are present. *Prevention* magazine published a letter from a reader who offered this inside glimpse of the pet food industry.

I once worked in a chicken-butchering factory in Maine. Our average daily output was 100,000 chickens.... Directly ahead of me on the conveyor line were the United States Department of Agriculture (USDA) inspectors and their trimmers. The trimmers cut the damaged and diseased parts off the chickens and dropped them in garbage cans, which were emptied periodically. These parts were sent to a pet food factory.

So the next time you hear a pet food commercial talk about the fine ingredients they use in their product, don't you believe it.

Similarly, a story appeared in a local paper revealing that dead animals found on the highway are sent to rendering plants where they are used in pet food.

I don't think it takes much imagination to realize the poor quality of such an ingredient source. Theoretically, a healthy opossum killed by a car, unless it is left lying in the sun for several hours, might provide acceptable nutrition in pet food. However, animals killed by cars because they are ill and can't move fast enough to avoid being hit might not.

It is difficult to determine which pet food makers are using products like these, or mixing in tumorous tissues, hooves, hair, feathers and some of the unsavory fillers we occasionally hear about. But it is common knowledge that the pet food industry is built on the undesirable remnants of the human food industry. And common sense suggests that the cheaper the food, the more suspect its quality.

According to the USDA, there is no

mandatory federal inspection of ingredients used in pet food manufacturing, though some states may oversee the canning processes. (However, even this minimal inspection is not assured for dry pet foods.) In all but two or three states, the laws allow pet food makers to use what are called 4-D sources—that is, tissues from animals that are dead, dying, disabled or diseased when they arrive at the slaughterhouse. Other pet food ingredients include food rejected by the USDA for human consumption, such as moldy grains or rancid animal fats. (Manufacturers can, however, voluntarily submit to continuous government inspection of their product's ingredients and their plant facilities. Such products bear a label saying that they have been packed under continuous inspection by the USDA.)

What effect might these substandard food and wastes have on animals? From his experience as a veterinarian and federal meat inspector, P. F. McGargle, D.V.M., has concluded that feeding slaughterhouse wastes to animals increases their chance of getting cancer and other degenerative diseases. Those wastes, he reports, can include moldy, rancid or spoiled processed meats as well as tissues severely riddled with cancer.

These meat scraps can also contain hormone levels comparable to those that have produced cancer in laboratory animals. Dr. McGargle attributed these high levels to two causes: synthetic hormones routinely fed to livestock to stimulate rapid growth, and meat meal whose source is often glandular wastes and fetal tissues from pregnant cows. Both are naturally high in hormones. When livestock is slaughtered and the meat is processed, the hormones are still active. High hormone levels have the most severe effect on cats, who are extremely sensitive to them. The tissues or pellets that are used to fatten steers and caponize chickens, for example, are considered toxic to cats, even in very low levels.

WHY SOME PET FOOD SMELLS THAT WAY

Although USDA inspectors are only allowed a few seconds to examine each carcass, there are many animals with obvious signs of disease or abnormality, according to Deborah Lynn Dadd, author of *The Nontoxic Home and Office*. Dadd's research shows that:

Each year about 116,000 mammals and nearly 15 million birds are condemned before slaughter. After killing, another 325,000 carcasses are discarded and more than 5.5 million major parts are cut away because they are determined to be diseased. Shockingly, 140,000 tons of poultry is condemned annually, mainly from cancer. The diseased animals that cannot be sold are processed into ... animal feed.

Perhaps consumer turnoff was one factor that led to the development of ever more "convenient" pet foods. Since they were first introduced, the popularity of "burgers," soft-moist chunks and dry kibble has grown, while the popularity of canned foods has diminished. Unfortunately, this trend means the average pet is eating more "junk food," because these new foods are full of sugar and preservatives to keep them fresh without canning or refrigeration.

THE ADDITIVES IN YOUR PET'S FOOD

Since I graduated from veterinary school in 1965, I've noticed a general deterioration in pet health. We now see very young animals with diseases that we used to see only in older animals. It is clear to me that an accumulation of poor health is being passed on from generation to generation; this accumulation increases with each step. Without the perspective of several decades, veterinarians just coming out of veterinary school think these degenerative conditions in younger animals are "normal." They do not realize what has happened over the passage of time.

I believe that, along with poor quality nutrients, the *chemical additives* in pet food play a major part in that decline. Just look at the label of a typical burger product for dogs. The ingredients are listed in order of their prominence. (For example, if water is the first ingredient, the product contains more water than anything else.) A popular soft-moist burger lists corn syrup as its third major ingredient. But what is this common sweetener doing in a burger at all? It's providing the soft-moistness! The FDA approved the use of corn syrup in its hydrogenated form as a "humectant and plasticizer"—that is, an ingredient that gives the product dampness and flexibility. Food scientists trying to develop similar products for people have acknowledged that despite the American sweet tooth, soft-moist dog food is so sweet that "humans just wouldn't like it."

Chemically derived from cornstarch, corn syrup produces the same energy highs and lows that table sugar does and causes the same stress on the pancreas and adrenals, a condition that may result in diabetes. It's easy to see that corn syrup is an undesirable ingredient, especially when you consider the other shortcomings of such an isolated refined sugar. Not only does it dilute other nutrients in the food by providing "empty calories" devoid of vitamins, minerals, proteins or fats, but it can overstimulate the production of insulin and acidic digestive juices as well. These interfere with a dog's ability to absorb the proteins, calcium and other minerals that *are* in the food. Moreover, corn syrup can inhibit the growth of useful intestinal bacteria.

The following common ingredients have appeared in soft-moist and other pet foods.

- *Propylene glycol.* This compound, known to cause illness in dogs, is also used to maintain the right texture and moisture and to tie up the water content, thus inhibiting bacterial growth.
- *Potassium sorbate.* Here's a commonly used preservative chemically similar to fat.
- *Ammoniated glycyrrhizin.* Add this to the list of sweeteners. It is also considered a potent drug that should be tested further for safety.
- *Sucrose.* This is simply table sugar.
- *Propyl gallate.* Manufacturers add this chemical to retard spoilage, but it is suspected of causing liver damage.
- *Ethoxyquin.* Originally developed for use in the production of rubber, this common preservative is among the compounds most suspect as causes of severe health problems in dogs.

◆ *Butylated hydroxytoluene (BHT).* This poorly tested preservative is implicated by some scientists as a cause of liver damage, metabolic stress, fetal abnormalities and serum cholesterol increase.

◆ *Sodium nitrite.* This compound is widely used as both a preservative and a red coloring agent. Sodium nitrite used in food can produce powerful carcinogenic substances known as nitrosamines.

Another class of common additives usually listed simply as *artificial coloring* does not require specific labeling. In pet food the class typically includes the following coal-tar derivative dyes, all allowed without adequate lifetime feeding studies.

◆ Red No. 3
◆ Red No. 40 (a possible carcinogen)
◆ Yellow No. 5
◆ Yellow No. 6
◆ Blue No. 1
◆ Blue No. 2 (shown in studies to increase dogs' sensitivities to fatal viruses)

Similar dyes that were banned from both pet and human foods in the mid-1970s included Red No. 2 (which appeared to increase cancer and birth defects) and Violet No. 1 (a suspected carcinogen that can also cause skin lesions).

Although concerned citizens have petitioned the FDA to ban artificial colors in pet foods, their use continues. In a crowded marketplace where all the major competitors use these colorings to make their products look more like fresh red meat, a company trying to sell a pet food in its true colors—various unattractive shades of gray—would put itself at a serious disadvantage. Since dogs and cats don't see colors as we do, it's clear that these dyes are added to please humans. However, some pet food products sold in natural food stores have no artificial colors, preservatives or flavors in them.

The largest class of food additives used in pet foods, *synthetic flavorings*, are called safe with little or no testing. Then they are added under the general term *artificial flavorings*, without need for FDA permission. Since consumers have no way of assessing the safety of what is used, anyone seriously concerned about health would be wise to avoid buying food products—for themselves or their pets—that contain this mysterious group of ingredients.

THE HIDDEN CHEMICAL CONTAMINATION

Aside from the chemicals intentionally added to pet food, others sneak in on their own. Chemical contamination of the food chain is increasing and becoming a major factor in chronic disease, particularly among animals. It is difficult to comprehend the extent to which these chemicals appear in food. The process starts with the herbicides, insecticides and fungicides used in growing crops. The process continues with antibiotics, growth stimulants, hormones, tranquilizers and other drugs given to livestock that consume these crops. Then, after these animals are slaughtered and processed into meat, more chemicals are added to the meat itself for coloring, softening, preserving and other purposes.

The problem the pet faces is threefold.

First, to eliminate toxic substances, the body is forced to expend energy and nutrients that could be put to better use. Second, anything the body cannot expel accumulates in the tissues. Third, those accumulated substances can interact with each other in unexpected, harmful ways.

Depletion of energy and nutrients. The body uses several natural mechanisms to detoxify and eliminate harmful substances. These processes occur primarily in the liver (detoxification), kidneys (elimination), skin (additional elimination especially through deposits in the hair) and immune system (reactions against harmful substances). Certain enzymes and their associated vitamins assist this process. The more toxic the chemical, the harder the body must work to get rid of it—and the more these enzymes and vitamins are depleted. This strain alone would be significant in a polluted world—but there is more.

Toxic accumulation. The body is incapable of detoxifying all substances because detoxification mechanisms were fine-tuned over many thousands of years to deal with the natural poisons an animal encountered during its lifetime. The last few decades, however, have seen the introduction of vast quantities of substances never before encountered in a natural setting. As of 1989, some 70,000 different chemicals were in use in our society, with nearly 3,000 new ones being introduced annually.

When you consider the huge numbers of these substances being produced and used each year, the reason our government can't adequately test for harmful effects becomes obvious. As of 1990, only about 2,000 (approximately 3 percent) of all the chemicals in everyday use had been tested for their ability to cause cancer in animals (and half were found capable of doing so). So is it any wonder that some of these chemicals cannot be processed by the body? Most were never encountered before.

If the body can't detoxify a chemical, it must store the compound in its tissues. And once it's inside those tissues, the chemical can interfere with normal function. The greater the amount, the more the interference.

Interactions among stored chemicals. If two different synthetic chemicals—substance A and substance B—are stored in the same body tissue, four possibilities are present.

◆ No interaction at all.
◆ A acts on B, possibly making B more toxic.
◆ B acts on A, possibly making A more toxic.
◆ Each acts on the other, possibly increasing each other's effects.

Now if we consider three substances, A, B and C, the possible interactions go up to nine. (The number of possible interactions is the square of the number of substances present.) Reflect on the quote at the beginning of this chapter—that assays have detected over 100 chemical contaminants in our tissues. Now the complexity of all their interactions—which can follow 10,000 possible pathways—begins to impact on you.

So when scientists studying a single chemical pronounce it harmless at a certain level, they may be right. But they can't predict the effects of its interaction with other contaminants in the body. Furthermore, they will probably never know such things. If the best our scientists have done up to now is to test only about 2,000 of our 70,000 industrial chemical substances for their cancer-causing potential, it's unreasonable to think they will ever decipher all the possible interactions of the chemicals we encounter.

CHEMICAL CONTAMINANTS IN MEAT

Because it's on a higher rung of the food chain, meat contains much more pesticide residue, heavy metals and other toxic pollutants than food from plant sources.

Contamination with lead, for example, can be very severe. In one study, a sampling of canned pet foods revealed levels ranging from 0.9 to 7.0 ppm (parts per million) in cat foods and 1.0 to 5.6 ppm in dog foods. Daily intake of only six ounces of such foods could exceed the dose of lead considered potentially toxic for children.

Much of this contamination comes from using bonemeal in pet foods. Though they are otherwise an excellent source of calcium and other minerals, the bones of American cattle contain high levels of lead from the long-term use of leaded gasoline in our cars. (The lead pollutes the air and the grazing land and the fodder we feed the cattle.) The only safe bonemeal today comes from cattle raised in South America or in other parts of the world with far fewer automobiles than are found in the United States.

Even meat approved by the USDA adds significantly to the accumulation of toxic materials, aside from lead. According to a study published in the *New England Journal of Medicine*, the chemical pollution of breast milk in the average American woman is 35 times higher than that of a strictly vegetarian American woman. Yet fewer than one out of every quarter million animals slaughtered in the United States is tested for toxic chemical residues. When you also consider that the condemned 4-D meats used in pet foods are more likely to come from unhealthy livestock weakened by environmental stress and toxins, you can see even more clearly why pet foods can be a concentrated source of health problems for pets.

This creates a very difficult feeding situation. Natural carnivores like dogs and cats need a certain amount of meat in their diets. This is especially true for cats, animals that cannot survive on vegetarian diets. Yet meat is one of the most contaminated foods available in America.

HOW CAN WE PROTECT OUR PETS?

Must we stand by as our pets get sick from eating unhealthy diets? What can we do to improve this situation?

For one thing, it is clearly time for each of us to take a role in reducing our society's use of untested, potentially dangerous synthetic chemicals—not just for the sake of animals, but for humans, too—those living now and those yet to come. This will surely call for many changes in our patterns of consumption.

Among the most important of these changes are the daily choices we make about what we feed our pets as well as what we eat ourselves. We can't expect to maintain good health on overprocessed, denatured, contaminated foods. (There is also a great deal of evidence that our society can't keep growing sufficient food if we rely on the nonsustainable, petroleum-based agriculture we have now. We'll have to make some changes.)

That's the bad news. The good news is that there are practical, affordable ways to make the necessary healthy changes in how you feed your pet. The next few chapters show you, step-by-step, practical and affordable ways to introduce fresh, even organically grown foods into your dog's or cat's diet.

First, we share some stories about animals that found a new lease on life when their owners switched them to fresh, natural diets. Then, we show you how to do the same—how to select the best ingredients and put them together in a variety of carefully formulated, nutritionally balanced recipes in response to different needs. For those not quite willing or able to switch completely, we also provide formulas for fresh foods and supplements that can be added to higher-quality kibbles. Throughout, we include time- and money-saving tips. Most animals will love the new food. But, for those that persist in their habits (like a few cats we all know!), we show how to help your pet make the transition to a new way of eating that's as old as the hills.

CHAPTER THREE

Try a Basic Natural Diet— With Supplements

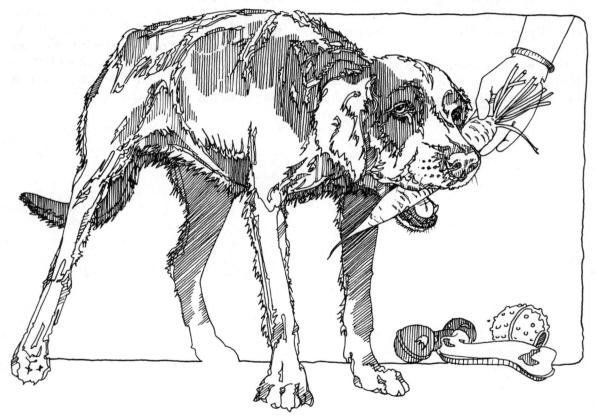

Feeding your pet a fresher, more natural diet takes a little time and effort. It's certainly not as easy as opening a bag of kibble. But once you understand which ingredients to use and how to put them together, you'll see that it's not so difficult. Also, you'll be rewarded by seeing your pet's health improve.

Countless clients, along with readers of this book's first edition, have switched their pets to more wholesome diets and have rejoiced at the results. For example, a grateful

New Jersey woman wrote to thank me for a big change in a little dog.

The health of my little dog Noel was declining very fast two years ago. She was eight. Her coat was dull and it smelled awful. Her breath had a foul odor. Noel's eyes were dull and she slept all day under a chair. She had always been friendly, but her temperament changed. She would try to bite me and growled if I tried to get her to come outside and play. I bought pet vitamins and they stimulated her appetite, but she was still so sick-looking.

Well, thanks to your wonderful book there's been a big change. Noel's on a natural diet now. No more dry and canned food. What a difference! Her coat and her breath don't have an odor. At ten years of age, her eyes shine and she prances around like a puppy. Noel loves whole grains, tofu, beans, eggs, cheese and all vegetables. (I also give her the supplements you recommend.) Another change: Her muzzle was turning gray, but now the hair is coming in black again, the color it was when she was a puppy. Thank you so much for saving Noel's life.

It is always gratifying to see animals spring back to health because of a good diet. It is even more encouraging to hear about the remarkable health of a pet fed a natural diet from an early age.

How to Balance the Homemade Diet

We've all heard a veterinarian or a pet food manufacturer warn against feeding pets table scraps or homemade diets. Such diets, they contend, have not been scientifically formulated to meet an animal's needs and may ruin a pet's health. And this could certainly happen if you just scraped junk-food leftovers into your pet's bowl.

But even if you're more conscientious than that, it's still easy to be misguided by your own tastes and needs, not realizing that what's good for you may not be good for your pet. (For example, because they are carnivores, dogs and cats need far more protein and calcium on a pound-for-pound basis than humans require.) However, do-it-yourself animal feeding has been with us since the first dog and person crossed paths at least 10,000 years ago. And generation after generation of animals got by just fine on the scraps and extras of our ancestors. So we need not worry about providing a "perfect" balance of nutrients with every meal we feed our pets.

Yet we do have the benefit of modern dietary analysis and research, so I believe it makes sense to use that information and adhere to it in formulating a pet's diet. Why do I say that, when few of us bother to calculate the exact nutrients in our own meals? The reason is that, unlike humans or wild animals with free access to natural and varied food supplies, our pets have little choice about what they eat. Rarely, if ever, do they get to follow their instincts in selecting individual foods; usually, a number of ingredients are mixed together and it's a matter of eating all or nothing. Moreover, the instincts of homebound pets are not so finely tuned as the instincts of wild animals. Like us, pets can easily develop a taste for the strong flavors of junk food.

The recipes in this book are palatable, easy to make and nutritious. Using a computer, we have been able to analyze the contents of each recipe and its suggested variations. Relying on standard data for 16 of the most important food constituents (given in the *USDA Handbook on the Composition of Foods*), we adjusted the recipes to make sure the amount of each nutrient met or exceeded the minimal amounts recommended for dog and cat foods by the American Association of Feed Control Officials. But first, let's talk about the best basic foods to use, along with some nutritional supplements that should be added to the basic food groups as a necessary part of the diet.

CHOOSE THE RIGHT FOODS

The first important principle in this do-it-yourself way of feeding animals is to aim for variety because that helps to ensure the best balance of nutrients. One meat or grain differs considerably from another in nutritional details—not only in the amino acid makeup of the proteins, for example, but in the presence and amount of various vitamins, minerals and trace minerals. So it's best to vary the recipes and to try some of the suggested ingredient substitutions. Soon you will find several combinations that are best suited to your lifestyle and your animal's preferences.

Another worthwhile principle is to stick to the recipes fairly closely. They've been carefully formulated to provide the best combination. Sometimes people try to take shortcuts by omitting the calcium supplement, for example, but that will cause a deficiency problem if done regularly.

Third, we strongly encourage you to use organically raised and minimally processed foods whenever possible. It's best for the immediate health of your pet, and it's best for the long-term health of the Earth and everything on it. Fortunately, it's possible for people throughout most of the United States to find organically raised grains. When bought in bulk in natural food stores, they are usually priced comparably with the chemically grown grains sold in supermarket packages. (See "Best Ingredient Choices for Feeding Your Pet," on page 32, which will also help you find the best protein buys.) It may be difficult, however, to find and/or afford other organic foods, especially meats. So just do what you can, and try to use the best whole, fresh ingredients you can afford. When these are made into balanced recipes, they are still a big improvement over commercial pet food products, which we know can be laced with everything from cancerous tissue to sugar, dyes and moldy grains.

The fourth general principle is to be patient yet persistent as you gradually introduce these new foods to your animal friend. Most people find their pets love these foods, but some animals hesitate to eat them at first, simply because the foods are unfamiliar. Also, any change of diet—even a switch from one commercial brand of food to another—means the pet's digestive system has to adapt. So take time to introduce the new foods, maybe a period of weeks, substituting ever-greater proportions of natural foods for commercial foods. (See chapter 6 for more discussion on making the switch.)

THE BASIC FOOD GROUPS

Now let's consider each of the basic food groups used in our recipes—and how best to buy, store and prepare them.

MEATS

Despite its high levels of chemical contamination and its great cost to the environment (see the discussion in chapter 5), meat is the most natural food for carnivores. It contains the most protein and is rich in many other nutrients as well. In our recipes we try to balance these issues. That's why most of the recipes in this book include some fresh meat combined with high-protein grains, legumes or dairy products to produce a total amount of protein that exceeds the recommended standards. The resulting protein levels are comparable to (or greater than) the crude protein levels found in commercial foods, which use a similar process of combining plant and animal proteins to boost the total protein level. In chapter 5 we also include some meatless recipes that are suitable for feeding dogs.

Another criterion we used when choosing meats was convenience. That's why our recipes use meats that are widely available, usually ground up, which makes it easier to mix them in with the recipe and harder for finicky eaters to pick them out. Most of the recipes in this book call for lean meats, which are considerably higher in protein and lower in fat.

The following meats are roughly interchangeable within each group. This means that you can, on occasion, substitute one meat for another in a recipe, pound for pound or cup for cup. The meats are listed in approximate order of best values, with the first ones representing the most protein for the typical price paid.

Lean meats (interchangeable): Turkey and/or giblets, liver (beef, chicken or turkey), mackerel, most chicken and/or giblets, tuna, heart (beef, chicken or turkey), lean hamburger, lean chuck, duck (without skin), rabbit or various fishes.

Fatty meats (interchangeable): Roaster chicken (with skin), fatty beef heart, brains, regular hamburger, fatty chuck, sirloin steak, lamb or pork.

Occasionally, you can use any of these fatty meats where the recipe calls for a lean meat. When you do, reduce the amount of oil in the recipe by about a tablespoon for every cup of meat. Cuts of meat vary, so use your best judgment in evaluating the degree of fat in a meat.

Note: 1 pound of ground meat equals about 2 cups.

Here are some guidelines for selecting and preparing meats.

Use variety. Feed more than one kind of meat in a meal, using different cuts. Include some muscle or flesh meats, such as hamburger, chicken and turkey as well as some organ meats, such as heart, liver or kidneys or giblets.

Note: Some people have seen great health benefits in their animals from regularly feeding them small amounts of raw liver. Just be sure that you don't go overboard with liver. Limit it to less than 10 percent of the meat you feed overall. Not only does the liver concentrate and store many pollutants, but it could overdose your pet with vitamin A, which is one of the few vitamins known to cause problems if consumed in excess.

Emphasize purer sources. One veterinarian I know who worked as a meat inspector has observed that turkeys, ducks and sheep have lower cancer rates than chickens, cattle and hogs. He attributes this difference to the amount of meat meal fed each species. So you would probably do well to emphasize turkey and lamb, for example, unless you can obtain quality-raised chicken or beef. Some natural food stores carry meats described as organically raised or chemical-free (meaning that no drugs, hormones or the like were used in the livestock feed). Also, it's a good idea to look for free-range chickens, rather than those stressed by being raised in the intensely crowded confines of factory farms.

Try ground meats. This is especially good for cats, because you can readily blend in other ingredients, and the cats can't pick out the meat and leave the rest. If you have a food processor, you can grind chunks of meat along with the other ingredients to make a nice texture; otherwise, buy it already ground or ask the butcher to grind it for you. (Chunks of meat have benefits, too, because chewing them exercises an animal's jaws and that helps condition the gums.)

Feed meat raw whenever possible if the animal will accept it. I make this recommendation on the basis of research, clinical practice and the natural habits of predators since the beginning of time. My clients have been feeding their pets this way successfully for years. All the meats listed in the recipes in this book may be fed raw. However, if you substitute by using a little fish, rabbit or pork now and then, you should cook them first to kill parasites like tapeworms or trichinosis organisms, which these foods can carry.

You should be aware that most veterinarians oppose feeding raw meat because of concern about diseases like salmonella or

Escherichia coli. However, after 17 years of experience in recommending this practice, I can attest to seeing no problem with infections from these diseases. On the contrary, I observed an improved level of health. This is not to say that animals never become ill from eating raw meat, but they certainly seem to be less susceptible to it than people are. Perhaps this is because dogs and cats are natural carnivores and raw meat is their natural food. If you are uncomfortable about feeding raw meat to your pet, feel free to cook it, of course. But remember, the nutritional values (given for raw meats) will not apply.

Freeze extra meat (or the whole recipe). We have tried to formulate the recipes in this book to utilize convenient quantities of meats, as purchased in pounds. If you're feeding a large dog or several animals, you will probably use up all the meat you can buy before it spoils. But if you have one small animal, you will need to take a different tack: Either divide the meat into recipe-size portions and freeze them for future preparation, or make up the whole recipe now and freeze any part of the mixture that your pet won't eat in the next two to three days. This reduces the time spent in preparing your pet's diet.

Undoubtedly, freezing the meat destroys some of its fresh qualities, but defrosted raw meat is still better than cooked meat and far superior to the meat by-products in commercial food.

You will probably need to freeze extra meat more often for cats than for dogs. Because dogs are natural scavengers, they can tolerate, and even relish, meat that is too gamy for human consumption. Cats, however, are truer carnivores. That's why they are very selective about the freshness of their meat and will readily let you know when their daily fare has aged beyond its time.

Tip: Reuse your soft plastic dairy and deli containers to freeze extra portions when you make up a recipe. Thaw each container in the refrigerator 24 hours before you want to serve it. If the food is not completely thawed, simply add a little hot water and use a fork to break it up in the serving bowl. Hot water can increase the palatability of any food just removed from the refrigerator. Try to use up frozen meat within three to four months.

Dairy Products

Besides meat, dairy products are good sources of protein. We recommend raw eggs and cottage cheese in the diets because they are economical, convenient sources of dairy protein. Yogurt and cheese are relatively expensive and less-concentrated protein sources than eggs. However, they are fairly balanced foods, so feel free to feed them (and milk, too) on the side.

About eggs: Eggs are a complete protein and are a good source of preformed vitamin A. I recommend the no-hormone, no-drug, free-range eggs often sold in natural food stores. The slight extra cost is worth it. Eggs are such a good protein source that the cost for the "natural" variety is about the same per gram of protein as that of most factory-farm-raised meat in supermarkets, in some cases even cheaper.

Opinions are divided about whether adult dogs and cats can digest raw eggs properly. For example, one study concluded that raw egg whites can cause a biotin deficiency. But this condition surfaced in experiments in which eggs were fed to rats in great excess. Personally, I have never seen the biotin problem. I think it's important to remember that predators in the wild rely on raw eggs as part of their diets. As a change, you can lightly scramble or boil the eggs occasionally. It also works well to add eggs to freshly cooked grains; the heat sets the egg just enough to give the food a better texture.

The threat of salmonella poisoning is also a common worry where raw eggs are concerned. However, in all my years of practice, I have not seen a dog or cat affected by this organism in connection with eating raw eggs.

Digestion of milk products: Some people believe raw milk and raw cheeses should form the bulk of a cat's diet. Others say that cats, especially Siamese, do not digest lactose (milk sugar) properly and that drinking milk causes gas and diarrhea in cats. Based on the feedback from my clients, I find that milk seldom causes such problems. (In addition, my experience is that if cats are sensitive to milk, proper treatment can eliminate the sensitivity.)

Pasteurization, however, does alter the chemical structure of protein and can destroy beneficial enzymes and bacteria found in milk, making it less digestible. So if your animal has a problem, try feeding it raw milk. Ordinarily, cottage cheese, yogurt and goat's milk are also easily digested. But if your cat still has difficulty, omit milk products from the diet.

Also, please do not presume that feeding your pet milk with every meal means you can omit the bonemeal or other calcium supplements in the recipes. To be used properly in the body, calcium must be provided in a certain ratio to phosphorus. Cats and dogs require such high amounts of calcium that the amount in milk is just about enough to balance the phosphorus in the milk itself. But that level of calcium is not enough to balance the high phosphorus levels in meats and grains. Bones provide much more extra calcium, and they are the natural way that predators achieve this balance.

GRAINS

Whole grains are a very cost-effective and environmentally sensitive way to provide the mainstay of your pet's diet. Not only do grains supply carbohydrates and an array of vitamins and minerals, they are inexpensive sources of protein as well. When a grain is combined with other grains, the biological effectiveness of its protein is greatly enhanced because the balance of amino acids is more complete. According to official standards, carbohydrates may properly supply over half of the diet for dogs and cats, on a dry weight basis.

Grains are one group of foods that definitely should be cooked. Usually, wild carnivores eat these foods only if they appear in the stomach of their prey, thus the grains are partially digested already. Because the intestinal tracts of dogs and cats are much shorter than those of cereal-eating animals like cows and horses, grains fed to dogs and cats need some predigestion (in the form of cooking).

To save both time and energy, we emphasize quick-cooking and economical grains—

Recommended Grains

Here are cooking directions for our recommended grains, including the amount of water to use per cup of dry grain. Caloric and protein content is also shown.

Grain (1 cup dry)	Water (cups)	Cooked Yield (cups)	Cooking Time (minutes)	Calories	Protein Amount (g.)
Barley	2–3	2½–3	30–60	696	19
Brown rice	2	2½	30–45	720	15
Buckwheat	2–3	2½–3	20–30	570	20
Bulgur	2	2–2½	10–20	602	19
Cornmeal	4	3½–4	10–30	462	12
Millet	3	3	20–30	641	19
Rolled oats	2	2	10	312	11
Wheat berries	3½	2½	60	652	20
Whole-wheat couscous	1½	2½	3–5	602	19

NOTE: Another good source of grain protein is whole-wheat bread. Two slices, which contain 122 calories, have three grams of protein. Crumble up the bread before mixing it in the recipes.

oatmeal, cornmeal, millet and bulgur. They are well-accepted by most dogs and cats and are high in nutrition. For example, oats and bulgur are loaded with protein, and millet is rich in iron. Larger grains like rice and whole wheat berries or barley are best used with dogs. Unless these larger grains are mashed, cats tend to pick them out. Crumbled whole-wheat bread is a quick and convenient ingredient when preparing food for a cat or small dog, but it's too expensive to use regularly for feeding large dogs. Amaranth, whole-wheat couscous, buckwheat, quinoa and spelt—all highly nutritious grains—are beginning to make their way into the American diet. They are usually costlier, but use them if you wish, substituting them in amounts similar to those of bulgur.

In the next chapter the recipes each suggest several grain substitutions that provide comparable or greater nutritional value. Amounts are given, but you may need to refer to "Recommended Grains" for cooking instructions.

LEGUMES

Beans and other legumes are emphasized in several of our recipes for dogs. That's because they provide a great deal of protein at less cost than any other food, allowing you to reduce your dog's meat consumption if you wish. It takes more time to prepare legumes, but when you fix large quantities of food, a little planning about including legumes will be well worth it. Here are some tips for saving time and/or energy when cooking legumes.

Use quick-cooking legumes such as split peas and lentils. If your time is really limited, you might substitute tofu, which is also easier for your pet to digest. It does, however, cost more per gram of protein than most commercial meats. With a little flavoring like soy sauce or meat drippings, most dogs accept tofu.

Presoak longer-cooking beans overnight. Soaking beans at least three hours helps reduce intestinal gas after they're consumed. It also helps to boil the soaked beans for 30 minutes, discard that cooking water and finish the cooking with fresh water. (Beans are done when you can easily lift off the outer "skin" of the bean.)

Use a pressure cooker. If you have one of these appliances, you can cook beans in 35 to 45 minutes.

Precook a large quantity of beans and freeze them in recipe-size portions for future use. The recipes list amounts for both dry and cooked beans for this reason.

Suggested legume-for-legume substitutions that provide adequate nutritional value are given with the recipes in the next chapter. Amounts are provided, but you may need to refer to "Recommended Legumes" on page 30 for cooking instructions.

PUTTING IT ALL TOGETHER

Now that we have considered the four major food groups that make up the bulk of the recipes, let's take a moment to put them in perspective.

"Best Ingredient Choices for Feeding Your Pet," found on page 32, gives you a quick way to compare the major ingredients, considering the following factors: cost per gram of protein, relative cost of organic versus commercial items, cooking time and best nutrients.

The foods are grouped by basic categories: grains, legumes, meats and dairy products. Based on a price survey of organic, natural and conventional foods in our local natural food stores and a national supermarket chain, we sorted the various choices within each category of food into price groups. The price groups start with the least expensive— foods from any growing method that cost less than half a penny per gram of protein; next, foods that cost about a penny per gram of protein; then, foods costing three cents and four cents per gram of protein. Those that cost more are excluded.

The table also shows the method of growing or processing—Organic, Natural or Conventional/Commercial. Whether organic or commercial, we used the cheaper bulk prices for most of the grains and legumes. So if you buy grains at a supermarket (where grains and legumes are seldom offered in bulk), figure a little more for the price.

The chart shows, for example, that most organically grown grains and legumes are priced close to what their commercially grown counterparts cost. Turkey is one of the best protein buys in meats. (Even the natural chemical-free version is cheaper per gram of protein than regular commercial chuck and comparable in value to most other meats.) Processed foods such as tofu, bread, cheese and yogurt are relatively expensive.

Now let's look at some of the secondary foods, snacks, flavorings and nutritional supplements that are part of a recommended pet diet.

Recommended Legumes

Use this table to find cooking instructions, yields and calorie and protein values for recommended legumes.

Legume (1 cup dry)	Water (cups)	Cooked Yield (cups)	Cooking Time (minutes)	Calories	Protein Amount (g.)
Kidney, red beans	3	2½	90	645	42
Lentils	4	2¾	30	578	42
Pinto beans	2	2½	90	628	41
Soybeans	5	2¾	180	806	68
Split peas	4	2½	30	696	48
White or black beans	4	2½	45–60	629	41

NOTE: Tofu, which is made from soybeans and doesn't need cooking, is also very high in protein. A pound of tofu has 35 grams of protein and 654 calories.

VEGETABLES

Despite their image as exclusive meat-eaters, the wild cousins of dogs and cats do consume plant foods—sometimes these are found in the stomach contents of their plant-eating prey (often the first part of a kill a wolf eats). Sometimes wild animals eat plant foods directly. Dogs, especially, like vegetables, which are valuable for adding vitamins, minerals and roughage to the diet. Most vegetables are so low-calorie that you can add them to the recipes in modest quantities with little effect on the proportions of the major nutrients. Some vegetables must be cooked to help carnivores digest them properly, but others may be fed raw, much like the grasses they sometimes nibble in the backyard.

These are the best-liked veggies that can be fed raw.

- ◆ Chopped parsley
- ◆ Alfalfa sprouts
- ◆ Finely grated carrots
- ◆ Finely grated zucchini

These vegetable favorites should be cooked before being fed to pets.

- ◆ Corn
- ◆ Peas
- ◆ Green beans
- ◆ Broccoli

Carrots may also be cooked, especially for cats.

Whole raw carrots are favored by many dogs that enjoy chewing on them much as they do bones. Such foods help exercise and clean teeth and gums.

Avoid feeding pets vegetables high in oxalic acid, a compound that interferes with calcium absorption. These include spinach, swiss chard and rhubarb.

In contrast to most vegetables, potatoes provide plenty of calories in the form of both carbohydrates and protein. Fortunately, they are also well-liked by many pets. So it's okay to use leftover cooked or mashed potatoes occasionally in place of some lower-protein grains such as rice, cornmeal and barley. Some people think their animals have trouble digesting potatoes, but others find that their pets relish spuds. Try using potatoes and judge your animal's reaction for yourself. (Be sure to cut out all green or sprouting parts, which contain large amounts of solanine, a toxic substance.)

A word of caution about fresh produce: In our community, several employees of a national supermarket chain revealed that insecticide was routinely but illegally sprayed directly onto many vegetables and fruits on display in an effort to control fruit flies and other pests. In spite of denials by the management, the employees insisted that this was a common practice throughout the country. Though this may not be done in your market, most likely the plants and fruits were sprayed at some point during production. (This is another reason to select organically grown vegetables whenever possible. With organically grown vegetables you are also sure that the produce has not been dyed, waxed or irradiated.) Be sure to wash nonorganic produce thoroughly. If you think it's appropriate, use a bit of dishwashing detergent (a way to reduce pesticide residues significantly).

Organic produce may be hard to come by in your area, but you can always grow your

(continued on page 34)

Best Ingredient Choices for Feeding Your Pet

Use the table below as a confidence builder when you begin to prepare healthful homemade food for your pet. At a glance you have all the information you need for choosing the most desirable ingredients—the least costly, quickest to prepare, most additive-free and richest in nutrients

Approx. Cost per Gram of Protein	Grains	Features*	Legumes
+/- ½ cent	—	—	Soybeans (CO)
	—	—	Split peas (C)
1 cent	Oats (CO)	Ca, I, P, S	Split peas (O)
	Cornmeal (CO)	**A**, S	Pinto beans (CO)
	Millet (CO)	**B**, I, P, S	Red kidney beans (CO)
	Barley (CO)	—	White navy beans (CO)
	Brown rice (CO)	—	Lentils (CO)
	Wheat berries (O)	I, P	—
2 cents	Brown rice (O)	—	—
	Bulgur (CO)	I	—
	Buckwheat (CO)	**Ca**, P	—
	Nutritional yeast (O)	**B, I**, P	—
	Potatoes (C)	B	—
	—	—	—
	—	—	—
3 cents	—	—	—
	—	—	—
	—	—	—
4 cents	Whole-wheat bread (C)	I, P	Tofu (O)
	—	—	—
	—	—	—
	—	—	—

*High nutrients are given in comparison to equivalent calorie portions of other items listed in the same food group. Boldface signifies remarkable values of unusually nutritious ingredients in their category.

KEY

C = conventionally grown, using pesticides, synthetic fertilizers and so forth

N = natural, i.e., no additives, no drugs or hormones fed to livestock

O = available organically grown

A = high in vitamin A

B = high in B vitamins

vital to cats and dogs. Because protein is basic in planning a meal for these pets (much more important than for humans), cost counts. Check the first column on the left for the approximate price per gram of protein in various foods—½ cent for soybeans, for example, and 1 cent for oats.

Features*	Meats	Features*	Dairy Products	Features*
A, Ca, I, P	—	—	—	—
P	—	—	—	—
A, P	Ground turkey (C)	**P**	Cottage cheese (C)	A, Ca, **P**
Ca	Beef liver (C)	**A, B, I, P**	Eggs (C)	**A, I, P**
I	Canned mackerel	**Ca, P**	—	—
I	—	—	—	—
A, I, P	—	—	—	—
—	—	—	—	—
—	Ground turkey (N)	**P**	Cottage cheese (N)	B, Ca, **P**
—	Ground chicken (C)	**P**	Eggs (N)	**A, P**
—	Regular hamburger (C)	—	Powdered milk (CN)	**B, Ca, P**
—	Lean hamburger (C)	A, I	Milk (CN)	A
—	Beef heart (C)	B, I, **P**	Cheddar cheese (C)	A, Ca
—	Chicken liver (C)	B, I, **P**	—	—
—	Canned tuna	**A, P**	—	—
—	Chuck roast (C)	—	Cheddar cheese (N)	Ca
—	—	—	Eggs, free-range (N)	P
—	—	—	Low-fat yogurt (C)	**B, Ca**
Ca, I, P	Ground chicken (N)	**P**	Low-fat yogurt (N)	**B, Ca**
—	Regular hamburger (N)	I	—	—
—	Chuck roast (N)	—	—	—
—	Canned salmon	A, **Ca, P**	—	—

Ca = high in calcium
I = high in iron
P = high in protein
S = short cooking time (saves time, money, natural resources)

own. Even apartment-dwellers can raise high-nutrition vegetables in the form of sprouts and potted greens.

Here's how to grow fresh, nutritious sprouts. First, buy one or two sprouting jars, or make your own by putting a piece of screen or cheesecloth inside a canning jar ring on a one-quart jar. Add two table-spoons alfalfa seeds or ½ cup lentils or mung beans (both available at natural food stores). Cover with water and soak for eight hours or overnight.

Afterward, drain off the water onto some thirsty houseplants. Rinse the sprouting seeds three or four times a day and place the jar mouth angled slightly down so the water can drain into a bowl or sink. After a couple of days, flood the jar and wash off excess seed coats through a coarser screen, if desired. In three to five days the sprouts will be ready to eat. If your pet won't eat the sprouts at first, you might try chopping them up.

Many dogs and cats also relish wheat grass. They'll even "graze" directly from the pots, if allowed, in the same way they go for lawn grass. This is part of a natural cleansing instinct, so you shouldn't try to discourage it. If herbicides and synthetic fertilizers have been applied to your lawn or if your pet is housebound, growing wheat grass can provide your animal with a safe, healthy source of greens.

Here's how to grow wheat grass. Soak one to two tablespoons of wheat berries (available at natural food stores) overnight. Drain the water onto some thirsty houseplants. Almost fill a flower pot or tray with potting soil and sprinkle the seeds evenly on top, spacing them about one berry apart. Cover with ¼

inch of potting soil. Water daily, just enough to keep the soil slightly moist.

When the shoots are about four inches high, offer them to your animal friend for grazing or "mow" some of the grass down to about an inch with a pair of scissors. Chop the trimmings and mix them into a meal occasionally.

Herbs are special plants. In addition to being excellent sources of minerals, they also possess mild medicinal qualities. Occasionally, add a pinch of any of the following to your pet's food: alfalfa, parsley, thyme, dandelion, red clover, raspberry or black-berry leaves, basil, comfrey, linden flowers or fenugreek.

SNACKS AND FLAVORINGS

Healthful natural snacks, flavorings and supplements help to round out a pet's diet, adding both appeal and nutrition. A good general rule for feeding snacks is to allow your animal fairly ample amounts of any healthful food it really likes, up to 20 percent of the diet. The following snacks, which can also be used as training rewards, are healthy alternatives to the kinds of human junk food that pets sometimes get hooked on.

BONES

Both cats and dogs, but especially dogs, have a high calcium requirement. That's why bonemeal or other calcium supplementation is an important component in my recipes. You may also let your pet gnaw on bones occasionally. It's the animal's most natural way to get calcium, and many pets relish bones. (If you do this fairly often, you may reduce the calcium supplementation as much as 25 percent.)

Be careful about feeding chicken, turkey, fish or pork bones to your pet, however, because they splinter easily and can cause injury. Some cats can manage these little bones quite well, but dogs do better with large, meaty ones. Feed your pet raw bones only, because cooked bones can splinter into sharp fragments.

Save the bones you can't give directly to your animal, and simmer them in water into a mineral-rich stock, which you can use for cooking your pet's grains. Adding a little vinegar and salt to the brew helps to extract the minerals.

One word of caution: If your dog is not used to eating bones, he may go crazy with delight when he is introduced to one. As a result, he may eat too much bone at one time, irritating his digestive tract. The result can be either constipation or diarrhea. Also, if your animal's health is not the greatest, digesting bones may be difficult at first. I believe this problem is related to weak stomach acid that develops because of a nutritional deficiency. So go easy at first and limit the time you allow your pet to gnaw on bones. A 15-minute trial period is a good start. As your pet's health improves, digesting bones will be easier. Also note that it is not unusual for a dog's stool to be hard and white after eating a lot of bones.

Both dogs and cats benefit from an occasional bone fast (one or two days a month in which they are given nothing but water and raw bones). These regular short fasts mimic natural conditions in which predators have both lean and fat times. They give the animal's digestive tract an opportunity to put aside regular duties and get at some overlooked "housecleaning." The practice of fasting also has the added benefit of keeping your pet's teeth and gums strong and healthy.

A similar idea is to occasionally feed your cat nothing all day but a small whole Cornish game hen, uncooked, or a piece of raw chicken.

BISCUITS

Homemade biscuits are another great treat for pets. (See recipes in "Additional Recipes" on page 350.) If you don't have the time to make your own, look for the additive-free commercially made biscuits that are found in many health food stores. Read the labels carefully and watch out for meat meal and meat by-products, sugar (sucrose) and any artificial colors, flavorings and preservatives.

By including some hard foods in the diet, such as biscuits, bones or even whole carrots, you will give your pet a good way to exercise and clean its teeth and gums.

FRUIT

Many dogs have a sweet tooth, and they enjoy an occasional piece of fruit as a snack. They like dried fruits such as figs, dates, prunes, raisins and apricots as well as fresh fruits like apples and berries. Like vegetables, fruits are great storehouses of vitamins, minerals and vital energy. For best digestion, feed such foods apart from the regular mealtime. Dried fruits are especially good natural sources of potassium, an important mineral that can sometimes be in short supply; other good sources are peanuts, potatoes and tomato sauce. Dates are extremely rich in folic acid, an important B vitamin.

NUTS AND SEEDS

We don't include nuts and seeds in our recipes because they are often expensive and contain more fat than protein. However, I have heard a few reports of healthy dogs who have eaten no form of concentrated protein other than nuts for many years. One of my clients gives his dog peanut butter sandwiches as a snack when they go on picnics. Nuts and seeds are best digested raw, either when made into a nut butter or finely ground. Now and then, you can include some in your pet's diet in place of fatty meats, if you like.

VEGGIE BURGERS

Have you ever tried any of the meat-substitute burgers made especially for vegetarians? Many of them are quite delicious, and we've found that a lot of pets think so too. We discovered this one day when our cat was going through a period of "finicky-ness," turning up his nose at what seemed to us like a perfectly acceptable rendition of what he usually eats. (Maybe "usual" was the problem and he just wanted a little more variety.)

In any case, when we decided to share a little of the "Gardenburger" we were eating, he snarfed it up in nothing flat. We pulled another one out of the freezer, popped it in the toaster, and he demolished it as well. We knew we were on to something, and since then, we've found these make excellent taste-tempters, both for mixing in with his usual fare and for an occasional meal in itself.

Not all meatless burgers are created equal, so you may need to try several brands. The tastiest ones seem to be those that incorporate some dairy products and that aren't too heavy on the soybeans or tempeh (a soybean product).

If your cat or small dog relishes them, you may even be tempted to feed meatless burgers as a major part of its diet; they are convenient and often use organic ingredients. However, we wouldn't recommend using them for more than, say, a third of the diet. We don't have any way to know how well their nutritional content meets the special needs of dogs and cats. Nor do we know how much calcium, vitamin A, taurine and so on to add to make any needed adjustments. We'd advise ⅛ to ¼ teaspoon bone-meal per burger when you serve it. Crumble up the burger and mix in the powder.

FLAVORINGS

Nutritional yeast and other items in our recommended nutritional supplements section (see "Supplements" below) also serve to add flavor to food. In addition, you can experiment with moderate amounts of the following flavorings: tamari (naturally brewed soy sauce), miso, tomato sauce, butter, garlic, mild chili powder, natural broth powders and herbed sea salt mixtures. Broken-up corn chips (organic, if you can get them) coated with nutritional yeast are also a hit with many pets. Just don't get carried away! Look to your animal for preferences. It's interesting that dogs, given a choice, usually prefer unsalted food. It appears that they have some natural good food sense, doesn't it?

GARLIC

Not only is garlic tasty to many pets, it also helps to tone up the digestive tract and discourage worms and other parasites, including fleas. Garlic is particularly potent when it's added fresh. Besides crushing a clove or two directly into a recipe, there's a tasty condiment you can add to your pet's daily fare as you serve it. Simply crush a clove of garlic into a small amount of tamari soy sauce. Let it sit about ten minutes, then remove the garlic. Use about ⅛ teaspoon to each cup of food.

YEAST SPRINKLE

Besides the nutritional yeast that is included in the "Healthy Powder" supplement (see page 39), many animals love to have a little yeast sprinkled on top of their meals, much the way we enjoy a little Parmesan cheese on top of pasta. Large-flake torula (nutritional) yeast is one of the best flavored. If you use it often, mix some up in a jar with a little powdered calcium supplement for optimal calcium/phosphorus balance. If your pet likes garlic, you can also add a little in powdered form. Here's the formula: two cups nutritional yeast plus three tablespoons bonemeal (5,600 milligrams calcium) plus one to four teaspoons unsalted garlic powder (optional).

A note on yeast and allergies: Some people say that yeast should not be used as food for animals because it may cause allergies. I can only report that my experience is to the contrary. I find that yeast is an excellent food without any such side effects. Granted, an occasional animal may be allergic to yeast. But I find that this is a very rare phenomenon. Instead, I find that pets are most often allergic to foods like beef, chicken, corn, soy and such.

SUPPLEMENTS

In addition to the basic natural food groups mentioned earlier, I always recommend including several nutrition-packed food supplements—such as bonemeal, nutritional yeast, lecithin, kelp, vegetable oil and several vitamins—in the diet. Part of the purpose of these supplements is to fortify the diet with plenty of important vitamins and minerals. Unfortunately, these are often inadequately represented even in fresh foods today because of loss during storage and cooking, soil depletion and forced-growing methods. Even the complication of acid rain has been causing a decrease in the ability of plants to take up essential minerals from the soil. For animals that are not in the best of health, supplements are an essential part of the diet.

Another reason why I recommend supplements is simply to balance the ingredients of the recipes given in this book so that they meet the nutritional standards for dogs and cats set by the Association of American Feed Control Officials for such important nutrients as calcium, iron, linoleic acid, vitamin A and B vitamins. So don't think of supplements as something optional, they are an integral part of each recipe, unless noted otherwise.

The basic supplements described below are usually included in each recipe. Here's a summary of the purpose of each supplement as well as various sources and how to prepare the supplement for inclusion in the diet.

CALCIUM SUPPLEMENT

Some supplemental source of calcium is an essential ingredient in every recipe. Also, every recipe should have a proper calcium/phosphorus ratio. This ratio should be between 1:1 and 2:1 for dogs and between 1.1:1 and 1.3:1 for cats. Here are some ways to add this calcium.

BONEMEAL

Buy the powdered bonemeal that is sold for human use such as Schiff Bone-all and Kal. It comes from sources less contaminated than the bonemeal sold in garden-supply departments. Bonemeal is the most natural calcium source for carnivores and provides many trace minerals. It is also convenient and easy to use. It contains lots of phosphorus, but in the recommended amounts there is still plenty of extra calcium to balance out the phosphorus. Bonemeal is the best choice when feeding large dogs, especially those with bone problems or signs of hip dysplasia.

DI-CALCIUM PHOSPHATE

For those people who prefer not to use animal products but who want a higher combined amount of calcium and phosphorus in the diet than provided by a calcium product alone, substitute di-calcium phosphate for bonemeal. This product is sometimes available in pet stores. You should use about two-thirds the amount stated for bonemeal in any recipe.

CALCIUM TABLETS OR POWDER

Besides bonemeal, each recipe gives a suggested dose of calcium, expressed in milligrams. Unlike bonemeal, this choice provides no additional phosphorus. This means less total calcium is needed to balance the total amount of phosphorus. The result is a lower-ash diet.

You can supply "plain" calcium through calcium carbonate, chelated calcium, calcium gluconate or calcium lactate. Except for the calcium carbonate, these are also considered the best assimilated forms of calcium. Avoid products that also contain phosphorus or magnesium.

Just look on the label to see how much powder or how many tablets you must use to equal the milligrams of calcium called for in a recipe. If you buy tablets, use a blender, mortar and pestle or pill crusher to grind them to a powder before mixing into the food.

EGGSHELL POWDER

This is the cheapest route, because you can make the supplement yourself from egg shells, which are very high in calcium carbonate. Here's how to make eggshell powder. Wash the eggshells right after cracking and let them dry until you have accumulated a dozen or so. (Each whole eggshell makes about a teaspoon of powder, which equals about 1,800 milligrams of calcium.) Then bake at 300°F for about ten minutes. This removes a mineral-oil coating sometimes added to keep eggs from drying out. It also makes the shells dry and brittle enough to grind to a fine powder with a nut and seed grinder, blender or mortar and pestle. Grind well enough that there are no sharp, gritty pieces.

"HEALTHY POWDER"

This rich mixture of nutrients is used in all the recipes. It contains several important food supplements, which are available at most natural food stores: nutritional yeast (rich in B vitamins, iron and other nutrients); lecithin (for linoleic acid, choline and inositol, which help your animal emulsify and absorb fats, improving the condition of its coat and digestion); powdered kelp (for iodine and trace minerals); enough calcium to balance the high phosphorus levels in yeast and lecithin (this enables you to add this powder in any reasonable quantity to any recipe or other diet) and vitamin C (not officially required for dogs or cats because they synthesize their own, but clinical experiences suggest its value).

HEALTHY POWDER

2   cups nutritional (torula) yeast

1   cup lecithin granules

¼   cup kelp powder

¼   cup bonemeal (or 9,000 milligrams calcium or 5 teaspoons eggshell powder)

1,000 milligrams vitamin C (ground) or ¼ teaspoon sodium ascorbate (optional)

Mix all ingredients together in a 1-quart container and refrigerate.

Add to each recipe as instructed. You may also add this mixture to commercial food as follows: 1 to 2 teaspoons per day for cats or small dogs; 2 to 3 teaspoons per day for medium-size dogs; 1 to 2 tablespoons per day for large dogs.

Variations:

Yeast substitution: The yeast is optional, but if you omit it, reduce the calcium in the Healthy Powder formula to 5 teaspoons bonemeal or 3,200 milligrams calcium or 1¾ teaspoons eggshell powder. Use half the usual amount of Healthy Powder specified in each recipe. To replace the lost nutrients, add a complete multi-vitamin-mineral supplement to the daily food, using the amount recommended on the label. Do not use additional vitamin A, C or E, because they should be adequately supplied by the pet vitamin.

Kelp substitution: If your animal doesn't like the flavor of kelp or you can't find it, substitute ¾ teaspoon of iodized salt plus ¼ cup of either alfalfa powder or montmorillonite (a natural trace mineral powder). Alternatively, you can use a complete pet multi-vitamin-mineral supplement as instructed on the label.

VEGETABLE OIL

Vegetable oils are all excellent sources of linoleic acid and other important unsaturated fatty acids needed by both dogs and cats. Dry foods are often low in fats to minimize rancidity during storage. Deficiencies of unsaturated fatty acids in the diet lead to dry hair coats and hair loss.

Use cold-pressed safflower, soy or corn oil and refrigerate it in a well-sealed container. If you like, you can premix vitamin E (see below) into the oil. Use 1,600 to 2,100 IU per cup. (Don't premix vitamin A into it, however, as this could create excesses in some recipes.)

Note: You may substitute butter for up to 50 percent of the oil in the cat recipes. Cats normally have high levels of animal fat in their diets and do well with it.

VITAMIN A

This important vitamin is included in many of the recipes, especially for cats. Most of the dog food recipes don't call for it because dogs can make their own vitamin A from carotene found in vegetables. (But if you leave out the vegetables in your dog's diet, add about 1,000 IU of vitamin A for every cup omitted.) Cats, on the other hand, require a preformed animal source of vitamin A. They are also sensitive to either too little or too much in their diets, so adhere to the amount listed in each recipe. There are four ways to provide the vitamin A in each recipe.

- Cod-liver oil. Because it is also an excellent source of unsaturated fatty acids, cod-liver oil is highly recommended, if your pet accepts it. Seal well and refrigerate it to prevent rancidity. Read the label to see how many teaspoons provide the amount of vitamin A called for in the recipe.

♦ Vitamin A and D capsules. Buy the lowest potency. This will probably be 10,000 IU per capsule. Break open the capsule to use.

♦ Liquid vitamin A and D. These drops are more convenient than capsules, if you can find them. Get the kind sold for humans in nutrition stores. The typical potency is about 1,600 IU per drop. Use the number of drops closest to the total amount called for.

♦ Pet vitamins. These tablets will also add extra vitamins and minerals to the diet. If you use pet vitamins, you may omit both vitamins A and E from the recipes. Instead, simply add the vitamins directly to each meal as suggested on the product label. (Or, if you prefer, you may crush several tablets into the recipe when you make it, adding an amount that will provide a level of vitamin A comparable to that called for in the recipe.)

Note: Some pet supplements supply large amounts of calcium without phosphorus, as you'll discover from the label. If this is the case, decrease the calcium supplement in the recipe a bit. Further, it is important to avoid any pet supplements containing the preservative sodium benzoate, especially for cats, for whom this preservative is a poison.

VITAMIN E

I include extra vitamin E in the diet for several reasons. Not only does it aid important body functions, such as fighting disease, but it also helps minimize the effects of pollution.

An antioxidant, vitamin E helps to preserve and protect the vitamin A and fatty acids in other supplements and foods. There are two ways that this supplement can be provided.

♦ Natural-source vitamin E capsules. Look for products containing the d-alpha tocopherols. (The dl-alpha tocopherols are a synthetic form.) The gelatin capsule variety provides a good "storage container." Open a fresh capsule for the recipe or premix it into the vegetable oil (see above). It's okay to use more vitamin E than the amount called for, if that's more convenient.

♦ Wheat-germ oil. Here is a good way to provide vitamin E in a natural complex. But be careful not to feed your animal rancid wheat-germ oil, which is detectable by a slightly bitter or burning aftertaste. Buy wheat-germ oil in capsule form. Read the label to determine the appropriate amount to use.

IRON (OPTIONAL)

You may choose to supplement your dog's diet with a source of iron. (Our cat diets, overall, do not require any supplementation to meet the latest official standards for pet foods because these diets contain a higher portion of meat.) After many years in which it was considered adequate to feed dogs iron in the amount of 0.003 percent of the total diet (by dry weight), the standards were raised in 1992 to 0.008 percent. As you can see in "Nutritional Composition of Recipes for Dogs" and "Nutritional Composition of Recipes for Cats" on pages 54 and 56, our unsupplemented dog diets provide 0.006 to 0.007 percent iron, which is slightly below the new standard.

But in my clinical experience, lack of iron in dogs is not a problem. Animals on my natural, home-prepared diets have shown very healthy blood values with no deficiencies of iron. Therefore, I am cautious about recommending iron supplementation. A similar controversy has arisen lately in the human nutrition field. Some major vitamin manufacturers are concerned that too much iron in their products may be causing problems. As a result, they now offer customers a choice between supplements with or without iron.

Though many diets in this book are adequate without supplementation, you may wish to add extra iron.

- Include an iron supplement from a health food store. Use iron asporotates or chelated iron, forms which are best assimilated. Either empty the contents of a capsule into the recipe or crush a tablet to a powder and mix it in. Add 10 to 15 milligrams of iron to any dog recipe that doesn't include heart, liver or millet. This supplementation will bring the levels up to the current recommended standards.
- Include plenty of heart and millet. Both of these are high in iron. Occasional use of liver also boosts the iron content of the diet.

TAURINE (OPTIONAL)

When preparing cat food, pet food manufacturers have been adding taurine. Unlike most animals, cats cannot synthesize this amino acid themselves, so they have to get it from their diets. And taurine is necessary, because a deficiency is known to cause degeneration of the retina and possible blindness as well as cardiac problems. Apparently, some shortages in the taurine level of pet foods developed because of processing procedures. For example, studies have shown that up to 80 percent of the taurine that occurs naturally in meat can be lost in the cooking process.

As a result of this information, the new standards call for taurine to comprise 0.1 percent of the diet on a dry weight basis. This amounts to 60 to 80 milligrams per day for the amount eaten by a ten-pound cat. If the meat is fed raw, as recommended, our chicken- and beef-based diets contain 30 to 50 milligrams of taurine per day's serving, which is a bit below the new standard. If it's cooked, the level drops to only 12 to 35 milligrams per day. Surprisingly, I found that even my pure meat recipe, Quick Feline Meatfest, falls slightly low, providing about 48 milligrams per day when made with beef and 76 when made with chicken.

Investigating further, however, I learned that the daily taurine content of the wild feline diet is only 25 to 50 milligrams and that this amount has been found adequate in most experimental studies. In conclusion, I am not concerned about the taurine content of my cat diet if the meat is fed raw. However, if you feed the meat cooked (e.g., from your own leftovers), use a partly vegetarian diet (see chapter 5) or just want to err on the safe side, there are two ways to address this issue.

- Add capsule(s) or tablet(s) of taurine in the amount stated in the recipes as an optional ingredient. Pills or powdered capsules of taurine can be purchased at many stores that specialize in nutritional products. Also, many vitamin-mineral supplements for cats now contain taurine. Just look at the label to see how many units are needed to provide the amount of taurine indicated in the recipe, rounding the figure upward if necessary. Be sure to add the taurine to the recipe only after the cooked grain has cooled down, or the heat might destroy it.

◆ Include tuna, mackerel, clams and heart in the diet. All are naturally high in taurine. (Maybe that's why most cats love them!)

Now that you have a good understanding of what goes into a fresh, natural diet for your pet, learn how to put it together in practical, tasty, balanced recipes!

CHAPTER FOUR

EASY-TO-MAKE RECIPES FOR PET FOOD

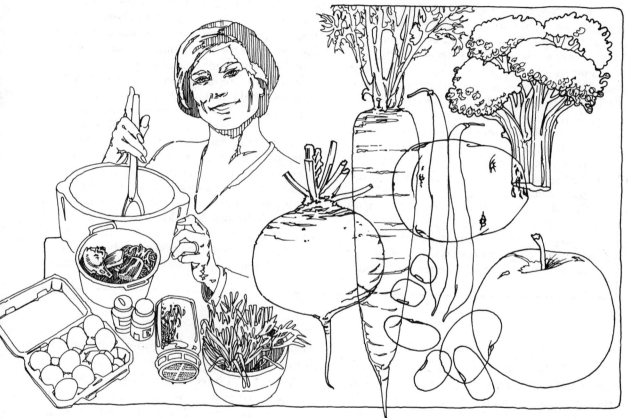

Now it's time to really talk turkey—to show you a variety of delicious, well-balanced recipes for feeding your animals. Fixing fresh, nutritious meals for pets is very little trouble once you get the hang of it. Many people even find it fun, especially when the concoction meets with the enthusiastic approval of an eager eater.

To ensure the best nutritional content, I

again remind you to follow the recipes fairly closely. Do, however, use a variety of grains, meats and vegetables rather than stick to the same formula every time.

I will give you an idea of how much to feed your pet, but you can generally give your dog or cat as much as it wants, unless overweight is a problem. A simple indicator: You should be able to feel your pet's ribs eas-

Streamline Your Pet Food Preparation System

Follow these tips for easier preparation of your pet's meals, preserving extras and adding appetizing touches when serving.

Keep recipes and supplies handy. Once you work out a basic routine, copy the recipes on cards or durable cardstock, adding notes if you care to. Store them with your pet's supplements in a cupboard or some other spot convenient to your food preparation area. That way they'll always be right at hand while you're mixing the chow.

Use quick-cooking grains. These include rolled oats, bulgur, cornmeal, whole-wheat couscous and quinoa. For a small pet it even makes sense to use crumbled whole-wheat bread sometimes.

Coordinate pet food preparation with cooking your own food. Unless you're fixing very large quantities of animal food, it's often convenient to prepare it while waiting for your own food to cook. Better yet, coordi-nate both meal plans, using the same basic grains— maybe rice or cornmeal—and other ingredients, such as tuna or lean hamburger.

Freeze extras. For small animals make up one to two weeks' worth of food at a time, freezing extras in plastic dairy and deli con-tainers. Thaw the frozen meals in the refriger-ator 24 hours in advance of feeding time.

Warm up prepared food. Since you will probably make enough chow to last for sev-eral days at a time and refrigerate the extras, here's how to warm up cold food to make it more palatable for your pet and easier to di-gest. Rinse the bowl with warm water. Dish the food into the bowl and pour a little hot water over it. Use a fork or shake the bowl to lightly mix the food in the water without making it mushy. Sprinkle a little yeast or other flavoring on top, if you wish. Mi-crowaving is not recommended because it would defeat the purpose of using raw meat.

---

ily as you slide your hand over his sides; if you can't, he's probably too heavy. Visible ribs usually mean the opposite. In cases of obesity, use the weight-loss recipes in the next chapter. If you have a number of ani-mals, you will, of course, need to multiply the recipe amounts accordingly.

BOOSTER MIXES FOR DOG KIBBLE

Let's start with something simple: three fresh food combos that you can add to a good-quality dog kibble, such as those sold at natural food stores. If you're not ready to jump whole hog into the home-prepared diet, or if you have several large dogs, these shortcuts offer a convenient way to provide many of the benefits of fresh foods and nu-tritious supplements and still maintain nutri-tional balance. By adding fresh meat, dairy products, vegetable oil and food supple-ments, you boost your dog's intake of qual-ity protein, fatty acids, lecithin, B vitamins and minerals—all helpful for skin and coat problems.

Resist any temptation to simplify these additions by just throwing a slab of meat or a dash of oil on the kibble rather than following the recipe as given. Meat is dramatically low in calcium as compared with its phosphorus content, so using meat alone could result in a net dietary calcium deficiency. That's why a calcium supplement is added to the recipes. Extra oil by itself is also counterproductive as it will lower the overall percentage of protein and every other nutrient in the kibble, which may already contain a marginal amount of the essentials.

As with other recipes, you can always pre-mix larger amounts of these supplements and freeze extras, thawing and using them as needed.

FRESH MEAT SUPPLEMENT FOR DOG KIBBLE

- 4 teaspoons vegetable oil
- 4 teaspoons Healthy Powder (page 39)
- 1¾ teaspoons bonemeal (or 1,100–1,200 milligrams calcium or ⅔ teaspoon eggshell powder)
- 50–200 IU vitamin E
- 5,000–10,000 IU vitamin A (or alternate regularly with Fresh Egg Supplement, below)
- 1 pound (2 cups) chopped or ground raw turkey, chicken, lean hamburger, lean chuck or lean beef heart

Mix the oil, powder, bonemeal and vitamins together. Then combine the mixture with the meat, coating it well.

Yield: Slightly more than 2 cups.

At mealtime, feed ¼ cup of this mixture for every cup of dog kibble served. You can either mix the meat supplement and kibble together or serve each separately.

COTTAGE CHEESE SUPPLEMENT FOR DOG KIBBLE

Cottage cheese is an inexpensive, convenient and palatable source of protein that can boost the nutritional value of kibble.

- 2 teaspoons vegetable oil
- 2 teaspoons Healthy Powder (page 39)
- ½ teaspoon bonemeal (or 300 milligrams calcium or ⅛ teaspoon eggshell powder)
- 50–10,000 IU vitamin A
- ¾ cup creamed cottage cheese
- ¼–½ cup vegetables (optional)

Mix the oil in kibble. Toss in the powder and bonemeal, coating the kibble; add the vitamin A. Serve the cottage cheese and vegetables together on the side, or mix them into the kibble.

Yield: Enough to supplement 2 to 3 cups of dog kibble.

FRESH EGG SUPPLEMENT FOR DOG KIBBLE

- 1 teaspoon vegetable oil
- 1 teaspoon Healthy Powder (page 39)
- ⅓ teaspoon bonemeal (or 200 milligrams calcium or ⅛ teaspoon eggshell powder)
- 50–200 IU vitamin E
- 2 eggs

Mix everything but the eggs into 1 to 2 cups of dog kibble. Break the eggs over the top.

Multiply the recipe accordingly when you are feeding more animals or large dogs. For 5 to 6 cups of kibble this would be: 1 tablespoon oil, 1 tablespoon powder, 1 teaspoon bonemeal (or about 600 milligrams calcium), 200–400 IU vitamin E and 3 eggs.

BASIC RECIPES FOR DOGS

The following recipes are meant to form the mainstay of the fresh, home-prepared diet for dogs. See "Nutritional Composition of Recipes for Dogs" on page 54 for nutritional data on each recipe. Each recipe indicates how many cups to feed adult dogs of different breed sizes. The weight range for each group is defined as follows: toy—2 to 15 pounds; small—15 to 35 pounds; medium—35 to 55 pounds; large—55 to 85 pounds; giant—85 to 165 pounds or more. These amounts will vary with many factors—activity level, ingredient substitutions, weather and so on. Let your dog's appetite and weight be the ultimate gauge.

DOGGIE OATS

Oats are a good choice of grain in cooking for pets. Not only are oats quick-cooking, but they contain more protein per calorie than any other common grain. It's best, though, to add some variety by substituting other grains at times (as recommended). That's because each grain varies in its amino acid composition and its vitamin and mineral levels. This versatile maintenance recipe for adult dogs ranges in protein value from about 22 percent (using fattier meats or tofu with bulgur) to 30 percent (using turkey with oats).

8   cups raw rolled oats (or 16 cups cooked oatmeal)

2   pounds (4 cups) raw ground or chopped turkey

½   cup Healthy Powder (page 39)

¼   cup vegetable oil

1   cup cooked vegetables (or less if raw and grated) (may be omitted occasionally)

3   tablespoons bonemeal (or 5,400–6,000 milligrams calcium or 1 tablespoon eggshell powder)

10,000 IU vitamin A (optional if using carrots)

400 IU vitamin E

1   teaspoon tamari soy sauce or ¼ teaspoon iodized salt (optional)

1–2   cloves garlic, crushed or minced (optional)

15 milligrams iron (optional)

Bring 1 gallon (16 cups) of water to a boil. Add the oats, cover and turn off the heat, letting the oats cook for 10 to 15 minutes, or until soft. Don't stir while cooking or the oats will become mushy. Then combine with the remaining ingredients and serve.

Yield: About 22 cups, with 205 kilocalories per cup.

Daily ration (in cups): toy—⅔ to 2⅔; small—2⅔ to 5⅓; medium—5⅓ to 7; large—7 to 9¾; giant—9¾ to 14⅔+.

Grain substitutes: Instead of oats, you may use 4 cups of bulgur (+ 8 to 12 cups water). If you're using poultry or lean cuts of beef, you may also use these lower-protein grains: 4 cups millet (+ 12 cups water); 3 cups brown rice (+ 6 cups water); 4 cups cornmeal (+ 16 cups water); 4 cups barley (+ 8 to 12 cups water). The higher-protein grains are necessary to provide adequate amounts of protein.

Meat substitutes: Instead of turkey, try chicken, hamburger, chuck or beef heart; lean or medium grades are okay, but don't use fattier meats.

If you use oats or bulgur, you may occasionally substitute either of the following for the meat: 2 pints cottage cheese plus 4 eggs, or 32 ounces of tofu plus 8 eggs. Add the eggs while the grain is still hot so they'll set slightly and give the best texture. See the next chapter for more vegetarian recipes suitable for dogs.

MINI DOGGIE OATS

For your convenience, here is the same recipe, divided by ¼.

    2   cups raw rolled oats (or 4 cups cooked oatmeal)
    ½   pound (1 cup) raw ground or chopped turkey
    2   tablespoons Healthy Powder (page 39)
    1   tablespoon vegetable oil
    ¼   cup cooked vegetables (or less if raw and grated)
    2   slightly rounded teaspoons bonemeal (or 1,400–1,500 milligrams calcium or ¾ teaspoon eggshell powder)
        2,500–5,000 IU vitamin A (optional if using carrots)
        100 IU vitamin E
    ¼   teaspoon tamari soy sauce or dash of iodized salt (optional)
    1   small clove garlic, crushed or minced (optional)
        5 milligrams iron (optional)

Yield: About 5½ cups, with 205 kilocalories per cup.

Daily ration: Same as for Doggie Oats (opposite page).

Grain substitutes: 1 cup bulgur (+ 2 cups water = 2½ cups cooked). With lean meats only: 1 cup cornmeal (+ 4 cups water = 4 cups cooked); 1 cup millet (+ 3 cups water = 3 cups cooked); ¾ cups brown rice (+ 1½ cups water = 1¾ cups cooked); 1 cup barley (+ 2 to 3 cups water = 2½ to 3 cups cooked); 5 cups boiled potatoes.
Meat substitutes: With oats only: 8 ounces tofu plus 2 eggs.

DOG LOAF

This recipe uses egg as a binder, so that you can either serve it raw or bake it like a meat loaf, with bread crumbs or other grains. It ranges from 24 to 30 percent protein, depending on which meat and grain you use. The egg provides adequate vitamin A, plus there is vitamin A in the vegetables.

    ¼   pound (½ cup) fairly lean beef heart
    6   slices whole-wheat bread, crumbled (about 3 cups)
    1   cup whole milk
    2   large eggs
    ¼   cup corn or other vegetables (can be omitted occasionally)
    1   tablespoon Healthy Powder (page 39)
    1   tablespoon vegetable oil
    1½ teaspoons bonemeal (or 1,000 milligrams calcium or ½ teaspoon eggshell powder)
        100 IU vitamin E
        10 milligrams iron (optional)
    ¼   teaspoon soy sauce or dash of iodized salt (optional)
    1   small clove garlic, crushed or minced (optional)

Combine all ingredients, adding water, if needed, to make a nice texture. Serve raw. Or press the mixture into a casserole dish so it's 1 to 2 inches thick and bake at 350° for 20 to 30 minutes, or until set and lightly browned.

If you use a moist grain and don't bake the mixture, you may choose to serve the milk separately rather than combine it in the mix. Another alternative is to mix ¼ cup powdered milk right into the recipe.

Yield: About 5¾ cups, with 190 kilocalories per cup.

(continued)

Daily ration: About the same (or slightly more) as amounts for Doggie Oats (above).

Grain substitutes: Instead of wheat bread, you may use 1¼ cups oats (+ 2½ cups water) or ½ cup bulgur (+ 1 cup water). With lean meats only you may use: ¾ cup cornmeal (+ 3 cups water); ½ cup millet (+ 1½ cups water); ½ cup barley (+ 1½ cups water); or 2½ cups boiled potatoes.
Bean substitutes: Try ground or chopped chicken, turkey, lean or medium chuck or hamburger instead of beef heart. Beef or chicken liver may be used once in a while, but not on a regular basis.

One-on-One

Now here's a truly inspired recipe, easy to remember and easy to multiply because it uses exactly one unit of each ingredient! It is also economical and ecologically sound, deriving part of its protein from beans. The protein levels vary from 22.2 percent (using beef heart) to 23.2 percent (main version) up to 28.5 percent (using turkey and oats). The calcium to phosphorus ratio is consistently excellent throughout the many variations.

The key to convenience in this recipe is to cook large quantities of beans in advance. Follow the cooking directions on the package. Freeze extra quantities in 1-cup containers (or appropriate multiples if you increase the recipe) and thaw as needed. The main version uses rice because it's a grain many people use in their own menus, but the other grain choices listed are higher-protein and, for the most part, faster-cooking.

1　cup brown rice (or 2½ cups cooked)

1　cup (½ pound) lean hamburger (or turkey, chicken, lean heart or lean chuck)

1　cup cooked kidney beans (half of a 15-ounce can)

1　tablespoon Healthy Powder (page 39)

1　tablespoon vegetable oil

1　tablespoon bonemeal (or 1,600 milligrams calcium or 1 scant teaspoon eggshell powder)

1　5,000 IU vitamin A and D capsule (or part of a larger capsule)

1　400–800 IU vitamin E capsule

1　teaspoon soy sauce or dash of iodized salt (optional)

1　small clove garlic, crushed or minced (optional)

1　10–15 milligram iron capsule (optional)

Bring 2 cups of water to a boil. Add the rice and simmer for 35 to 45 minutes. Mix in the other ingredients and serve.

Yield: About 4¾ cups, with 348 kilocalories per cup.

Daily ration (in cups): toy—⅓ to 1⅔; small—1⅔ to 3¼; medium—3¼ to 4+; large—4+ to 5¾; giant—5¾ to 8½+.

If you want to boost the protein content about 1 percent, add one egg or one tablespoon of nutritional yeast.
Grain substitutes: Instead of rice, you may use (with the highest protein versions listed first) 2 cups rolled oats (+ 4 cups water = 4 cups cooked); 1 cup bulgur (+ 2 cups water = 2½ cups cooked); 1 cup millet (+ 3 cups water = 3 cups cooked); 1½ cups cornmeal (+ 4 cups water = 4 cups cooked); or 1 cup barley (+ 2 to 3 cups water = 2½ to 3 cups cooked).
Bean substitutes: You may use one cup, cooked, of soybeans, pintos, black beans or white (navy) beans instead of kidney beans. Soybeans have the most protein.

FAST AND FRESH: DOGS

Here are three really simple recipes for those inevitable occasions when you have an eager eater nudging you, and you suddenly discover that you're all out of dog food, both home-prepared and commercial. These recipes are not meant to serve as regular fare, but they do provide a fairly complete meal made of basic items you're likely to have on hand. You can feed them to your pooch up to two or three times a week.

Note: You may also use any of the basic cat recipes (below) for dogs. They contain more protein than dogs require, but that's no problem unless your dog is on a low-protein diet because of old age or kidney problems.

QUICK CANINE OATS AND EGGS

- 1 cup raw rolled oats (or 2 cups cooked oatmeal)
- 3 eggs
- 1 teaspoon bonemeal (or 600–700 milligrams calcium or ⅓ teaspoon eggshell powder)
    Healthy Powder (page 39) or nutritional yeast (optional)

Bring 2 cups of water to a boil. Add the oats, cover and turn off the heat, letting the oats cook in the hot water for about 10 minutes, or until soft. (Use extra oatmeal from your own breakfast or else make some up.) Then stir in the eggs and bonemeal. Let the eggs set slightly from the heat, then cool for a few minutes before serving. You may mix in a little Healthy Powder or nutritional yeast if you wish.

Yield: About 2¾ cups, with 205 kilocalories per cup.

Daily ration: Same as for Doggie Oats, above. (Makes one meal or a half-day's ration for a medium-size dog. Double the recipe to make breakfast for a giant-size dog.)

Grain substitutes: Instead of oats, you may use ½ cup bulgur (+1 cup water = 1¼ cups cooked) or ½ cup whole-wheat couscous (+ ¾ cup water = 1¼ cups cooked).

Here's another simple recipe that uses only one egg and may resemble your own breakfast.

QUICK CANINE OATMEAL

- ¾ cup raw rolled oats (or 1½ cups cooked oatmeal)
- ¾ teaspoon bonemeal (or 300 to 350 milligrams calcium or ¼ teaspoon powdered eggshell)
- 1 cup 2 percent milk
    Healthy Powder (page 39) or nutritional yeast (optional)
- 1 egg

Bring 1½ cups of water to a boil. Add the oats, cover and turn off the heat, letting the oats cook in the hot water for about 10 minutes, or until soft.

Put the oatmeal into your pet's food bowl. Mix in the bonemeal and top with the milk. Before serving, sprinkle with Healthy Powder or yeast, if desired. In a separate small bowl, stir the egg slightly to mix the yolk and white, and give it to the dog.

Yield: A little less than 3 cups, with about 160 kilocalories per cup.

Daily ration (in cups): toy—¾ to 3½; small—3½ to 6¾+; medium—6¾ to 9; large—9 to 12½; giant—12½ to 18¾+.

QUICK CANINE HASH

1   cup bulgur or whole-wheat couscous (or 2½ cups cooked)

1   cup (½ pound) chuck, hamburger, turkey or chicken

1½ teaspoons bonemeal (or 1,200 milligrams calcium or ¾ teaspoon eggshell powder)

Healthy Powder (page 39) or nutritional yeast (optional)

For the bulgur, bring 2 cups of water to a boil, add the bulgur, cover and simmer 10 to 20 minutes. For couscous, use 1½ cups water and cook 3 to 5 minutes. Add the meat or poultry and bonemeal and serve. You may sprinkle a little Healthy Powder or nutritional yeast on top if you wish.

If you use this recipe more than occasionally, it's nutritionally best to use bonemeal rather than other sources of calcium.

Yield: A little over 3½ cups, with about 340 kilocalories per cup.

Daily ration: Same as for One-on-One (above).

Grain substitutes: Instead of bulgur or couscous, use 1½ cups rolled oats (= 3 cups cooked) or, with poultry or other lean meats only: 1 cup millet (+ 3 cups water = 3 cups cooked); or 1 cup brown rice (+ 2 cups water = 2½ cups cooked).

BASIC RECIPES FOR CATS

Now let's look at some recipes for cats, starting with basic maintenance recipes that you can use as the foundation of your cat's new diet. See "Nutritional Composition of Recipes for Cats" on page 56 for information about the nutritional composition of these recipes.

Daily rations are given after each recipe for small (4 to 6 pounds), medium (7 to 9 pounds) and large (10 to 15 pounds) adult cats. Increase amounts for more active cats. Many factors can affect the quantity needed, so the best guide is your cat's appetite and whether the food maintains the cat at a normal weight.

The next two recipes use the smallest proportions of meat to grain. Thus, they are the most economical and ecologically sound ways to feed your cat a fresh diet and still provide a little more than the recommended minimum amount of protein.

BEEFY OATS

4   cups raw rolled oats (or 8 cups cooked oatmeal)

2   eggs

2   pounds (4 cups) ground lean beef heart (or lean chuck, lean hamburger, liver, kidney or other lean red meats)

4   tablespoons Healthy Powder (page 39)

2   tablespoons bonemeal (or 4,000 milligrams calcium or 2¼ teaspoons eggshell powder)

2   tablespoons vegetable oil or butter (or 1 tablespoon each)

10,000 IU vitamin A

100–200 IU vitamin E

1   teaspoon fresh vegetable with each meal (optional)

500 milligrams taurine supplement (optional)

Bring 8 cups (2 quarts) of water to a boil. Add the oats, cover and turn off the heat, letting the oats cook in the hot water for about 10 minutes, or until soft. Then stir in the eggs, letting them set slightly from the heat for a few minutes. Mix in the remaining ingredients.

Yield: About 12¾ cups, with around 220 kilocalories per cup. Immediately freeze whatever cannot be eaten in the next 2 to 3 days.

Daily ration (in cups): small—½ to ¾+; medium—1 to 1⅓; large—1½ to 2¼.

Grain substitutes: 2 cups millet (+ 6 cups water = 6 cups cooked millet) or 2 cups bulgur (+ 4 cups water = 5 cups cooked bulgur).

POULTRY DELIGHT

This recipe is similar to the preceding one, except that here poultry is combined with millet. The two ingredients complement each other because poultry is lower in iron than red meats, but millet is high in iron compared with other grains. The two also balance each other in relative protein levels: Poultry is high in protein and millet is low.

2   cups millet (or 6 cups cooked)

2   eggs

2   pounds (4 cups) ground turkey or chicken (or lean chuck, lean heart, lean hamburger, liver, giblets, fish or other lean meats)

4   tablespoons Healthy Powder (page 39)

2   tablespoons bonemeal (or 4,000 milligrams calcium or 2¼ teaspoons eggshell powder)

2   tablespoons vegetable oil or butter (or 1 tablespoon each)

10,000 IU vitamin A

100–200 IU vitamin E

1   teaspoon fresh vegetable with each meal (optional)

500 milligrams taurine supplement (optional)

Bring 6 cups of water to a boil. Add the millet, cover and simmer 20 to 30 minutes or until the water is absorbed. You may need to add a bit more water during cooking. When the millet is soft, stir in the eggs to let them set a bit from the heat. Then mix in the remaining ingredients.

Yield: About 11 cups, with 275 kilocalories per cup. Immediately freeze whatever cannot be eaten in 2 to 3 days.

Daily ration (in cups): small—½ to ⅔; medium—¾ to 1; large—1 to 1¾.

Grain substitutes: 4 cups rolled oats (+ 8 cups water = 8 cups cooked) or 2 cups bulgur (+ 4 cups water = 5 cups cooked).

FELINE FEAST

Corn is the grain of choice for many cats, so that's the grain I used in the main version of this recipe. Try polenta, which is more coarsely ground than the flourlike meal usually called cornmeal, for the best texture. It's commonly sold in natural food stores. Yummied up with extra yeast for even more flavor, this high-protein formula is a sure winner. It's excellent for pregnant or nursing cats and their growing kittens.

Since this recipe contains a higher proportion of meat than the others, you can substitute many kinds of grains and meats, both low- and high-protein types, because there is still plenty of protein to spare. If you use lean meats, the dry weight percentage of protein ranges from a low of 41 percent (lean beef heart with rice or potatoes) to a high of 52 percent (turkey with oats). If you use fattier meats, the protein value ranges from a low of 30 percent (fatty beef heart with rice or potatoes) to a high of 40 percent (regular hamburger with oats). Alternate the use of poultry and red meats, or combine both in the same recipe to ensure plenty of iron and other nutrients that vary in different cuts.

(continued)

1 cup cornmeal or polenta (or about 4 cups cooked)

2 eggs

2 tablespoons vegetable oil or butter (or 1 tablespoon each)

2 pounds (4 cups) ground turkey or chicken (or lean chuck, lean heart, lean hamburger, liver, giblets, fish or other lean meats)

4 tablespoons Healthy Powder (page 39)

2 tablespoons bonemeal (or 3,200 milligrams calcium or 1¾ teaspoons eggshell powder)

10,000 IU vitamin A

100–200 IU vitamin E

1 teaspoon fresh vegetables with each meal (optional)

500 milligrams taurine supplement (optional)

Bring 4 cups (1 quart) of water to a boil. Add the cornmeal or polenta, stirring rapidly with a fork or whisk to keep it from getting lumpy. (It's easier to avoid lumping if you use polenta.) When it is thoroughly blended, cover and simmer on low 10 to 15 minutes. When the cornmeal or polenta is creamy, stir in the eggs and oil or butter. Mix in the remaining ingredients.

Yield: About 8¾ cups, with 250 kilocalories per cup. Immediately freeze whatever cannot be eaten in 2 to 3 days.

Daily ration (in cups): small—½ to ¾; medium—¾ to 1+; large—1¼ to 2.

Meat substitutes: It's a good idea to use fattier grades of meat sometimes, but eliminate the oil or butter from the recipe when you do. You can use 2 pounds of beef heart with fat showing, regular hamburger, poultry with skin, or choice chuck roast.

Grain substitutes: 2 cups raw rolled oats (+ 4 cups water = 4 cups cooked) or 10 slices whole-wheat bread or 4 cups cooked and mashed potatoes or 1 cup (dry) of any of the following: bulgur, millet, buckwheat, barley, brown rice, couscous, amaranth, spelt or quinoa.

MACKEREL LOAF

Canned mackerel makes a good seafood to use for cats occasionally. Not only is it an economical protein source, but it comes from deep waters and is less likely to be polluted than those fishes from areas closer to the coast. Cats can sometimes get addicted to seafood. If yours shows signs of addiction, hold firm; it's important to keep feeding a variety of foods.

4 eggs

3 cups milk (or less, as needed for moisture)

4 tablespoons Healthy Powder (page 39)

2 teaspoons bonemeal (or 1,200 milligrams calcium or ⅔ teaspoon eggshell powder)

5,000 IU vitamin A

100–200 IU vitamin E

500 milligrams taurine supplement (optional)

1 teaspoon fresh vegetables with each meal (optional)

2 tablespoons vegetable oil

2 15-ounce cans of mackerel, undrained (or 3 6-ounce cans tuna in oil or ½ pound cooked cod or other whitefish)

8 slices whole-wheat bread, crumbled

Blend the eggs, milk, supplements, vegetables and oil together. Add the mackerel and bread and mix well. Serve raw or bake in a shallow dish at 350°F for about 20 minutes.

Yield: About 11⅓ cups, with 275 kilocalories per cup. Immediately freeze whatever cannot be eaten in the next 2 to 3 days.

Daily ration: Same as for Poultry Delight, above.

Grain substitutes: 1½ cups rolled oats (+ 3 cups water = 3 cups cooked) or about 1 cup cornmeal or polenta (+ 4 cups water = 4 cups cooked) or 1 cup whole-wheat bulgur (+ 2 cups water = 2½ cups cooked).

FATTY FELINE FARE

This dense, satisfying formula is rich in animal fat at a level comparable to the fat in the wild feline diet. Stick to the suggested grains and use only bonemeal for the calcium source to ensure adequate total amounts of protein, phosphorus and calcium. Many markets will grind beef heart for you, although they may prefer that you phone in advance.

- 1 cup millet (or 3 cups cooked)
- 1 egg
- 2 pounds (4 cups) raw chuck roast (or the regular, fattier grades of beef heart or hamburger, or roaster chicken with skin)
- 3 tablespoons Healthy Powder (page 39)
- 1½ tablespoons bonemeal
     10,000 IU vitamin A
     100–200 IU vitamin E
- 1 teaspoon fresh vegetable with each meal (optional)
     500 milligrams taurine supplement (optional)

Bring 3 cups of water to a boil. Add the millet, cover and simmer 20 to 30 minutes or until the water is absorbed. You may need to add a bit more water during cooking. When the millet is soft, stir in the egg to let it set a bit from the heat. Then mix in the remaining ingredients.

Yield: About 7½ cups, with 425 kilocalories per cup. Immediately freeze whatever cannot be eaten in 2 to 3 days.

Daily ration (in cups): small—⅓ to ½; medium— ½ to ⅔; large ¾ to 1+.

Grain substitutes: 2 cups rolled oats (+ 4 cups water = 4 cups cooked) or 1 cup bulgur (+ 2 cups water = 2½ cups cooked).

FAST AND FRESH: CATS

Here are two quick and easy recipes for those occasional times when you suddenly realize you forgot to thaw out the regular cat fare, or you just plain ran out of it—and there's a hungry feline standing at your feet who won't take wait-a-while for an answer. These recipes are not intended for regular use, but they do provide a fairly complete meal using items you probably have on hand. As noted above, you may also use these recipes occasionally for dogs that don't require a low-protein diet. In fact, all these mixtures are higher in protein than necessary for either dogs or cats, but they won't complain.

QUICK FELINE EGGFEST

This mix is among the simplest I know and is a very natural food for small predator types of cats. It is high in protein, vitamin A and iron as well as B vitamins.

- 2 eggs
- ⅓ teaspoon bonemeal (or 250 milligrams calcium or ⅛ teaspoon eggshell powder)
- ¾ teaspoon nutritional yeast

Use a fork to mix the egg yolks and whites, stirring in the bonemeal at the same time. Sprinkle the yeast on top and serve raw. Or, if you prefer, you may scramble this egg mix lightly.

Yield: One meal, or about half a day's rations for a 10-pound cat (or dog), with about 170 kilocalories. A smaller cat might eat just one egg at a meal.

Nutritional Composition of Recipes for Dogs

Recipe	Kcal.	Protein (%)	Fat (%)	Carb. (%)	Fiber (%)	Ash (%)*	Calcium (%)*
Kibble Supplements‡							
Meat Supplement: turkey	3,945	26.0	8.6	59.4	4.4	5.9 (5.2)	0.9 (0.7)
Egg Supplement	587	24.3	16.7	52.9	3.9	6.1 (5.1)	1.0 (0.7)
Cottage Cheese Supplement	1,219	23.9	10.3	59.9	4.4	5.9 (5.2)	0.9 (0.7)
Basic Recipes							
Doggie Oats: turkey	4,500	29.7	15.5	46.8	1.1	8 (4.4)	1.8 (1.0)
Doggie Oats: cottage cheese, egg	4,618	25.4	17.5	49.1	1.1	8 (4.4)	1.8 (1.1)
Dog Loaf: beef heart	991	26.9	20.7	44.7	1.5	7.7 (5.0)	1.4 (0.8)
One-on-One: lean hamburger	1,610	23.2	12.0	58.2	1.6	6.7 (3.2)	1.5 (0.6)
Fast and Fresh							
Quick Canine Oats and Eggs	561	26.1	19.6	47.6	0.8	6.7 (3.3)	1.5 (0.7)
Quick Canine Oatmeal	441	24.2	14.3	52.4	0.8	9.1 (6.1)	1.6 (0.8)
Quick Canine Hash: chuck	1,202	24.5	18.8	50.9	1.1	5.8 (2.5)	1.3 (0.5)
Standard recommendations:§	see chart on page 59	≥18 (more for higher fat rations)	≥5	≤67	—	—	≥ 0.6

*The second figures for calcium and phosphorus (in parentheses) result if you use pure calcium rather than bonemeal. This also makes a lower-ash diet.

†The second figures for iron (in parentheses) apply if you add the optional iron supplement. See discussion in chapter 3.

Phosph. (%)*	Calcium: Phosph. Ratio*	Iron (mg.)†	Vit. A/kg. (IU)	Thiamin (%)	Riboflavin (%)	Niacin (%)
0.7 (0.6)	1.2:1 (1.2:1)	.008	9,567	.0003	.0021	.0035
0.8 (0.6)	1.2:1 (1.2:1)	.008	12,858	.0004	.0020	.0016
0.7 (0.6)	1.3:1 (1.2:1)	.007	5,881	.0003	.0021	.0018
1.4 (0.8)	1.3:1 (1.3:1)	.007 (.006)	18,328	.0011	.0005	.0069
1.4 (0.7)	1.3:1 (1.5:1)	.006 (.007)	21,954	.0011	.0006	.0028
1.1 (0.7)	1.2:1 (1.3:1)	.006 (.011)	39,056	.0010	.0010	.0075
1.1 (0.5)	1.4:1 (1.4:1)	.006 (.009)	13,631	.0005	.0003	.0068
1.2 (0.6)	1.2:1 (1.3:1)	.007	14,909	.0005	.0005	.0008
1.2 (0.6)	1.3:1 (1.3:1)	.005	7,709	.0005	.0007	.0007
1.0 (0.4)	1.3:1 (1.3:1)	.006	19,969	.0003	.0002	.0071
≥ 0.5	1:1–2:1 (1.3:1 ideal)	≥.008	5,000–50,000 IU per kg. dry weight	≥.0001	≥.0002	≥.0011

‡The amounts for the kibble supplements assume that you use a kibble that exactly meets the minimum requirements for dog foods set by the AAFCO in 1992.

§Standard recommendations are percentage total dry weight unless otherwise noted and are for maintenance of adult dogs under normal conditions. Source: AAFCO Nutrient Profiles for Dog Foods: Report of the Canine Nutrition Expert Subcommittee, 1992.

Nutritional Composition of Recipes for Cats

Recipe	Kcal.	Protein (%)	Fat (%)	Carb. (%)	Fiber (%)	Ash (%)*	Calcium (%)*
Basic Recipes							
Beefy Oats: heart	2,799	36	16.7	38.8	0.8	8.6 (4.7)	1.8 (1.0)
Poultry Delight: turkey	3,015	35.5	13.8	42.6	1.9	8.1 (4.7)	1.6 (0.9)
Fatty Feline Fare: chuck	3,176	34.2	32.8	26.1	1.2	6.9 (3.8)	1.4 (0.8)
Feline Feast: turkey	2,215	47.8	19.1	24.2	0.8	8.9 (5.1)	1.9 (1.1)
Mackerel Loaf	3,151	41.5	25.7	24.8	0.7	8.0 (6.8)	1.3 (1.0)
Fast and Fresh							
Quick Feline Meatfest: chicken	452	54.9	35.4	0.8	0	7.2 (2.9)	2.0 (0.8)
Quick Feline Eggfest	171	45.9	38.1	6.7	0.3	9.3 (5.0)	2.0 (1.1)
Quick Feline Cottage Cheese	180	60.4	18.7	13.2	0	7.7 (5.0)	1.5 (0.8)
Standard recommendations:†	~350 kcal/ day for 10- lb. cat	≥26 (46 for wild cats)	≥9 (33 for wild cats)	— (16 for wild cats)	—	— (3 for wild cats)	≥0.6

*The second figures for calcium and phosphorus (in parentheses) result if you use pure calcium rather than bonemeal. This also makes a lower-ash diet.

†Except where noted for wild felines, standard recommendations are percentage total dry weight and are for

Phosph. (%)*	Calcium: Phosph. Ratio*	Iron (mg.)	Vit. A/kg. (IU)	Thiamin (%)	Riboflavin (%)	Niacin (%)
1.5 (0.8)	1.2:1 (1.3:1)	.011	18,232	.0016	.0016	.013
1.3 (0.7)	1.2:1 (1.2:1)	.008	15,748	.0010	.0007	.009
1.2 (0.6)	1.2:1 (1.3:1)	.008	18,400	.0008	.0005	.009
1.6 (0.9)	1.2:1 (1.2:1)	.008	24,768	.0013	.0008	.013
1.1 (0.9)	1.2:1 (1.1:1)	.006	12,917	.0007	.0010	.014
1.5 (0.6)	1.3:1 (1.4:1)	.006	11,483	.0002	.0003	.021
1.7 (0.9)	1.2:1 (1.3:1)	.011	38,893	.0015	.0014	.004
1.2 (0.7)	1.2:1 (1.2:1)	.002	7,531	.0001	.0011	.001
≥0.5	1.1:1–1.3:1 (1.25:1 ideal)	≥.008	≥5,000 IU per kg. dry weight	≥.0005	≥.0004	≥.006

maintenance of adult cats under normal conditions. Sources: AAFCO Nutrient Profiles for Cat Foods: Report of the Feline Nutrition Expert Subcommittee, 1992, and the *Merck Veterinary Manual*, 6th Edition, 1986.

QUICK FELINE MEATFEST

Along with ease of preparation, this recipe boasts a calcium-balanced way to feed your cat chunks of meat, which help exercise his teeth and gums. (If you were to mix chunks of meat with grains for your cat, he'd probably pick out the chunks, eat them and leave the grains.)

1 cup raw or cooked chicken or turkey with skin (or chuck, hamburger or heart)

1½ teaspoons bonemeal (or 600 milligrams calcium or ⅓ teaspoon eggshell powder)

Break up the poultry or meat only enough so you can mix in the bonemeal and so your cat can manage it.

Yield: 1 cup, with about 450 kilocalories.

Daily ration (in cups): small—¼ to ½; medium—½ to ⅔; large—¾ to 1.

If you're feeding dogs this meal, each cup of meat provides about half a day's needs for a 40-pound dog or one-third a day's needs for an 80-pound dog.

THE ROLE OF NUTRITIONAL STANDARDS IN OUR RECIPES

In formulating our recipes, we took several nutritional guidelines into consideration, drawing upon the recommendations of the Association of American Feed Control Officials (AAFCO), the *Merck Veterinary Manual* and several other sources. We calculated the nutritional content of the recipes based upon information in the *United States Department of Agriculture Handbook of Nutritional Composition of Foods* and other sources (see charts on pages 54 and 56). You should realize, however, that the nutritional contents of foods can vary considerably, depending on how it is raised, stored and prepared.

In most cases our formulations exceed the official standards, which represent the bare minimum considered necessary for adult maintenance. We tried to strike a balance between those minimal standards and the natural wild diet. For adult cats, for instance, the AAFCO industry standards currently advise a minimum of 26 percent protein and 9 percent fat. Other sources have stated that 25 percent fat is considered ideal. In the wild, cats consume about 47 percent protein and 33 percent fat. One might contend that the higher standards of the "wild" diet would be optimal. We also need to be concerned, however, about minimizing meat consumption, both because it contains the highest levels of pollutants of any food group and because it is the most environmentally destructive to produce.

So, weighing these factors, our basic cat recipes fall in between the minimal and the "wild" standards. The protein levels range from 34 to 48 percent, averaging about 39 percent. The fat levels vary from 16 to 33 percent, averaging about 22 percent. For healthy adult cats you can feel confident in emphasizing recipes at either end of the continuum, as you choose.

IDEAL DOG FOOD

For dogs the current AAFCO standards advise a minimum of only 18 percent protein for adult maintenance and 22 percent for reproduction and growth (previous recommendations have been as high as 28 percent for lactation). The minimal level for fat is 5 percent (8 percent for reproduction and growth), although feeding studies have shown dogs can tolerate rations up to 50 percent fat if otherwise adequately nourished.

There is a direct relationship between fat and protein in the diet. The more fat in the diet, the more protein is needed. There are metabolic interactions between the two and also when a diet is fattier, an animal will eat less to assuage its hunger. That's why an animal can become undernourished if you add oil or meat drippings to its food without increasing the protein, vitamin and mineral content accordingly. Dr. Ben E. Sheffy of Cornell University in Ithaca, New York, has developed detailed minimum protein standards for dogs that range from 13 to 37 percent, depending on how much fat is in the diet and upon special needs, such as those described in the next chapter. All of our dog recipes meet or exceed whichever of the standards is higher—Dr. Sheffy's or the AAFCO's.

Average Caloric Needs for Adult Dogs

Weight (lb.)	Kcal./Day
10	410
15	550
25	840
40	1150
50	1380
60	1555
70	1690
80	1890
100	2270

NOTE: Increase values for working dogs or during cold weather.

HOW MUCH TO FEED?

I believe that your animal's appetite is generally a good guideline for how much to feed. Here's some information, however, that will help you gauge quantities to prepare based on average caloric needs for dogs and cats and the caloric content (kcal.) stated in the recipe charts on the preceding pages.

In nature a cat eats on a 28-hour cycle and it is normal for them to decline food occasionally when we feed them according to our schedules instead of theirs.

Average Caloric Needs for Adult Cats

Weight (lb.)	Kcal./Day Inactive Cat	Kcal./Day Active Cat
6	191	218
7	223	254
8	255	290
9	286	327
10	319	363
12	383	463

CHAPTER FIVE

SPECIAL DIETS FOR SPECIAL PETS

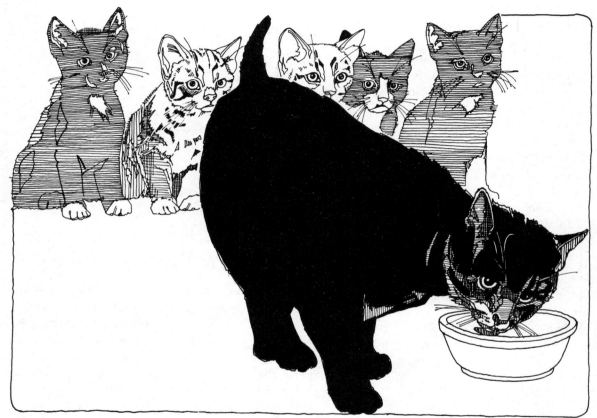

Most dogs and cats thrive on the basic maintenance recipes we just described in chapter 4, but certain others under distinct conditions do need special diets. Such animals include:

- Puppies and kittens. Extra protein and calories are needed for new tissue growth and youthful activity.

- Breeding, pregnant and lactating females. Conceiving, carrying, birthing and nursing offspring call for unusually high protein intake to grow new tissue.
- Animals undergoing strenuous exercise or stress. Such conditions signal the body to consume high amounts of energy and protein, which is needed for activity and tissue repair.

- Animals that need to regain strength after surgery, injury, illness or malnourishment. Higher-than-usual amounts of protein and energy are vital for healing.
- Animals exposed to extreme temperatures. Very hot weather calls for diets high in protein to compensate for decreased food intake caused by a sluggish appetite; cold weather exposure demands more calories just to keep the animal warm; these calories are best supplied by a high-fat diet.
- The pet of vegetarian families. Ethical, ecological or health considerations lead some people to eliminate meat from their diets. If they reduce their pet's meat intake as well, they must replace certain nutrients meat would provide.

Let's look at ways to satisfy each of these special dietary needs in turn. (See the "Quick Reference" section beginning on page 221 for diets created specifically to meet the needs of dogs and cats with disease problems such as kidney and urinary disorders.)

HIGH-ENERGY RECIPES FOR DOGS

In devising these power-plus recipes for dogs, we followed guidelines proposed by Ben E. Sheffy, Ph.D., of Cornell University in Ithaca, New York, which boost the recommended levels of protein beyond the usual standards as the energy density (or fattiness) of a diet increases. Extra protein is necessary because a dog eats less total food in a fattier, higher-calorie diet. So, in order to get the same amount of protein, a dog must eat a diet in which protein constitutes a higher portion of the total.

In a lower-fat diet with a caloric density of just 3.5 kilocalories per kilogram of dry weight, Dr. Sheffy suggests a minimum of 23 percent protein for proper growth. However, in fattier diets (5 kilocalories per kilogram) he recommends at least 30 to 33 percent protein. The three recipes below and their suggested variations approximate or exceed these guidelines. They are also suitable for adult cats under average conditions (not for reproduction and other special needs).

DOG GROWTH DIET A

The main version of this nutritious fare provides 30.4 percent protein, 15.4 percent fat and a calcium to phosphorus ratio of 1.28:1. (With oats and turkey, the protein level rises to 34.5 percent.) Caloric density: 4.5 Kcal./kg. dry weight.

    3 cups bulgur
    4 cups (2 pounds) lean hamburger
 2⅔ tablespoons bonemeal (or 4,400 milligrams calcium or 2½ teaspoons eggshell powder)
    2 tablespoons Healthy Powder (page 39)
    2 tablespoons nutritional yeast
    2 tablespoons vegetable oil
       10,000 IU vitamin A
       100–400 IU vitamin E
       15 milligrams iron (optional)
    ½ cup vegetables (optional)

Bring 6 cups of water to a boil. Add the bulgur, cover and turn down to simmer 15 to 20 minutes, or until it is soft. Stir in the remaining ingredients and serve.

(continued)

Meat substitutes: raw turkey, chicken or lean heart.

Grain substitutes: 3 cups millet (+ 6 cups water = 8–9 cups cooked); 3 cups whole-wheat couscous (+ 4½ cups water = 7½ cups cooked); 6 cups raw oats (+ 12 cups water = 12 cups cooked); or 2⅔ cups brown rice (+ 5½ cups water = 6⅔ cups cooked).

Yield: About 12 cups, with 320 kilocalories per cup.

DOG GROWTH DIET B

This recipe provides a little more protein. The main version provides 32.4 percent protein, 15.8 percent fat and a calcium to phosphorus ratio of 1.30:1. The highest protein version (turkey and oats) has 34.9 percent protein and 15.9 percent fat. Caloric density: 4.4 Kcal./kg. dry weight.

　3　cups rolled oats (or 6 cups oatmeal)

　2　large eggs

　2　cups (1 pound) lean beef heart

4½　teaspoons bonemeal (or 2,400 milligrams calcium or 1⅓ teaspoons eggshell powder)

　2　tablespoons Healthy Powder (page 39)

　1　tablespoon vegetable oil

　　　5,000–10,000 IU vitamin A

　　　100–400 IU vitamin E

　　　10 milligrams iron (optional)

　½　cup vegetables (optional)

Bring 6 cups of water to a boil. Add the oats, cover and turn down to simmer until they are soft, about 10 minutes. Stir in the eggs and let them set a bit from the heat. Then stir in the remaining ingredients and serve.

Meat substitutes: raw turkey, chicken, lean chuck or lean hamburger.

Grain substitutes: 1½ cups millet (+ 4½ cups water = 4½ cups cooked); 1½ cups bulgur (+ 3 cups water = 3¾ cups cooked); 1½ cups whole-wheat couscous (+ 2¼ cups water = 3¾ cups cooked); 2 cups cornmeal (+ 8 cups water = 8 cups cooked); or 1¼ cups brown rice (+ 2½ cups water = 3+ cups cooked).

Yield: About 8½ cups, with 210 kilocalories per cup.

DOG GROWTH DIET C

This nutritious recipe and its variations have the most protein and fat of the three growth recipes for dogs. That makes it optimal for nursing females and young pups. The main version provides 33.2 percent protein, 27.3 percent fat and a calcium to phosphorus ratio of 1.28:1. The highest protein version (made by using chicken and oats) provides 39.4 percent protein and 25.3 percent fat. Caloric density: 5.1 Kcal./kg. dry weight.

　1　cup bulgur

　2　cups (1 pound) chuck roast

　1　cup low-fat cottage cheese

　4　teaspoons bonemeal (or 2,400 milligrams calcium or 1⅓ teaspoons eggshell powder)

　2　tablespoons Healthy Powder (page 39)

　1　tablespoon nutritional yeast

　2　tablespoons vegetable oil

　　　5,000–10,000 IU vitamin A

　　　100–400 IU vitamin E

　　　10 milligrams iron (optional)

　½　cup vegetables (optional)

Bring 2 cups of water to a boil. Add the bulgur, cover and turn down to simmer until the grain is soft, about 15 to 20 minutes. Stir in the remaining ingredients and serve.

Meat substitutes: regular hamburger (not lean) or roaster chicken with skin.

Grain substitutes: 1 cup millet (+ 3 cups water = 3 cups cooked); 1 cup whole-wheat couscous (+ 1½ cups water = 2½ cups cooked); 2 cups raw oats (+ 4 cups water = 4 cups oatmeal).

Yield: About 6 cups, with 400 kilocalories per cup.

HOW MUCH SHOULD YOU FEED YOUR DOG?

The chart on page 64 shows which recipes to use for dogs with special needs. It also indicates the approximate amount to feed, using the main version of each recipe. Remember, however, that needs vary according to many factors, so, ultimately, you should just let your dog's appetite be the gauge. Feed half-grown pups and adult dogs with extra needs two or three times a day, allowing them to eat as much as they want. Younger puppies should be fed three or four times a day.

Several of the higher-protein variations of the basic dog maintenance recipes in chapter 4 may also be used for moderate growth needs, provided that you follow these guidelines.

Fresh Meat Supplement for Dog Kibble (page 45)—Use lean meats only.

Meatless Supplements for Dog Kibble (page 45)—Okay as stated.

Doggie Oats (page 46)—Only use variations calling for oats and lean meats.

One-on-One (page 48)—If you use oats, any lean meat is all right. With turkey, you may also use bulgur or millet. Often, but not always, a dog will eat as much as it

needs and no more. But if your dog is lethargic, always ravenous, pot-bellied or losing weight, you need to feed more. Also, try feeding a richer recipe (B or C in this chapter). If your dog is becoming overweight, feed less.

Note: Larger dogs require fewer calories per pound of body weight than smaller dogs. That's why a 55-pound dog isn't fed 11 times more than a 5-pounder.

RECIPES THAT CATER TO CATS' SPECIAL NEEDS

Most of the maintenance recipes for cats in chapter 4 contain enough protein and fat for felines with special needs. However, the chart on page 66 will help you select the best recipes for various conditions.

Variations of two of the maintenance recipes in chapter 4 are not quite high enough in protein for growth and development needs when used with fattier meats or lower-protein grains. So, for cats with special needs, *avoid* using Fatty Feline Fare (page 53) with millet (use oats or bulgur instead) or Feline Feast (page 51) with a fatty grade of heart.

CAT GROWTH DIET

This recipe is particularly high in protein compared with the other feline diets. It is especially useful for conditions that require the growth of new tissue but not necessarily the consumption of a lot of energy (calories). That makes it well-suited for a cat recovering from malnourishment or injuries as well as for pregnant cats and for kittens and mothers approaching weaning time. This nutritious fare provides 45.3 percent protein, 17.8 percent fat and a cal-

cium to phosphorus ratio of 1.2:1. Caloric density: 4.6 Kcal./kg. dry weight.

- 1   cup cornmeal or polenta (or 4 cups cooked)
- 2   eggs
- 4   cups (2 pounds) ground turkey
- 4   tablespoons Healthy Powder (page 39)
- 1½   teaspoons bonemeal (or 2,800 milligrams calcium or 1½ teaspoons eggshell powder)
- 2   tablespoons vegetable oil or butter (or 1 tablespoon each)
-    5,000–10,000 IU vitamin A
-    100–200 IU vitamin E
-    500 milligrams taurine supplement (recommended for growth)
- 1   teaspoon vegetables with each meal (optional)

Bring 4 cups of water to a boil. Add the cornmeal or polenta, stirring rapidly with a fork or whisk until smooth. When mixed, cover and turn down to simmer until soft and mushy, approximately 10 to 15 minutes. Then stir in the eggs. Allow the mixture to cool somewhat, then mix in the remaining ingredients and serve.

Meat substitutes: lean chuck, heart or chicken.

Feeding Dogs with Extra Needs

Special Condition Groups	Which Recipe to Use for Dogs in This Group
Pregnant female	A
Puppy, nearly grown	B
	C
Nursing female (past peak)	B
Puppy, half-grown	C
Nursing female (at peak)	C
Young puppy	C
Hard exercise	A
	B
	C
Stress	B
Cold weather	C
Convalescence	A
Malnourishment	B
Hot weather	C

Grain substitutes: 1 cup millet (+ 3 cups water = 3 cups cooked); 1 cup whole-wheat couscous (+ 1½ cups water = 2½ cups cooked); 2 cups rolled oats (+ 4 cups water = 4 cups oatmeal); or 1 cup bulgur (+ 2 cups water = 2½ cups cooked).

Yield: About 8½ cups, with 270 kilocalories per cup.

◆

Two of the fast and easy meals presented in chapter 4 (Quick Feline Eggfest on page 53 and Quick Feline Meatfest on page 58) may also be used occasionally for any of the conditions mentioned above. Both recipes are very high in protein and fat, approximating the contents of the wild feline diet. If you're taking a shortcut by using one of these meals, however, be absolutely sure to include the bonemeal or calcium supplement. Otherwise you could create a serious nutritional imbalance that might thwart the proper development of the kittens or damage the health of their mother.

Also, because taurine is especially important to the developing kitten, I suggest adding the optional taurine supplement when any of my fresh foods recipes are

How Many Cups to Feed Daily to Dogs of Different Weights

2 lb.	5 lb.	10 lb.	15 lb.	35 lb.	55 lb.	85 lb.	150 lb.
½	1	1½	2	4	5½	7½	11
¾	1⅓	2⅓	3¼	6	8	11	17
⅓	¾	1¼	1⅔	3	4⅓	6	9
1	1¾	3	4	7½	10	14	21
½	1	1½	2	4	5½	7½	11
⅔+	1¼+	2+	2¾+	5¼+	7¼+	10+	15+
⅔+	1¼+	2+	2¾+	5¼+	7¼+	10+	15+
½–1	1–2	2–3	2⅔–4½	5–12	6¾–11	9–15	14–23
1–1½	1¾–2	3–5	4–6¾	7½–19	10–17	14–24	21–36
½–¾	1–1½	1½–2½	2–2½	4–10	5½–9	7–12	11–19
1–1¼	1¾–2¼	3–4	4–5⅓	7½–10	10–14	14–19	21–28
½–⅔	1–1¼	1½–2	2–2¾	4–5¼	5½–7	7½–10	11–15
As needed to maintain normal weight. Add extra Healthy Powder, dog vitamins or nutritional yeast.							
As needed to maintain normal weight. Add extra Healthy Powder, dog vitamins or nutritional yeast.							
As needed to maintain normal weight. Add extra Healthy Powder, dog vitamins or nutritional yeast.							

used for growth. Many supplements for cats contain it.

FEEDING ORPHANED OR REJECTED KITTENS AND PUPPIES

Mother's milk is the best food there is, so use these recipes only if you have no choice. Sometimes a female cannot or will not nurse all her young adequately, and sometimes, unfortunately, the mother dies. In such cases you can keep the babies alive with a for-

mula designed to mimic as closely as possible the natural constituents of the nursing cat's or dog's milk. You can buy commercial products that do this (called KMR and Esbilac, respectively). But if you want to give your young charges the benefits of raw fresh foods, use the formulas below.

To boost the protein content of cow's milk to the level found in cat's and dog's milk, add protein powder. Buy an unflavored powder that contains at least 80 percent protein (dry weight basis) and lists its proteins from animal sources: casein, lactalbumin and egg albumin. Unlike powders based

Feeding Cats with Extra Needs

Special Condition Groups	Which Recipes to Use for Group
Pregnant female	Cat Growth Diet*
Kitten, nearly grown (30 wk.)	Cat Growth Diet*
Nursing female (past peak)	Cat Growth Diet*
Kitten, half-grown (20 wk.)	Feline Feast
	Mackerel Loaf
Nursing female (at peak)	Feline Feast
Young kitten (10 wk.)	Mackerel Loaf
Very active	Fatty Feline Fare
Cold weather	Feline Feast
Stress	Mackerel Loaf
Convalescence	Cat Growth Diet*
Malnourishment	Cat Growth Diet*
Hot weather	Cat Growth Diet*

*Or any cat diet in chapter 4, with the following two exceptions, which would not provide enough protein: Do not use a fatty grade of heart with Feline Feast, and use only oats or bulgur in Fatty Feline Fare. Feed about 1½ times the amounts suggested in chapter 4 for each weight group.

on soy proteins, animal protein powders will meet the special amino acid requirements of your young orphans. These powders are sold in many health food stores.

Supplement these formulas with vitamins made especially for adult dogs or cats, as suggested. Use a powdered formula or crush the tablet and mix it into the milk. If the formula contains calcium but not phosphorus, cut back a bit on the bonemeal or calcium supplement.

If you use a calcium source other than bonemeal, it's safest to use one based on calcium lactate or calcium gluconate. These are better absorbed than calcium carbonate, a common source that is also the basis of eggshell powder.

KITTEN FORMULA

This formula closely replicates the constituents of cat's milk, which are 42.2 percent protein, 25 percent fat, 26.1 percent carbohydrates and 6.7 percent ash. It contains 41.8 percent protein, 25 percent fat, 24.6 percent carbohydrates and 6.8 percent ash. The calcium to phosphorus ratio is ideal at 1.2:1. One serving has 566 kilocalories.

(continued)

How Many Cups to Feed Daily to Cats of Different Weights

1 lb.	2 lb.	3 lb.	4 lb.	5 lb.	6 lb.	8 lb.	10 lb.	12 lb.
¼	⅓	½	¾	1	1+	1½	1¾	2+
¼	⅓	½	¾	1	1+	1½	1¾	2+
¼	½	⅔	<1	1+	1⅓	1¾	2⅓	2¾
⅛	¼	⅓	½	½+	⅔	¾+	1+	1⅓
¼	½	½	⅔	¾	1	1⅓	2+	2½
½	<1	1⅓	1¾	2¼	2¾	3⅔	4½	5½
½	¾	1¼	1⅔	2	2½	3⅓	4+	5
—	—	—	⅓	<½	½+	¾	<1	1+
—	—	—	⅔	¾	1+	1½	1½+	1¾
—	—	—	½	¾	1	1⅓	1⅓+	2
As needed to maintain normal weight.								
As needed to maintain normal weight.								
As needed to maintain normal weight.								

2   cups whole milk

2   large eggs

5   teaspoons protein powder (from animal protein sources)

⅓   teaspoon bonemeal (or 200–300 milligrams calcium or ⅛ teaspoon eggshell powder)

1–2 days' worth of cat vitamins (adult dosage), powdered or crushed

100 milligrams taurine supplement (if not in cat vitamins)

Mix the ingredients well. Warm just to body temperature and feed with a pet nurser or doll bottle. Give each kitten just enough at each feeding to enlarge the abdomen slightly without distending it. Feed according to "Kitten Feeding Schedule."

After each feeding, gently massage the kitten's belly and swab the genital and anal area with a tissue moistened slightly with warm water. Mama cats lick the same areas to stimulate proper urination and defecation.

Start introducing solids (cat recipes mentioned above or high-quality canned food) when the kittens are 3 to 4 weeks old. Mix them with the formula to make a thin mush. Begin weaning the kittens from the bottle at about 4 to 6 weeks.

PUPPY FORMULA

Comparable in formulation to a dog's natural milk (33.2 percent protein, 44.1 percent fat, 15.8 percent carbohydrate and 6.9 percent ash), this mixture contains 33.7 percent protein, 40.9 percent fat, 15.8 percent carbohydrates and 9.6 percent ash. It has a calcium to phosphorus ratio of 1.3:1 and provides 486 kilocalories.

1   cup half-and-half (milk and cream)

2   large eggs

1   tablespoon protein powder

¾   teaspoon bonemeal (or 500 milligrams calcium)

1–2 days' worth of dog vitamins (adult dosage), powdered or crushed

Mix ingredients well and warm to body temperature. Using a pet nurser bottle, feed enough to slightly enlarge the abdomen but not to distend it. (Amount varies according to age and breed size. If in doubt, consult recommendations for the commercial formula.) Feed on the same schedule described for kittens. Clean each puppy after the feeding, as described for kittens. When the puppies are 3 to 4 weeks old, introduce solids (mixed with formula to make a gruel); wean them from the bottle at 4 to 5 weeks.

THE VEGETARIAN DIET: CAN WE CUT MEAT USE FOR PETS?

Now let's consider a special diet for normal, healthy dogs and cats whose vegetarian owners have qualms about feeding meat to their pets. Even if this is not a direct concern for you, I urge you to read this section because it raises important issues that affect everyone. I recall a lively discussion at a workshop I once gave on natural animal care that embodies this dilemma.

An earnest-looking young woman began, "I am a vegetarian because I love all animals and don't want to kill them. And I get along fine without meat. Yet, I feel that I have to feed it to my dog. After all, he's a carnivore and needs it . . . doesn't he?" She looked around the room and several people immediately smiled in recognition of a common problem.

One responded, "Well, I've been feeding my dog a vegetarian diet for the last three years. He eats mostly sprouts, seeds, grains,

Kitten Feeding Schedule

Age (wk.)	Weight	How Often to Feed	Total Amount/day (tbsp.)
0–2	4–8 oz.	every 2 hours	2–4
3	8–10 oz.	every 3 hours	4–6
4–5	10–24 oz.	every 4 hours	6–10
6	2+ lbs.	3 times a day	8–12

raw fruits, vegetables and dairy products and he's in great shape!"

"But what about the long run?" another interjected. "Here we've been talking today about the need for our animals to live and eat as naturally as possible, and a vegetarian diet is nothing like what a wolf eats! It seems to me that if we really wanted to follow nature, we'd feed our pets mostly raw meat and bones."

"But that's impractical," a fourth participant broke in. "It costs too much personally and it costs too much for the world. Meat production contributes to world hunger and to environmental problems because it takes a lot more land and other resources to produce it. To say nothing of the suffering it causes animals!"

Most of the complex issues involved with the question of pets living as vegetarians arose in that brief exchange. The possibility of no-meat diets for dogs and cats doesn't even occur to most of us because we have all been deeply conditioned by our culture to think that even we humans *must* eat meat.

Actually, that concept is relatively new in our country, and it results from an era of prosperity. In 1985 Americans ate one and a half times as much beef as they did in 1909. Poultry consumption increased by over 280 percent in that same period. Meanwhile, grain and potato consumption went down by about half. Furthermore, about half of

us keep predators as pets, far more than the number nature would support in the wild. These cultural patterns are taken for granted, and most of us live our lives without realizing what this high level of meat consumption actually means.

So let's discuss some reasons why more and more people are cutting down on meat and perhaps dairy products in their own diets and why they are interested in feeding their dogs or cats in the same way. The first group of reasons stems from health concerns, the second from global, ethical and environmental issues.

VEGETARIANS ARE HEALTHIER

Many of the people throughout history who chose a vegetarian diet did so because they believed it was a healthier way to eat. Now there is a body of scientific research that supports their views. Consider these facts, compiled by John Robbins, author of *Diet for a New America.*

◆ Women who eat eggs or meat daily face a breast cancer risk that averages more than three times higher than those who eat these foods once a week. Consuming butter and cheese just two to four times a week multiplies the risk by the same degree.

- Fatal ovarian cancer risk is three times higher for women who eat eggs frequently (three or more times a week, rather than once or less).
- Men who eat meat, dairy products and eggs daily triple their risk of fatal prostate cancer over those who eat these foods sparingly.
- While the average American man has a 50 percent chance of dying from a heart attack, that risk is only 15 percent for those who consume no meat and just 4 percent for men who eat no animal products at all.
- Americans who drop consumption of meat, dairy products and eggs by half reduce their heart attack risk by 45 percent.
- At age 65 the average measurable bone loss of female vegetarians is only about half that of female meat-eaters.
- Diseases that can be prevented, relieved and sometimes even cured by a low-fat diet that is free of animal products include: strokes, hypertension, diabetes, asthma, gallstones, osteoporosis, irritable colon syndrome and prostate, breast, colon and endometrial cancers.

Why these differences? For one thing, research indicates that meat fat favors the production of certain carcinogens in the intestines. But perhaps even more critical are the toxins that accumulate in animal tissues. The chemical pollution of breast milk in American women averages *35 times* higher than that of complete vegetarians.

Some of these differences might originate with the fact that we humans evolved to eat a largely meatless diet. Most other primates are basically vegetarians. Our teeth and digestive tracts seem best suited to such foods.

IS LESS MEAT BETTER FOR DOGS AND CATS, TOO?

For our pets *that* part of the equation is somewhat different. The cat is considered a true carnivore and clearly requires nutrients adequately supplied only by meat and animal products. Although the dog prefers meat, both its physiology and behavior indicate that it is better classed as an opportunistic omnivore—an animal that can meet its needs from a wide variety of sources. Wild coyotes and wolves, for example, consume vegetable matter including grasses, berries and other fresh material, plus predigested food found in the digestive tracts of their vegetarian prey. In fact, a three-generation test found that dogs fed meat as a sole source of protein, along with other essential elements, had difficulties producing adequate milk for their young, as compared with dogs fed a diet that included milk and vegetables.

So strictly from a health viewpoint it seems that the most natural diet for a dog or cat would be primarily fresh raw meat, eggs and bones (or bonemeal), supplemented with vegetables and fruits for dogs. Yet, such a diet may not be best for today's domesticated pets. Their needs may differ from those of their hunting ancestors who got more exercise, lived in purer environments and often, by necessity, fasted between large meals. Thus their bodies could cleanse themselves more easily, eliminating uric acid and other waste products of meat metabolism.

Our primary health concern about feeding meat to dogs and cats, however, is that meat is now the most polluted food source on the market. Even the highest-quality cuts approved for human consumption contain residues of antibiotics, synthetic hormones and toxic materials such as lead, arsenic, mercury, DDT and dioxin. There are also more pesticide residues in meat than in dairy products, grains, vegetables and fruits.

The long-term effect of all this toxic material—particularly the pesticides and heavy metals—may be increased cancer rates, allergies, infections, kidney and liver problems, irritability and hyperactivity for our pets.

Looking beyond the immediate personal health issues, what about the big picture? What about the impact of meat production on the environment, on the world's hungry and on factory-farm animals?

GLOBAL, ETHICAL AND ENVIRONMENTAL CONCERNS ABOUT MEAT

"A reduction in meat consumption is the most potent single act you can take to halt the destruction of our environment and preserve our precious natural resources," contends Robbins. And he makes the following points.

- If Americans were to adopt a meatless diet and stop exporting livestock feed, we could return 204,000,000 acres to forests—almost an acre for every American who would become vegetarian.
- Over two-thirds of the topsoil in the United States has been lost, with 85 percent of this loss associated with livestock production.
- It takes 78 calories of fossil fuel to produce 1 calorie of protein from beef. Only 2 calories will produce the same amount of protein from soybeans.
- The 5,215 gallons of water California uses to produce only *one* edible pound of beef would grow 209 edible pounds of wheat or 10 pounds of eggs or provide 300 five-minute showers.

It's clear that we can't continue with this pattern of inefficient consumption. For the sake of future generations, it would be wise for us to begin to rely more on plant sources for our daily food.

Even as we waste resources needed for the future, we contribute to the present world hunger problem. Some 20 million people a year die from malnutrition. Yet 15 vegetarians can be fed on the amount of land needed to feed 1 person eating a meat-centered diet. If Americans would reduce their intake of meat by only 10 percent, 100,000,000 people could be adequately nourished using the same land, water and energy no longer devoted to livestock feed. That's five times the number of people who now die of malnutrition.

Finally, let's consider the impact of meat production on the animals involved. When all we see is a neatly wrapped package in the supermarket and maybe a few cows out in the countryside, we may imagine that the meat came from animals who spent long, peaceful lives lazily scratching for bugs in a barnyard or grazing in sunny pastures. At the end of their idyll, we imagine, they are slaughtered quickly and humanely. Unfortunately, the reality is usually quite different.

I used to work with livestock and was often appalled at the crowded, stressful and uncomfortable conditions under which most chickens, pigs and cows actually live and die. Farming has become big business, and most animals are treated more like profit-making units than creatures capable of feeling pain and distress. To minimize costs and maxi-

Nutritional Composition of Growth Recipes and Vegetarian Recipes for Dogs

Recipe	Kcal.	Protein (%)	Fat (%)	Carb. (%)	Fiber (%)	Ash (%)*	Calcium (%)*
Growth							
Dog Growth Diet A: lean hamburger	3,858	30.4	15.4	47.0	1.2	7.2 (3.3)	1.6 (0.7)
Dog Growth Diet B: heart	1,807	32.3	15.8	43.4	0.9	8.5 (3.9)	1.9 (0.8)
Dog Growth Diet C: chuck	2,322	33.2	27.3	32.3	0.8	7.2 (3.6)	1.7 (0.8)
Vegetarian							
Polenta for Dogs	1,155	25.0	16.2	52.5	0.9	6.4 (4.8)	1.3 (0.9)
Beans 'n' Millet: millet	3,441	24.2	6.0	61.4	3.3	8.4 (5.0)	1.6 (0.8)
Mexi-Dog Casserole	5,061	25.3	14.8	52.5	3.0	7.4 (5.0)	1.4 (0.8)
Easy Eggs and Grain	1,151	23.7	14.7	54.3	1.4	7.3 (4.2)	1.6 (0.9)
Standard recommendations:‡	—	22–28 (growth) ≥18+ (normal)	≥8 (growth) ≥5 (normal)	—	—	—	≥1.0 (growth) ≥0.6 (normal)

*The second figures for calcium and phosphorus (in parentheses) result if you use pure calcium rather than bonemeal. This also makes a lower-ash diet.

†The second figures for iron (in parentheses) apply if you use the iron supplement as described in chapter 3.

mize profits, most of them are packed into crowded quarters like items in a production line, deprived of normal environments and relationships. They may never even see daylight or stand on the ground.

Those who enjoy the companionship of dogs and cats often have a special appreciation and caring for all sorts of animals. Knowing something about the realities of modern meat production understandably

Phosph. (%)*	Calcium: Phosph. Ratio*	Iron (mg.)†	Vit. A/kg (IU)	Thiamin (%)	Riboflavin (%)	Niacin (%)
1.3 (0.6)	1.3:1 (1.2:1)	.007 (.010)	11,833	.0008	.0005	.0096
1.5 (0.6)	1.3:1 (1.3:1)	.010 (.012)	9,266	.0014	.0013	.0104
1.3 (0.6)	1.3:1 (1.3:1)	.006 (.009)	11,411	.0009	.0006	.0083
1.0 (0.7)	1.3:1 (1.3:1)	.004 (.009)	10,118	.0006	.0008	.0023
1.2 (0.6)	1.3:1 (1.4:1)	.008 (.009)	11,151	.0012	.0006	.0041
1.1 (0.6)	1.3:1 (1.3:1)	.006 (.008)	14,687	.0009	.0005	.0026
1.2 (0.7)	1.3:1 (1.3:1)	.006 (.008)	10,097	.0009	.0005	.0049
≥0.8 (growth) ≥0.5 (normal)	1.1:1– 1.2:1 (1.3:1 ideal)	≥.008	≥5,000 IU per kg. dry weight	≥.0001	≥.0002	≥.0011

‡Standard recommendations are the percentage of total dry weight unless otherwise noted. Sources: AAFCO Nutrient Profiles for Dog Foods: Report of the Canine Nutrition Expert Subcommittee, 1992, and the *Merck Veterinary Manual*, 6th Edition, 1986.

causes many to wonder whether they can reduce or eliminate meat from their pets' diets. *Animal Liberation*, by philosopher Peter Singer, is an excellent book on the ethics of how we treat animals, with many graphic details about factory farming.

For these reasons, I recommend prioritizing the recipes in chapter 4 that use the least amounts of meat. While all of the basic dog recipes are tailored to use fairly low amounts of meat, the minimal-meat choices for dogs are (in this order): Quick Canine Oatmeal (page 49), Quick Canine Oats and Eggs (page 49) and One-on-One (page 48).

The best choices for cats are (in this order): Quick Feline Eggfest (page 53), Poultry Delight (page 51), Beefy Oats (page 50) and Mackerel Loaf (page 52).

In general, use more poultry, eggs and dairy products than beef, since their production consumes fewer resources. And whenever you have the choice, take turkey over chicken. Turkeys are often raised more humanely and with a more vegetarian feed.

Nutritional Composition of Growth Recipes and Vegetarian Recipes for Cats

Recipe	Kcal.	Protein (%)	Fat (%)	Carb. (%)	Fiber (%)	Ash (%)*	Calcium (%)*
Growth							
Feline Feast (turkey)†	2,215	47.8	19.1	24.2	0.8	8.9 (5.1)	1.9 (1.1)
Mackerel Loaf†	3,151	41.5	25.7	24.8	0.7	8.0 (6.8)	1.3 (1.0)
Cat Growth Diet (turkey)	2,306	45.3	17.8	28.1	0.5	8.7 (5.1)	1.8 (1.0)
Vegetarian							
Polenta for Cats	877	31.0	25.2	34.6	0.9	9.2 (5.2)	2.1 (1.2)
Standard recommendations:‡	—	26 (normal) 30–35 (growth)	9+ (normal) 9–16+ (growth)	—	—	~5	≥0.6 (normal) ≥1.0 (growth)

*The second figures for calcium and phosphorus (in parentheses) result if you use pure calcium rather than bonemeal. This also makes a lower-ash diet.

†See chapter 4.

They also produce the most protein.

For dogs, consider a predominantly lacto-ovo vegetarian diet (one that includes milk and eggs along with plant-based foods); for cats, a partial one. Vegetarian clients have often asked if you can safely exclude meat from a pet's diet. For dogs, the answer is yes, if you are careful in what you feed. Controlled research shows that dogs fed soy protein grow as well as those fed meat, and several meatless pet foods are now marketed through health food stores. For cats, the answer is with special supplements, maybe, but a diet that excludes meat is not the best for the cat.

The Vegetarian Society of the United Kingdom reports that meatless diets are successfully fed to both dogs and cats throughout Great Britain. Dogs do well, they say, on a breakfast of whole-grain cereal and milk and a dinner of high-protein food like cheese, eggs, ground nuts and textured vegetable proteins or legumes mixed with raw and/or cooked vegetables. They also suggest includ-

Phosph. (%)*	Calcium: Phosph. Ratio*	Iron (mg.)	Vit. A/kg. (IU)	Thiamin (%)	Riboflavin (%)	Niacin (%)
1.6 (0.9)	1.2:1 (1.2:1)	.008	24,768	.0013	.0008	.013
1.1 (0.9)	1.2:1 (1.1:1)	.006	12,917	.0007	.0010	.014
1.5 (0.8)	1.2:1 (1.2:1)	.007	13,807	.0010	.0007	.012
1.6 (0.9)	1.3:1 (1.3:1)	.008	18,881	.0024	.0011	.007
≥0.5 (normal) ≥0.8 (growth)	1.1:1– 1.3:1 (1.25:1 ideal)	≥.008	≥5,000 IU per kg. dry weight	≥.0005	≥.0004	≥.006

‡Recommended amounts are the percentage of total dry weight unless otherwise noted. Sources: AAFCO Nutrient Profiles for Cat Foods: Report of the Feline Nutrition Expert Subcommittee, 1992, and the *Merck Veterinary Manual*, 6th Edition, 1986.

ing whole-wheat bread, brown rice, sprouts, fruit and some hard foods, such as whole carrots and hard whole-grain biscuits, for exercising the teeth and gums.

The same British group reports that vegetarian cats thrive on a varied diet of high-protein sources that include textured vegetable proteins, wheat germ, oats, beans, yeast, milk, cheese, eggs, ground nuts, legumes and canned meat substitutes marketed for vegetarians. They also advise some vegetables (cucumbers, carrots, spinach and the like) as well as occasional melons.

In my own experience, however, I must say that I see some vegetarian animals that *aren't* so healthy. (Of course, it's the sick animals that people tend to bring to veterinarians!) My observation is that problems arise mostly when owners exclude *all* animal foods, including milk products and eggs, from their pets' diets. While people can do well on a carefully planned pure vegetarian (vegan) diet, I would not impose it on dogs—and certainly not on cats.

Cats have certain needs that can only be supplied from animal tissues. Unlike both humans and dogs, they cannot convert the beta-carotene found in vegetables to vitamin A; they require an animal source of vitamin A such as cod-liver oil, cheese or eggs. They also need a preformed source of arachidonic acid (also found in cod-liver oil) and ample levels of taurine, an amino acid not present in plant foods. Taurine is found in the highest concentrations in heart tissue and seafoods and to a lesser extent in meats and dairy products. And even in a meat-centered diet, up to 80 percent of the taurine in the ingredients can be lost through cooking. (Perhaps this is why so many cats on processed foods crave seafoods!)

Studies show that a taurine-deficient diet causes cats to suffer degeneration of the retina, leading to blindness and problems with their hearts (cardiomyopathy) and other functions. These changes can be prevented or reversed by using lactalbumin (from milk) or egg albumin as the dietary protein source.

Some vegetarians have experimented with a meatless or even a near-vegan diet supplemented with taurine for cats. However, I don't believe there is enough positive evidence at this point to recommend a vegetarian diet for cats, even if dairy products such as eggs are included. We just don't know all there is to know about the nutrients cats normally obtain from meat. Aside from the uncertainty of a meatless diet's health effects, there is also a palatability issue. Cats often turn down vegetarian recipes!

However, you can reduce your cat's meat consumption by alternating the following recipe with at least three or four feedings a week of Mackerel Loaf (page 52) or Beefy Oats (page 50). Use beef or poultry heart, which are both high in taurine, for at least half of the meat in these two recipes. Also, it's wise to add one to two teaspoons of unflavored protein powder derived from lactalbumin or egg albumin to any vegetarian recipe, along with a taurine supplement equalling 50 or more milligrams a day.

POLENTA FOR CATS

This recipe derives 71 percent of its protein from meatless animal sources. By comparison, the feline meat diets in chapter 4 derive 85 percent or more of their protein from animal sources. So be sure to add the taurine.

½ cup cornmeal or polenta (or about 2 cups cooked)

4 eggs, beaten

½ cup grated cheese

1 tablespoon Healthy Powder (page 39)

2 tablespoons nutritional yeast

1,000 milligrams calcium (or rounded ½ teaspoon eggshell powder or 1¾ teaspoons bonemeal)

50–100 IU vitamin E

200 milligrams taurine supplement (found in many cat vitamins)

1–2 teaspoons protein powder—from lactalbumin or egg albumin (optional)

1 teaspoon vegetables with each meal (optional)

Bring 2 cups of water to a boil. Add the cornmeal or polenta, stirring briskly with a fork or whisk. (Or mix the meal in ½ cup cold water first and add this to 1½ cups boiling water.) When blended, cover and simmer about 10 minutes or until the cornmeal is a smooth mush. While it is still hot, stir in the eggs and cheese. After the mixture has cooled, stir in the remaining ingredients. (Heat can destroy taurine.)

Grain substitutes: ½ cup millet (+ 1½ cups water = 1½ cups cooked); ½ cup whole-wheat couscous (+ ¾ cup water = 1¼ cups cooked); 1 cup raw oats (+ 2 cups water = 2 cups oatmeal).

Yield: About 3¾ cups, with about 240 kilocalories per cup. Feed 1 to 1½ cups a day, more if your cat is active.

◆

The version of polenta below is suitable for a "veggie" dog, and it is followed by three other canine vegetarian recipes. In these meatless recipes, it is probably best to include an iron supplement, as discussed in chapter 3. That's because dairy products and legumes contain less iron than meats do. To help counterbalance this deficiency, use plenty of millet, which is high in iron. Eggs are well-supplied with this mineral also.

POLENTA FOR DOGS

½ cup powdered milk + 4 cups water (or 4 cups low-fat milk)

1 cup cornmeal

2 eggs, beaten

½ cup grated cheese

600 milligrams calcium (or ⅓ teaspoon eggshell powder or 1 teaspoon bonemeal)

1 tablespoon Healthy Powder (page 39)

1 teaspoon vegetable oil

100–200 IU vitamin E

15 milligrams iron supplement

½ cup vegetables (optional)

Bring powdered milk and water to a boil. (If using all milk, scald and stir to avoid burning.) Add the cornmeal quickly with a whisk and blend until smooth. Cover and turn down to simmer until the cornmeal is soft and mushy, about 10 minutes. While the cornmeal is still hot, blend in the eggs and cheese. After some cooling, stir in the remaining ingredients.

Grain substitutes: 1 cup millet (+ 3 cups water = 3 cups cooked); 1 cup whole-wheat couscous (+ 1½ cups water = 2½ cups cooked); 2 cups raw oats (+ 4 cups water = 4 cups oatmeal).

Yield: About 5½ cups, with 210 kilocalories per cup.

(continued)

Daily ration (in cups): toy—²/₃ to 2¹/₂; small—2¹/₂ to 5; medium—5 to 6¹/₂; large—6¹/₂ to 9; giant—9 to 13¹/₃+.

MEXI-DOG CASSEROLE

Adapted from a delicious recipe for people, here's another bean-based dish. This one is topped with a cheesy layer of cornmeal. It makes a large quantity, so you might want to reserve some for yourself (minus the supplements) when you make it for your pet.

- 4 cups pinto beans (or 10 cups cooked or canned)
- 3 cups whole milk
- 1 cup cornmeal
- 2 cups grated cheddar cheese
- 4 eggs
- 2 tablespoons vegetable oil
- 2 rounded tablespoons bonemeal (or 4,200 milligrams calcium or 2¹/₃ teaspoons eggshell powder)
- ¼ cup Healthy Powder (page 39)
  10,000 IU vitamin A
  200–400 IU vitamin E
  20 milligrams iron supplement
- 1–2 cups vegetables (optional)

Soak the beans overnight. Drain, rinse and pick out any broken or damaged beans. Bring beans to a boil in 8 to 10 cups of water. Simmer, covered, for 1¹/₂ hours or until you can blow the skin off a bean. (To reduce gas, discard cooking water after the first half-hour and start over with fresh water for the final hour.)

Meanwhile, make the cornmeal topping. Scald the milk. Gradually add the cornmeal, stirring with a whisk or fork. Cover and steam until soft, about 10 minutes. Remove from heat and add the cheese and eggs. After the mixture has cooled, add the remaining ingredients and serve. Freeze anything that can't be eaten in 3 days.

Bean substitutes: You may use equal amounts (before cooking) of kidney, white or black beans.

Variation: You can omit the beans and serve the corn topping by itself. If you do, eliminate the vitamin A and change amounts as follows: 2 teaspoons oil, ¹/₂ teaspoon bonemeal (or 600 milligrams calcium or ¹/₃ teaspoon eggshell powder) and 2 tablespoons Healthy Powder. The resulting food (5.3 Kcal./kg.) would be good for active dogs.

Yield: 17 to 18 cups, with about 290 kilocalories per cup.

Daily ration (in cups): toy—¹/₂ to 2; small—2 to 3¹/₄; medium—3¹/₄ to 5; large—5 to 7; giant—7 to 10¹/₃+.

EASY EGGS AND GRAIN

This simple-to-make dish relies on eggs for its main protein source. Eggs provide an economical protein. They're also high in fat, but the protein powder helps to balance that. Look in a health food store for an unflavored powder that includes some of its protein from lactalbumin and egg albumin.

- 1 cup bulgur
- 4 eggs
- 1 tablespoon chopped parsley or sprouts or ¹/₂ cup cooked vegetables
- 3 tablespoons protein powder
- 2 tablespoons Healthy Powder (page 39)
- 2 teaspoons vegetable oil
  1,200 milligrams calcium (or ²/₃ teaspoon eggshell powder or 2 teaspoons bonemeal)
  100–200 IU vitamin E
  5 milligrams iron supplement (optional)
- 1 clove garlic, minced (optional)
- ¹/₂ teaspoon tamari soy sauce (optional)

Bring 2 cups of water to a boil. Add the bulgur, cover and turn down to simmer until the grain is soft, 10 to 20 minutes. Stir in the eggs while the bulgur is still hot. After it cools a bit, add the remaining ingredients and serve.

Grain substitutes: 1 cup millet (+ 3 cups water = 3 cups cooked); 1 cup whole-wheat couscous (+ 1½ cups water = 2½ cups cooked); or 2 cups raw oats (+ 4 cups water = 4 cups oatmeal).

Yield: About 4 cups, with about 290 kilocalories per cup.

Daily ration (in cups): Same as Mexi-Dog Casserole (above).

BEANS 'N' MILLET

Here's a well-balanced meatless recipe for dogs that makes use of beans and cottage cheese, both of which are high in protein and economical.

> 2   cups kidney beans (or 5 cups cooked or about 38 ounces canned)
>
> 2   cups millet (or 6 cups cooked)
>
> 2   cups low-fat cottage cheese
>
> 2   tablespoons vegetable oil
>
> 4   tablespoons Healthy Powder (page 39)
>
> 2½   tablespoons bonemeal (or 4,500 milligrams calcium or 2½ teaspoons eggshell powder)
>
> ½   cup cooked carrots, broccoli or peas (optional)
>
> 2   teaspoons tamari soy sauce or ½ teaspoon iodized salt
>
> 1–2   cloves garlic, crushed or minced (optional)
>
> 5,000 IU vitamin A
>
> 50–200 IU vitamin E
>
> 10 milligrams iron supplement (optional with millet; recommended with other grains)

Soak the beans overnight. Drain, rinse and pick out any broken or damaged beans. Bring the beans to a boil in 6 to 8 cups of water. Simmer, covered, for 1½ hours or until you can blow the skin off a bean. (To reduce gas, discard cooking water after first half-hour and start over with fresh water for the final hour). Meanwhile, prepare the millet. Bring 6 cups of water to a boil. Add the millet, cover and simmer on low for 20 to 30 minutes, or until soft. Combine when both are done; then add the remaining ingredients and serve.

Grain substitutes: You may use 2 cups (before cooking) of bulgur, brown rice or barley.
Bean substitutes: You may use equal amounts (before cooking) of lentils, pintos, soybeans or white or black beans. Or to save time you may use a 16-ounce package of tofu. In this case, it's okay to use creamed cottage cheese instead of low-fat, and you'll still have plenty of protein.

Yield: 13 to 14 cups, with about 250 kilocalories per cup.

Daily ration (in cups): toy—½ to 2¼; small—2¼ to 4½; medium—4½ to 6; large—6 to 8¼; giant—8¼ to 12⅓+.

◆

It's a good idea to include some hard foods for vegetarian dogs to chew on to keep their teeth and gums in top shape. Instead of bones you can offer raw carrots, apples or biscuits made from one of the recipes in "Additional Recipes" on page 350.

Even if you are not trying to feed a meatless diet to your animal, you can still use these vegetarian recipes now and then to decrease the level of pesticides and other toxic residues in your pet's diet and lower your costs. Besides, it's good to know that you can lighten your load on the planet by using less meat and reduce suffering for both humans and animals at the same time.

CHAPTER SIX

HELPING YOUR PET MAKE THE SWITCH

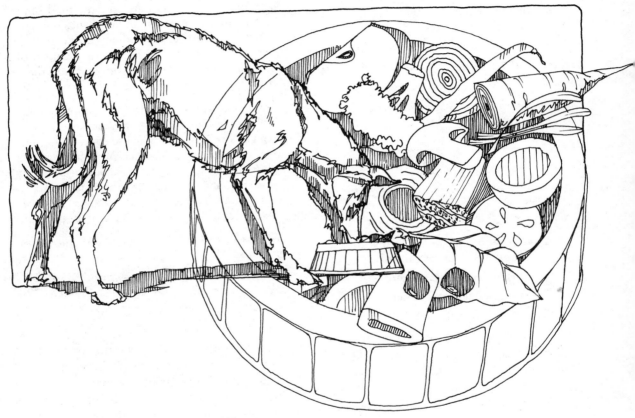

Most pets love their new diets. But some may run into a few snags along the way—snags that can be prevented or smoothed over. Here are some examples of common problems.

One reader phoned to tell me that her cats would not eat the foods in the diet I suggest.

"What have you given them?" I inquired.

"You name it! I've tried adding supple-

ments like bonemeal, nutritional yeast and wheat germ. I've offered them meats, dairy products, grains, vegetables, everything you can think of! But practically *all* they will touch, especially the older cat, is just canned tuna and chicken. Not only that, but it has to be one *certain* brand, if you can believe that!"

Similarly, a client reported back after following a course of natural foods and remedies for her dog's chronic problem: "Henry was doing okay and then suddenly he just stopped eating and began acting like he was sick. He just lay around and didn't seem to have any energy."

Another owner who had started to feed the natural diet called for reassurance and advice: "My dog liked the new food, and he's been on it a few weeks. But yesterday he just passed a whole bunch of worms! What do I do?"

In the first instance—a cat who turns up its nose at new foods—we are dealing with the fussy feline, star of cat food commercials. Many cats have become habituated ("addicted") to the particular foods they were given as kittens or foods they've been fed over a long period of time. Under such circumstances the body's natural instinct for selecting a healthy, balanced diet diminishes considerably. Similarly, among humans, narrow food preferences that were learned early in life often become deeply entrenched habits.

In cases like the last two—the dog that stopped eating and the dog that passed worms—I am actually happy to hear about these responses to the switch. It's not that I like to see an animal suffer or that I'm eager for more business. On the contrary, I know from experience that such signs can be favorable omens in terms of natural healing. After a brief period on a higher-quality diet, it is fairly common for an animal in suboptimal health to discharge accumulated toxic material or to undergo a brief aggravation of its symptoms (often called a healing crisis). These apparent setbacks are normal, often necessary bumps on the road to well-being.

Nearly all the snags your pet might encounter in a change of diet will be of these two types—getting a finicky eater to like nutritious food or helping an animal through the sometimes uncomfortable stages of a natural cleansing process.

THREE WAYS TO INTRODUCE THE NEW FOODS

When you have a finicky eater on your hands, first make sure you serve the food in an appealing manner. Rather than serving refrigerated food cold, warm it up a bit, which greatly increases aroma and appeal. Also, be sure to serve the food in a safe place, not in the middle of your path of movement around the kitchen. Beyond that, you can choose one of three strategies: Introduce new foods gradually until they're accepted, let your animal go without eating until it's hungry enough to try the new fare or compromise with a combination of the natural diet and your pet's old favorites.

The gradual transition. This not only helps your pet get used to the taste of new foods but also gives the animal's digestive system time to adjust. Whenever the diet is changed abruptly, even from one commercial brand to another, temporary diarrhea or loss of appetite might occur. That's because the bacterial flora in the digestive tract is still adjusting to the new material. So by switching over gradually, you can reduce or avoid acceptance problems and the possibility of discomfort for your pet. If the gradual method doesn't work, you probably have a food addict on your hands, and more drastic measures will be necessary.

Fasting your animal a few days. This stimulates a lagging appetite, helps cleanse the body and deconditions old taste habits all at the same time.

To fast, your pet needs a healthful setting—plenty of fresh air, quiet, access to the outdoors and some moderate exercise.

Here's the process.

1. Begin the fast with a break-in period of one to two days. Feed a smaller quantity of the usual food during this first phase, perhaps adding a little meat, cooked grain and/or vegetables.
2. Move to a liquid fast for the next two to three days. During that time give your animal only liquids, such as pure water, vegetable juices and broths.
3. To break the fast, add some solid foods to the liquid regime over a day or two, perhaps vegetables (for dogs) or eggs, yogurt or small amounts of fresh meat (for dogs and cats).
4. After a day or so, increase the amount of meat and add a grain, gradually adding other ingredients until the recipe is approximated; then add the supplements (often the least-accepted part of the diet, except for nutritional yeast, which many animals love).

In stubborn cases it often pays to continue fasting the animal a few more days. One client reported worriedly that her cat wouldn't eat any of the natural foods offered in the "breaking-out" period. I advised her to keep the cat on liquids for a while longer. She did, and in a few days she called back enthused to say that her formerly finicky cat was now eating all kinds of things it would never touch before—like vegetables, grains, meats, nutritional yeast and even soy grits! In addition to the longer fast, she found it helped to mix a little bit of fish (an old favorite) into the new diet.

Some people are frightened by the idea of fasting their pet. At first it does seem that some animals would rather starve to death than eat anything but the food to which they're addicted. But the instinct for survival is very strong. Sooner or later, the pet comes around. Somehow we have convinced ourselves that a day or two without food will take a cat or dog close to death's door. Not true. Cats, being true carnivores, actually prefer a 28-hour eating cycle. In fact, healthy cats trapped in moving vans and such have been known to survive without any food or water for periods of up to six weeks. They have adapted to eating two or even three times a day because they live with people. However, this eating schedule is not natural to them, or even desirable.

Obese dogs have been known to fast on just water and vitamins for as long as six to eight weeks without ill effect. Wild carnivores fast naturally since the prey they live on may elude them for days at a time. So don't worry about trying the fast on your pet for a few days.

How long should you let your animal go hungry before giving up and returning to the old diet? With cats, keep trying for up to five days. With dogs, two days should be enough. I use these figures because I have not seen healthy animals go longer than that before they become truly hungry.

Some cats or dogs, however, simply do not develop a normal hunger even after several days of not eating. A weak appetite like this is often a symptom of chronic illness. I do not mean that these animals are necessarily ill with symptoms or a defined disease. Rather, they are in a sub-optimal or low-grade state of health. In such cases I use individualized homeopathic treatment to improve the animal's overall level of health. Afterward, the animal begins to eat more normally. If your pet won't eat and you don't have access to a vet of this type, you may want to try the third approach.

"The compromise." Suppose you've tried a gradual transition and your pet just won't convert to a new diet. Or perhaps fasting just doesn't work for *you*. It is difficult for some people to let their animals get hungry. They can't handle the agitation that the animal shows in asking for food. And in other cases, the cat or dog is not healthy enough to undertake a fast. In such situations, it is best to compromise by mixing the old food into the new.

Sometimes even a small bit of the pet's familiar fare makes a difference. One woman I know finds that mixing just a spoonful of her pets' favorite canned cat food into the natural recipe does the trick. "There seems to be something about the sight and sound of the old familiar can-opening process that gets them excited," she told me. Another trick you might try is to pulverize some of the usual dry kibble in a food processor or blender and then sprinkle it over the natural food recipe, perhaps mixing some in as well. This is just the kind of catalyst that some finicky felines need to get them started eating a natural diet. Then nature takes over. It's likely that after eating a compromise mixture of both natural and commercial foods for a while, your pet will become so used to the new foods that the old ones will be forgotten. Eventually, many pets turn up their noses at their old favorite canned food or kibbles.

TAKING CHARGE

Don't allow your animal's habits to run your life. Remember, for the average healthy animal, the most important factor in accepting a new food is hunger. Many animals will not accept a change in diet simply because they are not really that hungry. They lack the motivation to try something new. Cats, in particular, are well-adapted to cycles of feast and famine, and it often takes several days for them to reach a state of true hunger. When food is available several times a day, they learn to just nibble, but seldom get a decent appetite.

Ideally, cats should be fed once a day. However, most people prefer feeding them twice daily. This can work out fine as long as the food is available for no more than 20 minutes at each feeding, morning and evening. Practitioners find that cats fed frequently during the day and those with constant self-feeding access to kibble are not in tip-top health, have a poor hair coat and tend to form "gravel" in the bladder with resultant cystitis (bladder inflammation). Carnivores need a certain interval between meals so that the body can digest food properly and eliminate the many toxins associated with a meat-based diet.

With dogs, things are simpler. By nature, the dog is a partial scavenger, so it is adapted to eat whenever the opportunity arises. It's okay to feed a healthy dog once or twice a day, or even more often.

CLEANSING REACTIONS

Some animals, particularly those in marginal health, may experience some physical difficulties even if the transition to a natural diet is gradual. They may seem out of sorts for a few days or even throw up hair balls or pass worms. Often, these are transient cleansing reactions. But not always. If you suspect that your pet is having excessive difficulty, a checkup, as described in "How to Give Your Pet a Quick Checkup," will let you know if your pet has an underlying health problem that is being aggravated by a change of diet.

If your animal really does not look healthy to you, it is time to get some help. Ask your local veterinarian to work with you on the diet switch. Explain what you are trying to do and why, perhaps showing the recipes and analyses. Ask your doctor to examine your pet periodically to make sure that there are no health problems of which you are unaware and to see that your pet responds to the diet as expected and does not lose weight or weaken.

If your veterinarian does not want to help as you switch your pet to a fresh foods diet, don't hesitate to seek help elsewhere. Veterinarians interested in nutrition and a holistic approach to medicine are growing in number. Most states have a few; some will consult by phone, which can be quite helpful.

How to Give Your Pet a Quick Checkup

Your animal might be in poor health without your realizing it. Perform this brief exam to get a much better idea of your pet's actual state. Then resolve any concerns that arise by consulting your vet.

1. Does the hair coat feel greasy? Is the skin color a normal gray-white or is it pink or red with inflammation? Do you see dandrufflike scales of dead skin among the hairs?
2. Use your fingers to brush the hair against the grain. Do you see numerous little black specks? These are the excreta of fleas.
3. Now smell your fingers. If the odor they picked up is rancid, rank or fishy, it's a sign of poor health.
4. As you examine the eyes, check for matter in the corners. Pull down the lower eyelids so you can see the underside. Are the lids red inside or irritated on the edges?
5. Look into the ear holes. Do you see a lot of wax? Do the insides look oily? Sniff to check for an offensive odor.
6. Inspect the gums for a red line on the gums along the roots of the teeth. To check the back teeth for that red line, raise the upper lip and push back the corners of the lips at the same time (it is not necessary to open the mouth).
7. Now check the teeth themselves, including the back ones. Are they gleaming white or coated with a brown deposit? Does the breath smell okay or are you overcome by it?
8. Last, feel the backbone in the middle of the back and run your fingers back and forth (sideways) over it. Do you feel definite bones there? Is there a prominent ridge sticking up in the middle? If your answers to these questions are yes, your animal is much too thin.

THE BODY RESPONDS

By examining your pet regularly, you can easily monitor its overall health. No matter what you've heard, it's *not* normal for a dog to have a "doggy odor" or a cat to have foul breath. Pets that have an unpleasant smell about them show signs of a chronic low health level. If your pet is in mediocre condition or it has a particular disease, starting the new diet may trigger a cleansing process.

What happens? For years your animal has been eating overprocessed food that was probably loaded with the harmful ingredients discussed in chapter 2. No doubt it has also been exposed to environmental pollutants and, perhaps, some strong drugs. So when your pet finally eats really fresh, nutritious food that is minimally polluted, strange things begin to happen. The body responds!

Your animal usually feels better at first. Energy and nutrients are flowing through the tissues. The quality of the blood and its oxygen-carrying capacity improves, so the animal starts to be more active. The added exercise in turn helps recharge lazy tissues.

After two to three weeks, the animal may feel perky enough to tackle some long-neglected interior housecleaning by throwing off debris it's been accumulating. For example, a mass of worms that, until now, have been existing comfortably may be swept out, leaving behind a clean intestine.

More often, the cleansing results in a lot of discharge from the kidneys, colon or skin, all important excretory organs. Thus, the urine might become dark and strong-smelling, the feces dark, temporarily containing mucus or blood, or the skin might erupt with sores or develop a lot of dandruff. Sometimes a lot of dead hair falls out as the skin becomes more active, getting ready to grow a new crop of fresh, healthy hair (much like a plant dropping dead foliage before putting out new leaves).

THE HEALING CRISIS

Appearances are deceiving. In spite of what you see, the body is getting *cleaner*. I know that's hard to grasp. Most of us expect that when a physical problem is being treated effectively, the condition will steadily improve until the disturbance just disappears. (Certainly, we don't expect it to look worse!) That's how antibiotics and other familiar drugs often work—at least for a while. Unfortunately, such drugs sometimes simply suppress the symptoms, leaving the underlying disorder that led to the illness just as it was. So the same problems or related ones may crop up again. One long-term effect of using drugs to control diseases is that the body tends to become lazy about attempting to keep itself healthy. That's when an animal gets the kind of symptoms described in "How to Give Your Pet a Quick Checkup."

In bygone times, people more clearly recognized the stages of healing—one of which was a period of crisis that might show up as a fever, inflammation or temporary exaggeration of symptoms. At such a point the patient either began to recover or died. This healing crisis, as it has been called, represents the point at which the body's defenses are mobilized to their maximum capabilities. It's an all-out effort.

When we interfere with this process by injecting antibiotics or cortisone, for example, the defense system is not utilized. That means it can't address the underlying weakness that gave rise to the disease in the first place. Like an underused muscle, the defense system gets weak. Soon resistance to any new disease is weak, and the body needs more drugs to cope with new problems. Poor nutrition makes things worse by lowering disease resistance even further, which then leads to the use of still more drugs. Weakened by infections and the toxic elements of drugs, the body demands more of the available nutrition, which overtaxes the supply and creates a deficit. Before we know it, we are caught in a vicious circle.

What will break this cycle? A good diet, for one thing. By supplying optimum nutrients we can increase disease resistance and help the body to eliminate the toxic effects of drugs. So don't be discouraged at signs of detoxification when you improve your pet's diet. You have things moving.

INTERPRETING REACTIONS

"But," you might ask, "how can I tell whether my pet's in the process of detoxification or is suffering from some serious disease?" This is a sticky point, of course. If you feel uncertain, consult your veterinarian. And if you favor a conservative approach (minimum drugs, maximum wait-and-see) tell the vet so. But here are some general clues to help you interpret what is happening.

- ◆ If your pet has a high-energy level and has a good appetite, temporary symptoms such as passing worms, mucus or a little blood are probably insignificant.

And bear in mind that it is also common for an animal switching from all-commercial to all-fresh food to undergo a lethargic period of a day or two, usually within two to four weeks of the diet change. This is a cleansing period that may result in a temporary energy drop and appetite loss plus more time spent sleeping.

- ◆ Returning symptoms of problems previously suppressed by drugs—such as skin eruptions, bladder irritation in cats and ear problems in dogs—mean the body is rallying its increased energies to try to heal underlying chronic disturbances that should have been dealt with long ago. If these problems persist or become intense, you will need help from a veterinarian who knows how to work with the body to bring this process to healthy completion. I use homeopathy, but there are other natural treatment methods that support the body in this process, including acupuncture and herbology.

- ◆ If your pet's energy level decreases steadily for more than a few days or if you see mental/emotional changes such as depression, irritability or forgetfulness *that were not present before,* your pet may have serious problems that should be checked out by a vet.

- ◆ If any symptoms—such as loss of appetite, abnormal stools or other problems of elimination—continue despite your precautions, food allergy is a likely possibility. Stop using the new foods. If the problem clears up, reintroduce vegetables, grains, meats, dairy products, brewer's yeast and legumes one at a time until you find out which one is causing the problem. When you identify the culprit, eliminate it from the diet permanently. Foods commonly known to cause allergic reactions in pets are described along with a special diet in the "Allergies" section on page 229.

Cats sometimes find it harder to metabolize unsaturated oils than saturated ones (animal fats). Choosing olive oil as your cat's oil source and adding ample vitamin E to the diet should allay this problem. Or else stick to animal fats like lard, butter or meat trimmings and drippings.

HERBS TO EASE THE PROCESS

Should your pet have some moderate distress in changing to a fresh diet, you can smooth the way (or try to prevent problems from the start) with some herbs that help cleanse the body and rebuild tissue. Use only one herb, rather than a combination. Pick the one that best matches the problems listed in the brief descriptions below.

Alfalfa (*Medicago sativa*) is an excellent tonic that stimulates digestion and appetite. It helps animals gain weight and improves physical and mental vigor. Alfalfa is best used for animals that are underweight, nervous or high-strung. It can also help those with muscle or joint pains or animals with urinary problems—especially where there is crystal formation and bladder irritation. Depending on your pet's body size, add 1 teaspoon to 3 tablespoons of ground or dry-blended alfalfa to the daily ration. Or make a tea by steeping 1 to 2 tablespoons

of the herb in 1 cup of water for 20 minutes. Mix it with food or administer it orally with a bulb syringe (or turkey baster), using the dry amounts as guidelines to judge how much to give.

Burdock (*Arctium lappa*) cleanses the blood and helps the body detoxify. It's particularly good for easing skin disorders. Soak 1 teaspoon of the root in 1 cup of spring or distilled water in a glass or enamel pan for 5 hours. Then bring to a boil, remove from heat and let cool. Give ½ teaspoon to 2 tablespoons per day, depending on the animal's size.

Garlic (*Allium sativum*) helps to eliminate worms, strengthen digestion and beneficially stimulate the intestinal tract. Use it to promote intestinal health. It is also indicated for animals that have been on a high meat or fish diet, and those that tend to be overweight or suffer hip pain from arthritis or dysplasia. Include fresh grated garlic with each meal, using ½ to 3 cloves, depending on the animal's size.

Oats (*Avena sativa*) are also a tonic, particularly for the animal whose main weakness is in the nervous system, as in epilepsy, tremors, twitching and paralysis. Oats also counter the weakening and exhaustive effects of heavy drugging and diseases. They help to cleanse the body and nourish new tissue growth. Use oatmeal as the chief grain in the diet.

Also, you can use oat straw to provide a healing bath: Boil 1 to 2 pounds of the straw in 3 quarts of water for 30 minutes. Add this to the bathwater or sponge on repeatedly as an after-bath rinse by standing the animal in a tub and reusing the solution. Such treatment is useful for skin problems, muscle and joint pain, paralysis and liver and kidney problems.

One of these herbs along with the benefits of the new diet should make the road to good health smoother and shorter. After a month or two give your pet another exam, and I bet you'll see a difference.

Above all, don't be discouraged from trying a change of diet for your pet. Remember, most animals that switch to natural foods do not experience the problems I have described in this chapter. The majority enjoy the new diet and digest it well. And if you follow the advice here about easing the transition period, in all probability your pet will simply be happier and healthier than ever before.

CHAPTER SEVEN

EXERCISE, REST AND NATURAL GROOMING

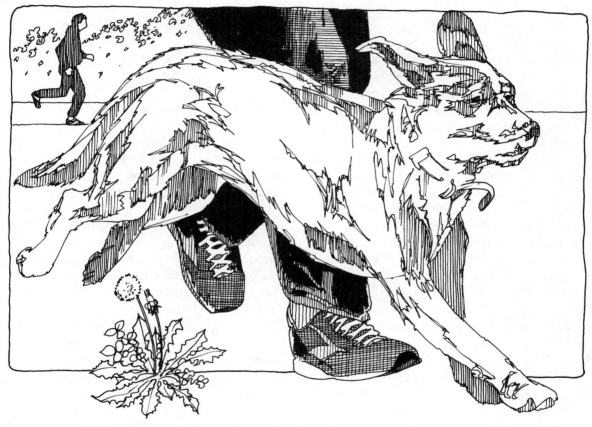

You can't expect to keep your car in top shape by merely filling the gas tank. You also have to change the oil, lube the joints, replace parts that wear and get an occasional tune-up. Without this kind of attention, even the best car eventually becomes a junker.

Certainly, animals can't be equated with machines. But, like machines, they need more than just the right fuel (food). Besides a healthy diet, animals need pure water, fresh air, sunlight, regular exercise, grooming, space of their own and much more.

So while good nutrition is essential for maintaining or improving your pet's health, you can't stop there. Many additional factors, both obvious and subtle, affect its well-being. What we must do is develop a broad view that allows us to see the many

89

diverse elements as a whole—a whole that can enhance your pet's life or threaten it.

Consider for a moment the difference between the lifestyle of our pets and the ways of their wild ancestors. For example, a typical city dog eats highly processed foods nearly all the time and never spends a fresh, sunny day investigating the path of a stream or running hard through sweetly scented woods on the trail of prey. Instead, she devotes most of her life to sleeping or pacing indoors on vinyl floors and carpets made from synthetic fibers. Her time "outdoors" is often spent in a stuffy parked car waiting while her owner does an errand.

She doesn't socialize much with her own kind, but does have an intense mutual attachment with one or more humans who often display complex and confusing emotions. But mostly the humans are at work or at school, and she is alone in the confines of an apartment, house or yard.

If she is lucky, every week or two she's treated to one of her great delights—a walk through the fields. But her fun is somewhat marred by painful foxtails that lodge easily in the abnormally long, curly hairs of her coat. When she gets home, she quenches her thirst with tap water that smells of chlorine. Sometimes, largely because of these conditions, she's a bit irritable and snappish or depressed and bored. But overall she's good-natured and takes each day as it comes.

Do our animal friends really have to lead lives lacking in so many basics? Let's examine an animal's real needs and see what we can do to meet them.

The circumstances that affect a pet's health are complex, of course, but we can understand them better if we remember one basic principle: The less we interfere with nature, the more life's processes flow healthfully. Not all of us are able to let our dogs run free in natural settings, even occasionally, but we can control many other important factors that affect the quality of a pet's life. Among these are exercise, grooming and exposure to environmental pollutants.

THE IMPORTANCE OF EXERCISE

For the wild cousins of domestic dogs and cats, regular exercise is an integral and necessary part of daily life. They *must* keep on the move because they *must* hunt for food. A walk to the food bowl is the only exercise many house pets ever get.

Yet regular exercise is essential for optimal health. Sustained, vigorous use of the muscles stimulates all tissues and increases circulation. Blood vessels dilate and blood pressure rises. As a result, tissues become oxygenated, which helps to clean the cells of toxins. Digestive glands secrete their fluids better and the bowels move more easily.

Join your pet in jogging, taking a walk, playing ball or chasing sticks and Frisbees. Nearly all dogs benefit from half an hour or more of daily vigorous exercise. If your pet is old and weak or has a bad heart, settle for slow walks around the block.

Cats, on the other hand, are not inclined to chase balls or jog, but they usually get enough exercise if they are allowed outside part of the time and have a suitable place to "scratch." The practice of removing their claws (which is equivalent to cutting off the last joint of each of your own fingers) is not only cruel and painful, but it also prevents

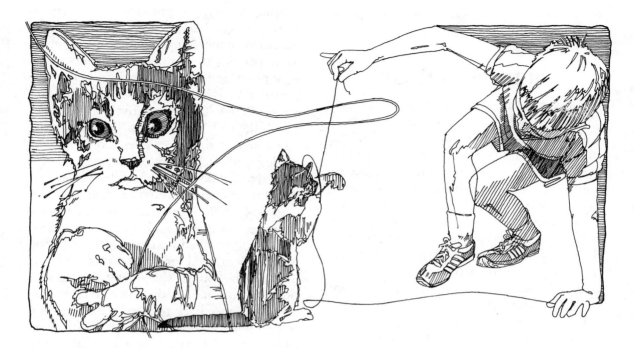

Thing-on-a-string, an irresistible game for cats, provides needed exercise for the "inside" pet.

the important feline exercise pattern of using the claws to knead and stretch—which benefits the muscles of the forelegs, backbone and shoulders. A cat that can't perform this ritual is likely to become weaker and thus more susceptible to illness and degeneration.

Most cats also love to play "thing-on-a-string," chasing and batting at a piece of string with a loop or mouse toy attached to one end. Pet stores sell many such toys for both cats and dogs. When playing games with a pet, however, do not use your bare hand as the "bait" or the object of teasing. This can teach your animal that it's all right to scratch or bite your hands, a lesson you will want him to "unlearn" in the future.

Make sure the toys you give your pet are safe for biting and chewing. Some of the best toys are those made of leather, rawhide and similar natural materials. Another word of caution: Don't leave your animal alone with a ball of yarn or string. Your pet might swallow some of the string or become dangerously entangled in it.

If your dog is temporarily unable to walk because of a sore foot or a partial paralysis, encourage him to swim in place in a bathtub, large trough, swimming pool or natural body of water to get exercise. Swimming strengthens the body in the same way running does. If your pet tends to sink, place a towel or cloth as a sling under the body for support. This exercise is especially good for dogs with back problems.

Quiet and Rest

Every creature needs a clean, quiet, private place to sleep and rest, a place where it will be warm in the winter and cool in the summer. Even if your pet sleeps in your bed some of the time, provide a suitable place or two of its own. A lot of animals—especially big dogs—are denied these havens. Many are left out in the elements, but unlike their wild cousins who have a cozy den to hide in, they must make do with a patch of dirt next to a noisy street or perhaps a drafty slab of cement beneath a porch roof. The difference is an important one.

Cats and smaller dogs are happy with a padded basket or even just a clean folded blanket or towel in a corner or on a chair. Large dogs don't necessarily require a bed such as a basket, but they do need some kind of secure, clean place that is comfortable in both winter and summer—such as a carpeted corner in a room or dog house, an old chair or a special rug of its own in a quiet spot.

Use natural fabrics and stuffings for the bedding, such as cotton, wool, feathers and kapok. Woven wool fleece, which resembles sheepskin, makes a warm, soft, washable natural cover for a pet to sleep on. Sold by the yard in many fabric stores, it provides the same healthy sleeping benefits as more costly sheepskin mattress pads sold for human use. Buy enough to cut two sheets a little larger than your pet's body. No sewing is needed. Pets love them and, besides, they look *so* cozy curled up on them!

Study your pet's preferences and try to provide several quiet sleeping spots, given the circumstances of your home and climate. Your pet might like one quiet, out-of-the-way place and another that's closer to the center of activity where it's easy to keep an eye on things. Cats instinctively gravitate to small, defined areas with a little elevation, which makes them feel safer. Commercially made window perches or carpeted shelves affixed to windows give cats a front-row seat on all their favorite shows on "cat TV" (see page 354). You might also consider carpeted cat houses on posts, sold at many pet stores.

Are you worried that your pet sleeps too much? It's normal for a pet that is left alone most of the day to sleep a lot during that time. But if your pet does not greet you on arrival or goes back to sleep soon after you come home, it could mean the pet's low on energy. This is especially true with dogs. Cats naturally sleep more than dogs and often take frequent naps throughout the day and night. My way of deciding if a cat sleeps too much is to learn if there are several active periods during the day and if the cat grooms himself several times a day. The healthy cat will alternate sleep with activity—looking out the window, going outside, exploring and grooming. If this activity is rare, there may be a problem.

Cleanliness Is Next to Healthfulness

A clean animal is a beautiful animal, and, more importantly, a healthy one. Every living organism is constantly breaking down and eliminating natural metabolic products and old cells. Ordinarily, about a third of the body's cells are dying at any one time. Each of these cells must be broken down and re-placed. In today's world, the body must work even harder to counteract the heavy load of synthetic chemicals in the air, soil, water and food chain.

These accumulated toxins, as well as external dirt and secretions, can encourage the growth of germs and parasites. They also sap general vitality by overburdening normal organ and glandular functions. A buildup of toxins may not cause a specific disease by itself, but it can make a pet more susceptible and set the stage for worse conditions—infectious disease, acute inflammation or gradual organ degeneration punctuated by occasional flare-ups. For ex-ample, an animal with chronically inflamed skin may de-velop a sudden moist eczema ("hot spots"); another may get an attack of nephritis (kid-ney inflammation) arising from a silent de-generation and loss of kidney tissue over years.

If you doubt that this load of toxins our pets face every day is a heavy one, take a closer look at some animals you know. Give them the checkup described in "How to Give Your Pet a Quick Checkup" on page 84. I see a lot of animals that show low-level signs of chronic excessive toxicity. Oily or smelly secretions on the skin, ears or eyes or deposits on the teeth are signs that the body is struggling to eliminate toxins.

Here are three natural ways you can as-sist the hard-working organs—the skin, liver, kidneys, digestive tract and lungs—that carry wastes out of your pet's body.

- Daily exercise stimulates waste removal through improved metabolism and cir-culation.

- An occasional day of fasting relieves the digestive tract of its usual duties and frees the organs to break down toxins stored in the liver, fats and other tissues. During a fast, the organs can also consume excess baggage, such as cysts, scars and growths. The process and the therapeutic uses of fasting are described more fully in chapter 15.
- Regular grooming not only removes dirt and secretions directly, but stimu-lates the skin's natural elimination pro-cesses as well. Let's take a closer look at this important aspect of pet care.

NATURAL GROOMING AND SKIN CARE

Nobody ever gives a wolf or a bobcat a bath and those animals seem to do just fine, so why should we have to groom our pets? For one thing, a wild animal moves from place to place, which means it can get away from a colony of parasites such as fleas. A pet, on the other hand, keeps getting rein-fested with these critters from the eggs dropped in its quarters.

Furthermore, a lot of domestic animals are bred to have abnormally long or curly or very fine hair, which can be too great a challenge for their limited self-grooming tools—tongue, paws and teeth. As a result, mats, stickers and dirt build up, predispos-ing the skin to irritation.

Also, dust and debris on your pet's fur can contain various toxic and unhealthful contaminants, such as lint from synthetic fibers, tiny flakes of paint or debris from au-tomobiles (including asbestos fibers from brake linings). Of course, it's better for the pet's health if you remove this debris from his coat than if the animal licks it off and swallows it. Because we humans have intervened in the natural order and changed the physical structure and environment of our animals, it's up to us to help care for the skin and coat of those pets that need it.

Long-haired pets need daily brushing with a special "slicker" pet brush made for picking up hair. Short-haired animals may need brushing less often. Another excellent tool for regular grooming is a flea comb (described below). Frequent brushing and combing stimulate hair and skin health, bringing normal secretions from oil glands onto the skin and discouraging fleas. It also keeps mats from building up and helps to remove stickers and other plant debris.

Make regular checks of the feet, ears, eyes and vagina or penis sheath to detect and remove foxtails and other plant stickers before they penetrate the skin's surface and cause harm, requiring removal by your veterinarian. If you live in a hot climate, it's also a good idea to have your dog's coat thinned by a professional groomer.

Bathing also plays a major role in pet grooming. It is one of the safest and most effective ways to control fleas, which are killed by the soap and water. But don't bathe your pets too often, because bathing can dry the skin. Unless your adult dog is unusually dirty, a bath every month or two is plenty. However, in the case of a bad flea infestation, skin problems or discharges, you may want to bathe the animal every week. If you do, be sure to use a gentle shampoo that will not strip all the natural oils from the hair.

Cats don't need frequent bathing since they generally do a good job of it by themselves. But if your cat has problems with bad skin or fleas, you can bathe it monthly; otherwise, once or twice a year is adequate.

Select a good-quality castile soap or a natural shampoo (see page 352). Don't use hair conditioners, sulphur-tar shampoos, shampoos containing dandruff suppressors or any other chemical medication. Avoid pet shampoos that contain synthetic insecticides unless the safer approaches described below have not been successful. If fleas are a problem, look for a natural pet shampoo containing flea- and insect-repellent herbs. Some contain d-limonene, a natural extract from citrus fruits that will kill fleas with minimal side-effects. Or you can make your own insect-repellent shampoo by adding a few drops of essential oil of pennyroyal or eucalyptus to a bottle of natural shampoo or castile soap. (Do not apply these oils directly to the skin. They are too irritating.)

Some pets resist bathing. If yours is one of these, be gentle and speak in soft, reassuring tones throughout the experience. Remove the collar and lower your pet into a laundry tub, bathtub or sink as you gradually fill it with comfortably lukewarm water. Wet and lather up your pet's neck first, to trap any fleas that might try to escape toward your pet's head. Shampoo the entire body and rinse lightly, using either a spray attachment or a container of lukewarm water. Then shampoo a second time, working the lather well into the skin and letting it stay on for five minutes or as long as your friend will allow. This assures the most complete treatment of fleas. Meanwhile, you can comb out and drown any critters making their way toward high ground.

Then rinse your animal thoroughly. It's nice to follow this plain-water rinse with a vinegar-water rinse (1 tablespoon white vinegar to 1 pint warm water). It removes soap residue and helps prevent dandruff. Pour on the solution, rubbing throughout the fur. Then rinse again with plain water.

At this point you might like to try this homemade herbal rinse.

ROSEMARY CONDITIONER

Rosemary tea, used by Anitra Frazier, author of The Natural Cat, *makes an excellent conditioner that promotes a glossy coat and helps to repel fleas.*

> 1 teaspoon dried rosemary (or 1 tablespoon fresh)
> 1 pint boiling water

Combine and steep for 10 minutes, covered. Strain and cool to body temperature. Pour it over your pet after the final rinse. Rub in and towel dry without further rinsing.

◆

When you're finished with the bath, use several towels to blot off excess water. Then let your pet do what comes naturally, shaking and licking off more of the water. Make sure she has a warm place to dry off.

For pets that just won't put up with water baths, try this simple dry shampoo.

Place ½ to 1 cup bran, oatmeal or cornmeal on a cookie sheet. Put the oven on low for 5 minutes to warm the grain. Removing a little at a time, so that the rest stays warm but not too hot, rub the grain into the fur with a towel. Concentrate on the greasy, dirty areas. Then brush these areas thoroughly to get the grain out.

Finally, here's a spot remover that will help you get rid of grease spots in your pet's fur between baths, especially those spots that cats get on their heads from prowling under cars. Rub a few drops of Murphy's Oil Soap and a small amount of warm water onto the greasy spots. Then rinse thoroughly with warm water.

FLEA CONTROL: BEYOND TOXIC CHEMICALS

Now we come to fleas, the bane of many a beast. Fortunately, there are safe alternatives to the toxic chemicals often used for controlling these pesky little creatures on your pet and in your home. And that's important, because the worst environmental pollutants that threaten pets are surely the poisons that well-meaning owners regularly dip, spray, powder, collar and shampoo directly onto and into their flea-bitten companions.

The labels of most flea products bear such odd cautions as "Avoid contact with skin." (I've never been able to figure out why it's all right to thoroughly drench a pet with something that's too nasty for humans to touch briefly and then wash off afterward. Skin is skin, after all.) In any case, animals and veterinary technicians alike are often poisoned from the application of insecticides and even from the "inert" ingredients in flea-control products, both of which are absorbed through the skin and by inhalation. In addition, pets may lick these compounds off while grooming, and we may pick them up while stroking our animals. Some flea collars and powders are so potent that they produce extreme skin irritations and permanent hair loss on pets.

The net effect of all this poisoning is to make the fleas stronger and ourselves weaker. Because fleas reproduce so rapidly, those that survive flea-control products are the ones that have developed resistance to insecticides. This is especially a problem in places like Florida, where warm winters facilitate year-round flea breeding.

It is a common observation among veterinarians that the animals in poorest health attract the most fleas. So the problem is not just the presence of fleas. It's that we have weakened our pets to the point where fleas can take advantage of them. Moreover, our excessive use of vaccines, antibiotics and cortisone-like drugs has created severe allergy problems so that many pets cannot tolerate fleas at all.

What's in all these flea-control products, anyway? Pet, house and garden products all contain one or more classes of insecticides, many of which are nerve poisons. "Common Ingredients in Flea-Control Products" on page 98 lists some of the more common pet insecticides, both synthetic and natural. Most of these, especially the organophosphates and carbamates, have caused poisonings as the result of misuse or overdose, particularly in young or sick animals and in cats. These symptoms are noted in the chart. However, I think that there are also more subtle delayed effects that we do not yet fully understand. For example, some studies show that organophosphates can cause permanent nerve damage to humans, including burning, tingling and weakness in the legs and arms starting 8 to 14 days after exposure.

Other dangerous chemicals sometimes found in pet products include: *sodium arsenite*, *boric acid*, *benzethonium chloride*, *napthalene* (used in mothballs), *oil of anise*, *para-cymene* (xylene), *pine tar* and *sodium cresylate*. Others considered less toxic but still dangerous include: *benzene hexacholoride*, *chloranil*, *DDD*, *dimethyl phthalate*, *depentene* and *menthols*.

SAFE, EFFECTIVE FLEA CONTROL

The best approach to controlling fleas is to start with the least toxic and most natural choices, resorting to stronger measures only if reasonable control is not achieved. As a prerequisite to any flea-control program, I recommend building up your animal's health and resistance as much as possible through a healthy diet and lifestyle. Along with that, it's important to practice thorough sanitation and cleaning.

Understanding the life cycle of the flea makes it clear why cleaning is so important. Adult fleas live about three to four months. During that time they are steadily laying tiny white eggs on your pet that look like dan-

---

Labels Reveal Lethal Levels

Individual labels are a guide to the product's relative danger. The terms below signify the ingested amount that would kill an adult human.

Label Term	Lethal Amount for Adults
Danger—Poison	Just a pinch
Warning	About a teaspoon
Caution	Two tablespoons to two cups
No label	Considered nontoxic

druff or salt crystals. Flea eggs hatch out into larvae that live in the cracks and crevices of rugs, upholstery, blankets, floors, sand, earth and the like.

Because these tiny larvae cannot jump or travel very far (less than an inch), they feed on the black specks of dried blood ("flea dirt") that fall off along with the eggs during grooming and scratching. After one to two weeks, the larvae go through a cocoon stage (pupa). A week or two later, they hatch out as small fleas that hop onto the nearest warm body passing by (usually your pet—sometimes you!), bite it for a meal of blood and then start the whole process all over again. This cycle takes anywhere from 2 to 20 weeks, depending on the temperature of the house or environment. During summer—flea season—the entire cycle is usually just 2 weeks long. That's why fleas increase so rapidly at that time.

The bad news is that, no matter how many adult fleas you manage to kill, numerous future fleas are developing in the environment simultaneously. The good news is that these eggs, larvae, pupa and the flea dirt they feed upon can be sucked up by a vacuum cleaner or washed away in the laundry. And because the developing fleas are so immobile, they are most concentrated wherever your pet sleeps, so you know where to focus your efforts.

Your important ally in the battle against fleas is cleanliness both for your pet and your home, particularly in your pet's sleeping areas. Regular cleaning interrupts the life cycles of the fleas and greatly cuts down on the number of adult fleas that end up on your pet, especially if you act before flea season begins. So start your program with these nontoxic steps.

Steam clean your carpets at the onset of flea season (or whenever you begin your flea-control program). Though it is somewhat expensive, steam cleaning is effective in killing flea eggs.

Thoroughly vacuum and clean floors and furniture at least once a week to pick up flea eggs, larvae and pupae. Concentrate on areas where your pet sleeps and use an attachment to reach into crevices and corners and under heavy furniture. If there is a heavy infestation, you may want to put a flea collar (or part of a flea collar) in the vacuum bag to kill any adult fleas that get sucked up and might crawl away. Or else immediately dispose of the bag or its contents because it can provide a warm, moist, food-filled environment for developing eggs and larvae. Mop vinyl floors.

Launder your pet's bedding in hot, soapy water at least once a week. Dry on maximum heat. Heat will kill all stages of flea life, including the eggs. Remember that flea eggs are very slippery and easily fall off bedding or blankets. So carefully roll bedclothes up to keep all the flea eggs contained on the way to the washing machine.

Bathe the animal with a natural flea-control shampoo. Use a nontoxic shampoo as recommended above, such as one containing d-limonene.

Use a flea comb to trap and kill fleas that are on your pet. Most pet stores carry special fine-toothed combs that trap fleas for easy disposal. Make a regular habit of flea-combing your pet while you watch TV or talk on the phone. Depending on the degree of infestation and the time of year, this might be daily (at the onset of the flea season), weekly or monthly.

Gently but thoroughly comb as many areas as your pet will allow, especially around *(continued on page 100)*

Common Ingredients in Flea-Control Products

Insecticides	Effects of Overdose and Possible Long-Term Effects
Organophosphates	
Chlorpyrifos, Cythioate, DDVP, Diazinon, Dichlorvos, Dursban, Endothion, Fenthion, Korlan, Malathion, Naled, Neguvon, Parathion, Phosmet, Propetamphos, Ronnel, Trichlorfon and Vapona.	*Initially:* salivation, involuntary defecation, urination, vomiting, wide stance. *Progresses to:* difficulty standing, weakness, convulsions, tremors, constricted pupils, teary eyes, slow heartbeat, labored breathing. May also cause dermatitis, aggravate heart and respiratory disease. Fenthion may cause chronic appetite and weight loss, depression, mild head and neck tremors. Vapona (DDVP, Dichlorvos), widely used since 1950s, may pose significant leukemia hazard.
Carbamates	
Aldicarb, Baygon, Bendiocarb, Bufencarb (BUX), Carbaryl, Carbofuran, Ficam, various Methylcarbamate compounds, Moban, Maneb, Propoxur, Sevin, Zectran, Zineb and Ziram.	*Initially:* salivation, involuntary defecation, urination, vomiting, wobbliness, wide stance. *Progresses to:* difficulty standing, weakness, convulsions, tremors, constricted pupils, teary eyes, slow heartbeat, labored breathing. Can cause depression of bone marrow, degeneration of the brain.
Organochlorines	
Dichlorophene, DMC, Endosulphan, Endrin, Heptachlor, Isobenzan, Lindane (Gamma BHC), Methoxy-chlor, Paradichlorobenzene, Toxaphene, TDE. Banned or restricted: DDT, DDE, Aldrin, Dieldrin and Chlordane.	Exaggerated responses to touch, light and sound. Spasms or tremors appear (usually first in the face), progressing to epilepsy-like seizures, often followed by death. No known antidote. Many members of this group have been shown to cause cancer in experimental animals. Because of concern about carcinogenic potential, Lindane was banned as an indoor fumigant in 1986.
Methoprene	Considered nontoxic, but usually combined with toxic chemicals to kill adult fleas.

Notes

Among the most common pet insecticides, found in all types of products. Some are used systemically (kill fleas through pet's blood). Can be extremely toxic. Considered responsible for most pet poisonings. Most are readily absorbed through the skin, eyes, stomach and lungs. Act by decreasing cholinesterase activity, which sends nerve signals, in effect paralyzing the nerves. Being studied for delayed neurotoxic effects. Fenthion and Cythioate should not be used for cats, puppies or sick dogs. Malathion and Ronnel are among the least toxic in this group.

Based on carbamic acid, found in all types of pet products. Like organophosphates, toxic effect is immediate, but carbamates are generally less severe. Sevin and Carbaryl do not accumulate in tissues and are said to be much less toxic than, for example, Parathion.

Less immediately toxic than the above, which have largely replaced them. But they accumulate in tissues and persist for years in the environment (e.g., DDT was banned in 1972, but it's still found in 55% of Americans). Insects have developed resistance to many. Cats are particularly vulnerable to this group, especially to Lindane, DDT and Chlordane. Dogs are susceptible to Toxaphene and DDE.

A growth regulator used in foggers or commercial sprays to inhibit fleas from hatching from the pupal stage. Only effective indoors.

(continued)

Common Ingredients in Flea-Control Products — Continued

Insecticides	Effects of Overdose and Possible Long-Term Effects
Rotenone and other cube resins	Skin irritation. Overdose can cause death through paralysis of respiration. Chronic exposure may injure liver and kidneys.
D-Limonene	Toxic signs in cats: excess salivation, weakness, muscle tremors. No toxic effects reported in dogs.
Natural Pyrethrins and Synthetic Pyrethroids Allethrin, Resmethrin and Permethrin.	Can cause allergic dermatitis and systemic allergic reactions. Large amounts may cause nausea, vomiting, ringing in the ears, headaches and other central nervous system disturbances, but rapidly detoxified in the intestines. Prolonged use may cause slight liver damage. Permethrin may be a slight carcinogen (according to mice studies).
Arecoline Hydrobromide	Vomiting, unconsciousness, diarrhea and depression. Though natural, it must be considered a potentially toxic substance.
Benzyl Benzoate	Nausea, vomiting, diarrhea and a slowing of the heartbeat and breathing rate.
Piperonyl Butoxide, N-octylbicycloheptene dicarosimide E	Large doses cause vomiting and diarrhea.
Boric acid derivatives (Fleabusters Rx for Fleas)	Ingestion may cause nausea, vomiting, diarrhea, rash, dizziness.
Microencapsulation Process	Reduces toxicity of insecticides to pets and people because the tiny capsules pass through intestines before all their contents are absorbed.

the head, neck, back and hindquarters. As you trap the little buggers, pull them off the comb and plunge them into a container of hot, soapy water (or dip the comb and pull the flea off underwater). Cover your lap with an old towel to catch extra clumps of hair and flea dirt and to wipe the comb off as you work.

Notes

Derived from a poisonous tropical legume. Considered fairly toxic to mammals. Loses much potency in presence of light and oxygen; has little residual action. Slower-acting, but more potent than Pyrethrin. Found in shampoos, dips and powders.

Natural citrus extract. Dissolves flea's waxy coating, causing dehydration and death. Kills 99% of fleas if shampoo lather left on for ten minutes.

Labeled nontoxic. Considered least toxic to mammals of all insecticides. Derived from chrysanthemums. Mostly in aerosol sprays, sometimes in flea shampoos and sprays. Causes rapid paralysis of insect nervous system (many die, but many also recover in a few hours, so repeat applications are necessary). Synergists may be added to inhibit flea's detoxification process and increase residual effect.

The active compound found in the areca nut, an Oriental folk remedy for worms, it has long been used in tapeworm control. Considered unsafe for cats. Can cause undesirable responses in dogs also.

Often used for mange control. Can be toxic if applied over too large an area or too often. Cats more susceptible, but dogs occasionally die from excessive use.

Not true insecticides. Added to other ingredients to block flea's detoxification process and increase effectiveness.

Mineral salts applied to carpets to kill developing fleas. Low toxicity. Reported to be very effective for up to a year.

Use of thin nylon or urea shell around minute bits of insecticide, used for sustained release and longer action. Less effective if used with flea repellents.

When you're finished flush the soapy water and fleas down the toilet.

If your pet goes outdoors, follow these steps as well.

Mow and water your lawn regularly. Short grass allows sunlight to penetrate and warm the soil, which kills larvae. Watering drowns the developing fleas.

Encourage ants. Perhaps I should say "do not discourage ants." They love to eat flea eggs and larvae. This is another reason not to use pesticides that kill all the insects in your yard.

"Sterilize" bare earth sleeping spots. If your pet likes to sleep or hang out in a certain bare or sandy area, occasionally cover the spot with a heavy black plastic sheet on a hot, sunny day. Rake up any dead leaves and other debris first. The heat that builds up under the plastic does an excellent job of killing fleas and larvae. Of course, this is not appropriate to use where you want to preserve live grass or plants.

Apply agricultural lime on grassy or moist areas. This helps to dry out the fleas. Rake up any dead leaves and grassy debris first.

Along with the above steps, you might try these methods to repel fleas that may try to jump back on your pet, especially those harder-to-kill ones hanging out in the back-yard.

Use an herbal flea powder. You'll find them in pet stores and natural food stores, or you can make your own. Combine one part each of as many of these powdered herbs as you can find: eucalyptus, rosemary, fennel, yellow dock, wormwood and rue. Put this mixture in a shaker-top jar, such as a jar for parsley flakes.

Apply the flea powder sparingly to your pet's coat by brushing backward with your hand or the comb and sprinkling it into the base of the hairs, especially on the neck, back and belly. To combat severe infestations, use several times a week. Afterward, put your animal friend outside for a while so the disgruntled tenants vacate in the yard and not in your house. Some herbal flea powders also contain natural pyrethrins, which are not strong flea-killers but do seem to greatly discourage them.

Use an herbal flea collar. These are impregnated with insect-repellent herbal oils. Some are made to be "recharged" with the oils and used again. Buy them at natural food stores.

Try a natural skin tonic. The animal herbalist Juliette de Bairacli-Levy recommends this lemon skin tonic, which many of my clients successfully use on their pets for a general skin toner, parasite repellent and treatment for mange.

Thinly slice a whole lemon, including the peel. Add it to 1 pint of near-boiling water and let it steep overnight. The next day, sponge the solution onto the animal's skin and let it dry. You can use this daily for severe skin problems involving fleas. It is a source of natural flea-killing substances like d-limonene and other healing ingredients found in the whole lemon.

Add ample nutritional or brewer's yeast and garlic to the diet. Some studies show yeast supplementation significantly reduces flea numbers, though others indicate no effect. My experience with using yeast is that it has some favorable effect, particularly if the animal's health is good. You can also rub it directly into the animal's hair. Many people also praise the value of garlic as a flea repellent, though so far studies do not support this.

If these methods do not control the fleas sufficiently, take the following steps.

Get your carpets treated with a special anti-flea mineral salt. There have been some developments in safe flea control. My clients report success with some companies that apply or sell relatively nontoxic mineral salts for treating carpets. (Fleabusters and Radar Rex are two of the companies recommended.) Effective for up to a year, the products safely kill fleas and their developing forms over a few week's time.

Once or twice a year, sprinkle natural, unrefined diatomaceous earth along walls, under furniture and in cracks and crevices that you cannot access with a vacuum. This product, which resembles chalky rock, is really the fossilized remains of one-celled algae. Though direct contact is harmless to pets and people, it is bad news for many insects and their larvae, including fleas. The fine particles in the earth kill insects by attacking the waxy coating that covers their external skeletons. The insects then dry out and die.

I do not recommend using diatomaceous earth frequently or directly on your animal—mostly because of the irritating dust that can be breathed in by both of you. It also is messy. Be careful about breathing it in. Wear a dust mask when applying. It is not toxic, but inhaling even the natural, unrefined form of this dust can irritate the nasal passages.

Important: Do not use the type of diatomaceous earth that is sold for swimming pool filters. It has been ground very finely, and the tiny particles can be breathed into the lungs and cause chronic inflammation.

Use a spray or powder containing pyrethrins or natural pyrethrum. These are the least toxic of all the insecticides used on pets, and they are found in both conventional and natural flea-control products. For a more lasting effect use a microencapsulated product, perhaps labeled "slow release." Repeat the applications as you simultaneously use the carpet treatment system or diatomaceous earth. This will help kill both adult fleas and developing fleas at the same time.

For more information concerning both external and internal parasites, as well as skin problems in general, see "Skin Parasites" on page 299, "Worms" on page 330 and "Skin Problems" on page 303.

CHAPTER EIGHT

CREATING A HEALTHIER ENVIRONMENT

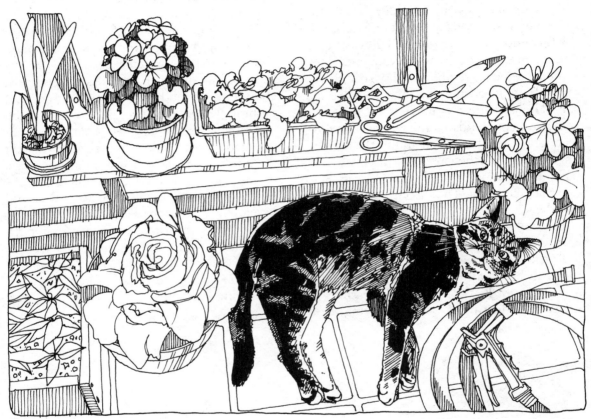

My husband and I are blessed with a good-size back yard, filled with many beautiful flowering shrubs and perennials, along with a small fish pond occasionally visited by a blue heron. Caring for this lovely spot often fills the better part of a weekend. We enjoy it, of course, or we wouldn't do it.

Yet somehow we get so busy snipping off branches, pulling up weeds or planting an-nuals that we tend to lose touch with the slower pace of life's mysteries constantly unfolding before us. When we get too wrapped up in our activity, it helps to take a lesson from our cat. Like all cats, he's quite adept at just sitting and looking.

Today was one of those times. Putting aside my projects, I (Susan) went out to the yard to just sit and look. Settling down in an out-of-the-way spot under a wisteria, I gazed down a seldom-used path. It was teeming with ants among the small, leafy weeds that thrive in shady places that are hard to hoe.

At first a glimmer of gardener thoughts passed through my mind. Were these carpenter ants? Should I destroy them so they don't destroy our home? Should I pull up some of those weeds before they go to seed? But, letting these thoughts pass on by, I calmed down and returned to just looking.

No longer filtering the scene through gardener eyes, I began to see more deeply. The weeds had a beauty of their own, as lush and diverse as a forest floor. Even the ants were admirable, so energetic and so enduring. They had crawled over this land long before we humans appeared. And despite all the wars we wage upon them, ants still thrive and will probably outlive us. It felt good to just let them be.

I felt humbled at how little I understood about the thousands of backyard plants and animals whose lives were affected by my actions.

A small moment. But without such moments in our busy lives we might gradually detach ourselves from nature and unwittingly accept the idea that we are free to tamper with the web of life.

With each passing year we humans dump innumerable tons of toxins into the web of life, destroy millions of forest acres and hasten the extinction of many species, some that we don't even know about! We further weaken the thin layer of ozone that protects us from the sun's radiation. We jam the airwaves with millions of electronic signals whose effects on our bioelectric fields we barely understand. Surely, we wouldn't tolerate these actions if we realized how profoundly they affect the fate of every living thing, including ourselves, our children and our animals.

A shocking national survey by the Public Health Service showed that Americans have hundreds of toxic chemicals stored in our fatty tissues. Nearly all of us have such harmful substances as dioxin, benzene, styrene and ethyl phenol. A significant majority have PCBs, radioactive isotopes, creosote, lead and other heavy metals, asbestos and numerous pesticides.

Surely, these are also contained in the bodies of our pets, perhaps in greater proportions because of their smaller sizes.

DIRT IS DIRTIER NOW

In evaluating the special impact of chemical pollution on our pets, it's essential to realize that dogs and cats live in close contact with the ground. They sit, play and sleep on it. Even indoors, pets are exposed to plenty of dust. A six-room urban house may accumulate as much as 40 pounds of dust in a year. And when our pets lick all this dust off their fur, they actually consume it. That used to be fairly safe—"you'll eat a peck of dirt before you die," moms used to say. But dirt is a lot "dirtier" nowadays. We need to take special precautions to protect children and pets from possible harm.

A scientific team of "dust busters" found that 25 out of 29 typical homes they studied in Seattle had rugs with excessive levels of toxins and mutagens. They also found that toddlers ingest more than twice as much dust as adults. And contaminated dust is probably more risky for pets than it is for children. Pets wear no protective clothes or

How to Protect Your Pet from Environmental Pollution: A Checklist of *Do's* and *Don'ts*

Do

- Brush and bathe your animal frequently to remove toxic particles from its fur.
- Use natural and least toxic methods of flea control instead of dangerous insecticides.
- Feed a fresh diet featuring organic foods whenever possible.
- Reduce pollutants by using low-meat recipes and minimizing liver, tuna and animal fats in the diet.
- Include these pollution protectors in the diet: Vitamins A, E and C, calcium and zinc.
- Use a water filter or bottled water for your pet's (and your own) drinking water. Change the water daily and keep the bowl away from dusty areas.
- Use natural fibers for pet bedding (organic cotton, wool, kapok and so forth).
- Vacuum and dust frequently.
- Remove shoes at the door, especially in homes that are near dusty industrial, high-traffic or farm areas.

- Avoid shag and deep-pile rugs; if you already have them, vacuum and steam clean often.
- Ventilate your house well to reduce indoor air pollution.
- Let your pet outdoors in moderation or provide sunny, open windows with screens; otherwise, purchase a full-spectrum light for the animal's usual daytime rest area.
- Close your windows and keep your pet inside on smoggy days or when pesticides are being sprayed nearby. Use air filters if you live in a polluted area.
- Reduce indoor air pollution by removing outdated and unwanted toxic chemicals and store others in ventilated areas away from pets and living space. Use nontoxic alternative products.
- Grow houseplants that filter the air, such as philodendrons, spider plants, aloe vera, chrysanthemums and gerbera daisies.
- Keep pets from chewing on poisonous plants and their fruits.

---

shoes and, like a shag rug, their fur attracts dirt (till they lick it off).

Because they settle to the ground, heavy metals are a particular hazard in dust. Lead is among the most widespread of these. It enters the environment from flaking layers of lead-based paint, auto exhaust, lead water pipes, batteries, colored newsprint and smelters. At typical levels lead primarily affects the blood and nervous systems. Symptoms can be vague, often including listlessness, loss of appetite, irritability, stupor, incoordination, vomiting, constipation and abdominal pain. Not surprisingly, lead poisoning has caused epileptic-like seizures in small urban dogs. Other dangerous metals polluting the environment include cadmium, mercury and arsenic.

Asbestos is another common ingredient in urban dust, with particles found in the lungs of virtually every city dweller who had an autopsy. It comes from brake lin-

- Guard against pets encountering solvents, paints, drugs, other chemicals and the dust from remodeling projects.
- Test your home and take recommended actions if radon gas is a risk in your area.
- Consider using a negative ion generator if you live in a large building with central heating ducts, a heavily paved city or in an area often subject to hot, dry winds or smog.

Don't

- Pet your animal with dirty hands.
- Confine your pet to a garage, basement or shed that contains household chemicals or lacks natural light.
- Keep your pet outside if you live by a busy roadway.
- Exercise your pet on smoggy days or along busy streets.
- Carry your pet in the back of a pickup truck.

- Allow your pet to roam near a toxic dump, old landfill or industrial/commercial area.
- Let your pet drink from or play in puddles or other contaminated waters.
- Apply or dump anything in your yard that you would not want to enter the water, food or air you consume—motor oil or paint, for example.
- Allow smoking inside your home.
- Let your pet sleep near or under house foundations that may have been treated with poison for termites.
- Use pesticides unless absolutely necessary.
- Let your pet sleep on or near an operating TV, microwave, computer monitor, electric blanket or heater, clock-radio or plug-in electric clock.
- Use medical x-rays unless needed.
- Overexpose your animal to the sun, especially if you live in an ozone-depleted area.

ings, ceilings, insulation, floor tiles, cement, shingles, paints and fabrics. Though commonly linked with lung cancer, asbestos can affect many body organs.

So what's a caring owner to do? Here are some simple suggestions supported by the Seattle study.

- Use entrance mats and remove or clean shoes at the front door.
- Houseclean thoroughly and often.

- Keep the entryway swept or hosed off to minimize sources of outdoor dirt. If possible, pave dirt or gravel driveways or entryways.
- Avoid shags and deep-pile carpets when you decorate. Consider a natural wood or tile floor with washable rugs instead.
- Brush and bathe your pet regularly.

Follow these suggestions when remodeling or repainting.

◆ Be especially careful about sanding or cutting into paint layers of homes built before 1960, because most of them contain lead paints. (Home test kits can confirm its presence.)

◆ Wear a dust mask while working on painted areas and keep pets and children away.

◆ Clean up thoroughly after each workday.

◆ If intact, old lead paint layers can be painted over or covered with drywall. Consider replacing old wood doors and windows because just operating them can create lead dust.

◆ Wipe the work area frequently with a solution of trisodium phosphate (sold at hardware stores). Be sure to wear gloves.

INDOOR AIR POLLUTION

Besides toxic dust, air can also carry unhealthy gases and vapors, such as formaldehyde, ozone, chloroform, radon and many more. These waft into the atmosphere from household products, furniture and many other common sources. A New Jersey study testing 20 common air pollutants showed that indoor levels were actually much worse than outdoor levels, in some cases a hundred times greater!

Reactions to indoor air pollution may show up as chronic headaches, fatigue, itchy or watering eyes, nasal or throat infections or dryness, depression, dizziness, nausea, colds, asthma, bronchitis and allergies. If any of these show up in your pets or family members who are usually indoors, note whether the symptoms have appeared after moving, remodeling or purchasing new furniture or carpets. Are the symptoms worse when the house is tightly sealed? If so, it makes sense to set about reducing the indoor pollution in your home. In any case, it's good preventive medicine for the whole family *and* your pets to take these steps.

Ventilate your home. If you're in an area of low air pollution, just open your windows as often as possible to ventilate. If outdoor air is smoggy or temperatures are too extreme, on the other hand, try using an electronic fiber or charcoal air filter. Further, scientists have learned that certain houseplants reduce pollutants, especially philodendrons (formaldehyde, benzene and carbon monoxide), spider plants (carbon monoxide), aloe veras (formaldehyde) and gerbera daisies and chrysanthemums (benzene).

Remove pollutants. Inventory all the household products tucked away in your kitchen, bathroom, laundry and garage that contain poisonous and sensitizing chemicals. Clear out any products that are more than a few years old and that you no longer use (they may contain chemicals that have since been banned), and those with rusting or leaking containers. Safer substitutes may be available.

Cats are particularly sensitive to phenols, which are contained in many disinfectants. Several books listed in "Recommended Reading and Tapes" on page 357 can point you to nontoxic cosmetics, cleansers, polishes, paints and home care products that are now available, or even show you how to make your own. For disposal call your local government to ask about special household hazardous waste collections. If there are none, tighten any loose containers, wrap them in several layers of newspaper, seal them in a heavy plastic bag and put them in the trash. Do *not* pour such substances down the drain or on the soil.

For those products you keep, tighten lids and update fading labels. If possible, store them in a well-ventilated area away from living space. Fumes can come out of even well-sealed containers, so don't confine your pet in the same space—a garage, for example.

Make sure that all gas, oil or wood furnaces and appliances are properly serviced and ventilated. This reduces levels of carbon monoxide and other combustion by-products. Seal boiler rooms from the rest of the house. When you replace units, buy electric models or choose gas furnaces with sealed combustion chambers and pilotless gas appliances.

Check for radon. This odorless radioactive gas may be responsible for up to 30,000 cancer deaths a year, particularly lung cancer. Produced by the natural decay of radium in underlying soil and rocks, radon enters the home from the foundation or from well water; then it gets trapped in the sealed air of the house, especially in wintertime. Call your state health department or regional office of the Environmental Protection Agency to find out if you live in a radon "hot spot." Inexpensive activated charcoal screening tests ($10 to $25), available through the mail, can help you find out if you should take further action. For an updated list of approved testing companies, write: EPA Office of Radiation Programs, Washington, DC 20460.

Be alert to toxic emissions from building materials and furnishings. One of the worst offenders is formaldehyde, which irritates the eyes and respiratory system and may even cause cancer. It is found in foam wall insulation, carpeting, upholstery, vinyl flooring, imitation wood paneling and furniture, plus many more items. If family members or pets have eye problems or respiratory problems and you live in a modern home built with many synthetic materials, consider moving to an older home with hardwood floors, original cabinets and no foam insulation.

Avoid preservative-treated timbers when building pens or other structures for pets. One of my clients traced behavioral and health problems of her cats to a new enclosure built with such wood. After she sealed the wood to prevent the fumes from reaching the animals, the cats returned to normal.

HOUSE AND GARDEN PESTICIDES

Besides the insecticides used in flea and tick products, pets may also be exposed to high levels of other household pesticides. The National Academy of Sciences reports that homeowners use four to eight times as many chemical pesticides per acre as farmers do. Many home and garden insecticides are the same as those used on pets. Additional risks come from herbicides, fungicides and rodent poisons. Because of their contact with the ground, pets are more likely to pick up residues. The National Cancer Institute found in 1991 that dogs whose owners used 2,4-D, a common broadleaf weed killer, had twice the rate of lymphoma (a cancer of the immune system) as dogs whose owners did not use it.

Even if you don't use pesticides, they may drift onto your property from neighbors' yards or from heavily sprayed areas such as nearby parks, campuses, power line corridors and orchards. Ask people to call you when they plan to spray so you can close your windows, since pesticides have a longer life indoors.

Also, poisonous residues may persist in your house from previous occupants. For instance, the termite insecticide chlordane has been detected in the air of some homes 14 years after application. It has been found in soil after 30 years.

"Recommended Reading and Tapes" on page 357 lists several excellent books that detail safer alternatives to dangerous pesticides and other household products and materials. If you must use a lawn or household pesticide, seek out a knowledgeable nursery salesperson to help you choose the least-toxic products. Some products, such as the herbicide glysophate, seem to be relatively harmless to animals if used as recommended. There are also non-toxic and organic products available. Follow label directions carefully, which often means keeping pets off areas that have been recently treated. Should you suspect a possible poisoning, call the National Pesticide Telecommunications Network, a toll-free service available 24 hours a day at 1-800-858-7378.

PET POISONINGS

A lot of the chemicals that are bad for pets, including pesticides, enter through an eager mouth attached to a curious nose. Poisonings account for 1 to 2 percent of veterinary cases, with a greater risk for dogs.

A prime danger is antifreeze poisoning, which causes vomiting, nervousness and coma, then death. Both cats and dogs may lap up spilled or uncovered antifreeze (which has a sweetish taste because of its chemical makeup) or lick it off their fur. Another risk is the consumption—usually by dogs—of poisons put out for snails, slugs and rodents. Cats sometimes eat a poisoned mouse.

Mischievous pets can get into all sorts of trouble. So keep the following out of reach of mouths and paws: automotive products, cleansers, cosmetics, art and photo supplies, solvents, pesticides, paints, disinfectants, medicines and, last but not least, spoiled garbage—a common source of pet poisoning.

Though it is rare, small animals have also been poisoned by eating parts of certain plants, including oleander, castor bean, dumb cane (dieffenbachia), chokecherry, jimsonweed, morning glory and others. Provide your pet with fresh greens such as sprouts, parsley or spinach to cut the temptation to nibble on toxic plants.

TOXIC CHEMICALS IN FOOD

Animals can develop subtler forms of poisoning just from eating what they're supposed to eat—their food! One survey showed that canned pet foods contain high amounts of lead, from 0.9 to 7.0 parts per million (ppm). A daily intake of six ounces of these foods (about what a cat or small dog eats) could give as much as *four times* the amount of lead considered potentially toxic for children.

Pet foods containing fish and fish by-products may contain high levels of mercury, a risk for cats addicted to seafood. Excessive mercury intake can damage the nervous system, causing tremors, irritability, anxiety, loss of appetite, lack of response and difficulty sleeping. It can also damage the kidneys.

Commonly added to public water supplies to prevent tooth decay, fluoride is considered safe at the level of 4 ppm in water or a maximum of 2.5 milligrams daily for children. But because of its accumulation in the food chain, 11 to 193 ppm have been found in leading pet foods (canned foods are worst). That means that a large dog could be consuming a whopping 21 to 368 milligrams daily.

Excessive exposure to fluoride may cause tiredness, mottling of the teeth, kidney and bladder disorders, arthritis, pain and crippling in the joints, stomach problems, hair loss, skin disorders, bronchitis, asthma and numerous other conditions. It can also reduce blood vitamin-C levels, weaken the immune system and cause birth defects and genetic damage. Ten European countries have banned fluoridation of water.

Hundreds of other toxic chemicals accumulate in the food chain, and it is very difficult to protect yourself and your pets from such unseen dangers. You *can*, however, reduce the risks by feeding a fresh, unprocessed diet that contains relatively little meat, especially liver and kidneys, which concentrate toxins. Many contaminants are stored in fats, so it's better to go with low-fat dairy products or lean meats. Corn oil is preferable to either soy or cottonseed oil because it's generally lower in pesticide content. When possible and practical, use organically grown foods.

You can also help your pet cope with pollutants by including certain vitamins and minerals in the diet. Calcium, for instance, helps protect against some heavy metals and radiation. Vitamin A and selenium also help combat radiation. Vitamin E counters the effects of many smog pollutants, and kelp helps the body resist radioactive strontium. Lecithin is also useful. These nutrients are included in our recommended diet.

If you live in a particularly polluted area, give your pet vitamin C (for pollutants in general and especially for cadmium, lead, copper and DDT) and zinc (for cadmium, lead and copper). Depending on your pet's size, use 100 to 500 milligrams of vitamin C and 5 to 20 milligrams of zinc. (For these vitamins, you can use regular supplements intended for human use.)

CLEANING UP THE WATER

Fluoride is only one of the questionable ingredients in many public water supplies. All told, more than 2,100 toxic chemicals have been detected in U.S. water. Some of the most common contaminants are: lead, cadmium, arsenic, insecticides, nitrates, fungicides, herbicides, benzene, toluene and dioxin. Many of these pollutants are known to cause cancer or damage the kidneys, liver, brain and cardiovascular system. Communities with particularly polluted sources of water have unusually high cancer rates of the gastrointestinal and urinary organs. In spite of these hazards, most utilities test for less than 30 chemicals and only a tiny fraction use modern technologies to remove them. That's because most treatment plants were built decades ago simply to kill bacteria and reduce sediment. Though it has served well as a disinfectant, the chlorine added to most municipal water also combines with organic debris to create a number of carcinogenic compounds, such as chloroform. Also, chlorine itself can be irritating to the mucous membranes of the eyes, nose, throat, airways and lungs, especially in sensitive individuals. As a result, lifetime users of chlorinated water have an increased rate of bladder cancer and possibly of colon and rectal cancers. Scientists are currently investigating alternative means of disinfecting water.

Since pure water is so important for your family, including your pets, we strongly recommend use of a good quality water purifier. Though initially costlier than bottled water, it is much cheaper in the long run, costing only pennies a gallon. Take your time to select a good-quality purifier that will do the job well. *Nontoxic, Natural and Earthwise*, by Debra Lynn Dadd, has an excellent discussion of the topic.

Also, change your pet's water daily. Keep the bowl clean and in a place protected from dust and debris. Most of all, make it available, so that your pet will not be as tempted to drink from a contaminated puddle, creek or pond. One woman living near a New York landfill (estimated to contain as much as a ton of dioxin) saw six of her cats die a few days after they visited the local stream.

ELECTROMAGNETIC EFFECTS ON HEALTH

Let's look now at some less familiar but potentially important environmental influences on health. All plants and animals operate by tiny electrochemical pulses that beat at about the same rate as the low frequency energy field of the Earth. Similarly, life has adapted over eons to a spectrum of other natural electromagnetic energies—light from the sun, background radioactivity from the Earth's crust and charged air molecules (positive and negative ions). In just a few decades, however, we have blanketed ourselves with an electronic smog of new frequencies created by our house wiring, power lines and appliances—radio, TV, microwave, beeper and cellular phone broadcasts—and radioactive nuclear blasts and leakages. Unknowingly, we have initiated a dangerous thinning of the ozone layer that shields us from destructive levels of ultraviolet radiation. And at the same time, we have retreated to a more indoor lifestyle, with reduced exposure to beneficial levels of sunlight and ionized air.

How do all these changes affect us? We aren't sure. But we are convinced there is cause for concern. For example:

- Studies show increased childhood leukemia and brain cancer in those living near high-tension power lines, which emit large fields of Extremely Low Frequency (ELF) energies. Also generated by house wiring and appliances, ELFs can trigger high blood pressure, nervousness, allergies and impaired sleep. They alter the heartbeats, blood chemistry and behaviors of lab animals.
- Proximity to video display terminals on computers is connected to miscarriages among female workers.
- Lab studies tie microwave exposure to fatigue, headaches, cataracts, tumors, birth defects and changes in blood cells, hormones and signals to the heart.
- The increased ultraviolet radiation from the thinning ozone layer is blamed for

doubling the world-wide rate of melanoma, a deadly form of skin cancer.

◆ Lab animals raised indoors under pink lights had smaller litters and developed behavioral problems, calcium deposits in the heart and increased tumor rates, plus inflammation and dead tissue on the skin of their tails. Ordinary incandescent light bulbs have more pink rays in them than natural sunlight—a potential hazard for housebound pets.

◆ Many people become depressed, tired and prone to gain weight when deprived of sunlight in winter. Full-spectrum lights provide relief for many who suffer from this Seasonal Affective Disorder (SAD).

◆ Urban dwellers and their pets often experience depleted levels of negative ions in favor of positive ions. This phenomenon can be traced to such factors as paving, smog, synthetic fabrics and building ductwork. Shortages and imbalances of ions can trigger insomnia, anxiety, depression, headaches, dizziness, tremors and heart palpitations. Lab animals deprived of all ions died young.

TAKING ACTION

Determining whether any of these environmental hazards are causing chronic health problems for your pet takes some careful detective work. Think about when the problem began and when it's better or worse. Consider any potential hazards in your home, neighborhood or region that may be linked with your pet's symptoms. Test kits and environmental consultants may help you pinpoint dangerous conditions (which may threaten your whole family) and lead you to take corrective actions.

Meanwhile, the best medicine is prevention. Do what you can to follow the "Do's" and "Don'ts" on page 106.

Environmental pollution and disturbances are a fact of modern life. Perhaps we will adapt to many of them eventually. Meanwhile, it's wise to use the many sensible ways available to make our homes healthier for both our pets and ourselves. Along the way, we can take a lesson from the animals. They can teach us how to feel our connection with nature and do what we can to care for our larger home, the Earth.

CHAPTER NINE

CHOOSING A HEALTHY ANIMAL

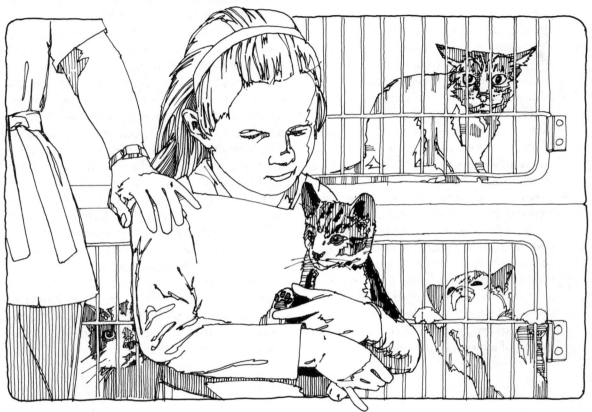

Selecting a pet with good genetic characteristics is one of the most important steps you can take to increase the chances that your animal will have a healthy, happy life. For one thing, that means overriding the temptation to decide on a particular breed just because you like its looks—or to pick out the most pitiful-looking pup in the litter because it elicits your sympathy. But it's not quite as simple as picking out the liveliest, friendliest and the most inquisitive one you find either.

Every type of dog or cat (pure or mixed breed) has physical characteristics—face, build, relative body proportions—that invite predictions about its potential well-being. Different breed types also have different behavioral tendencies. In this chapter you'll learn more about these indicators and how to use them to pick a quality animal. If you plan to breed a dog or cat, you'll also learn how to help prevent congenital problems and birth defects.

My work as a veterinarian has often led me to ponder these issues. For instance, one day someone brought in a lost miniature poodle to a clinic where I used to work. The poor dog was covered from head to foot with burrs, foxtails and tangled hair. One eye was closed and discharging pus, and the areas between his toes were red and swollen. Clearly, he was a victim of the "foxtail season."

Foxtails, or plant awns, are those stickery little things that attach to your socks when you walk across a field. They latch onto dogs, too. And because of their pointed ends, these burrs work their way not only into the coat but sometimes right through the skin, burrowing also into the eyes, ears, nose, mouth, vagina, rectum and between the toes.

Because our patient was so badly affected, we had to give him a general anesthetic before beginning the long process of removing the stickers. First we pulled and clipped the burrs out of his coat; then we worked them from between his toes. While my assistant, Dottie, attended to the feet, I found and removed two or three foxtails from deep in the ear canal. Careful examination revealed another lodged in the eye—the cause of the inflammation and discharge.

As we worked, Dottie and I began talking about how pets get into such a state after even a short trek in the fields.

"Here is the cause of the problem," I said, holding up some of the matted hair we had clipped off. "An animal with this kind of curly coat is like walking Velcro. Once the stickers brush against it, there's almost no place else for them to go but deeper in."

I pondered the matter for a moment. "You know," I went on, "people have unwittingly created this type of problem by deliberately breeding dogs to have such hair as well as floppy ears like these. Both are perfect traps for foxtails. Wild animals don't have anywhere near this difficulty with stickers."

Later that day the receptionist, Betty, showed us a news clipping describing an unusual breed of cat, the Scottish fold. "Isn't it cute?" she exclaimed. Sure enough, someone had found a way to breed cats guaranteed to have problems. Instead of having the upright ears typical of felines, this cat had bent ears that formed a short flap over the ear hole. Such cats couldn't help but be prone to ear mites.

Situations like these have led me to reflect on the many ways we have interfered with the natural reproductive patterns of domestic animals. In the process of selective breeding, we have created a host of abnormal body structures that increase the likelihood of health problems. In addition, drugs, synthetic chemicals, radiation and certain infectious diseases can damage the fetus and further increase the incidence of birth defects.

Animals born with defects can face lifelong health troubles despite excellent care and feeding. That's why it's so important to understand how these malformations are caused and what can be done to prevent or minimize them. First let's look at problems that have developed because of inbreeding and unwise selection.

THE EFFECTS OF BREEDING

When we humans began to domesticate animals, we took over many of nature's decisions about which animals were best suited to carry on the line. No doubt we made many good choices, often picking the strongest and the healthiest. But often animals were chosen for a unique appearance or some unusual behavior that pleased us or suited a particular need—horses with thick, beefy legs for pulling heavy loads; toy versions of dogs for lap companions; no-tail novelty cats. The inbreeding created new lines that had never before existed. And the result?

Consider the dog. As the first animal to be domesticated (some 10,000 to 20,000 years ago from wolves that began to associate with humans), the dog has probably been bred more than any other animal. Over thousands of generations, we developed dogs of every size and purpose. With a social structure and instinct similar to our own, they have served us well as hunters, herders, sled dogs, watch dogs, guide dogs, religious symbols, personal companions and even as a source of food.

Cats, by contrast, were the last animal to share the home life of humans. They were lured by the many mice in the granaries of ancient Egypt and stayed to become a religious symbol of that culture. Not easily trained, the cat was not bred for any further duties except companionship. Their natural talent as mousers made cats welcome in households all over the world.

Just page through a picture book on breeds and you'll see the different breeding histories of dogs and cats. Dogs show much more variety in size, shape and hair texture than cats. The difference in appearance between certain modern breeds of dogs and their wild ancestors is particularly striking when compared with the relatively minor changes in cats.

Surely this greater interference with natural selection explains why a clinical study of birth defects in cats, cows, dogs and horses showed that dogs had the most congenital malformations at birth and cats the fewest. This occurred despite the fact that cats are generally more sensitive to chemicals and other agents known to cause birth defects.

How does selective breeding lead to defects and malfunctions? An important factor in the creation of many breeds is *neoteny*, or a return to more primitive or undeveloped characteristics—either those that occurred early in the species' existence or those common to immature puppies or kittens: short legs and muzzles, silky hair, floppy ears and the tendency to bark (adult wolves rarely bark).

So, many of the features we find appealing in purebred animals are actually the products of arrested development—either physical or psychological. A desired trait is often a trade-off for a defect or loss of function. For instance, breeding dogs for a short muzzle (upper jaw) has spelled trouble for breeds like bulldogs, boxers and terriers. That's because separate genes determine other features that are closely related, such as the teeth and the soft palate (which separates the mouth and throat), and still size them for a normal muzzle. So the crowded teeth are forced to grow in crooked and sideways and the soft palate hangs so far back into the animal's throat that the threat of suffocation is ever present.

Inbreeding adds to the problem. To fix a given characteristic into a breed (so that it will breed *true*, that is, reappear consistently), selected brothers and sisters must be mated, or a parent crossed with its offspring. Such intensive inbreeding might ensure the desired trait, but it might also perpetuate basic weaknesses in the line, such as poor resistance to disease, low stamina, low intelligence, birth defects and inherited diseases that include hemophilia or deafness. For example, miniature poodles bred for just the right color have produced litters in which all the puppies had severely malformed lower jaws.

Breeding to meet market demand can also lead to disaster. During the 1920s, for example, the recently imported Siamese cat became so popular that breeders mated siblings as well as parents and offspring to meet the demand. The kittens born of these matings so weakened the breed that it almost died out entirely. Sobered by this experience, breeders began to make wiser selections. Many breeds of dogs—such as the collie, the cocker spaniel, the beagle and the German shepherd—have also suffered in this way as a result of surges in popularity.

The problem of genetic disease is particularly sad because animals undergo much unnecessary suffering simply because they're often bred for financial gain or for something considered "cute" or unusual (such as squat faces, long faces, curly or silky hair, hairlessness, wrinkly skin, floppy ears or missing tails) or useful (such as short legs for access to dens in hunting or massive size for fighting or guarding). The question rarely comes up whether the animal will have a comfortable, well-adapted, potentially healthy body. And we don't seem troubled by the high rate of defective pets. People rightly get alarmed at a human birth defect rate of one in a thousand, but many pet breeders simply accept statistics that predict 10 to 25 percent of their litters may be born defective, largely because of common breeding practices.

Another ethical issue involves producing countless litters to satisfy the demands of people who insist only on purebreds. At the same time, millions of mixed-breed animals that would make equally good pets go begging. Up to 75 percent of the dogs and cats born each year face death by accidents, star-

vation or euthanasia because they can't find permanent homes.

However, selecting a mongrel from the local animal shelter probably won't necessarily reduce the risk of acquiring a pet with congenital problems. Often an adopter chooses an animal that especially arouses pity, perhaps one with strangely colored eyes or drooping ears and eyes that look sad or a short, pushed-in, childlike face.

Sometimes pets just find their way into our homes and hearts (such as the deaf white cat that came to us as a stray), and we accept them as is. But at least we can decide not to breed an unhealthy animal or one with characteristics that interfere with normal functioning.

A CASE IN POINT: THE POODLE

Let's consider an example. Besides having floppy ears that encourage infections and foxtails and a longhaired, curly coat that attracts stickers (traits common to many breeds), the poodle's hair often grows into its ear canal causing problems that require regular hair removal. Plugged tear ducts cause eye secretions to run down the dog's face instead of the normal course (through the nasal cavity), leaving dark, moist tracks.

This popular breed also can carry defective genes that produce such problems as malformed leg bones, problem arteries near the heart, retina degeneration, dislocated shoulders, displaced kneecaps, epilepsy, abnormal behavior, bladder stones, diabetes, brittle bones, skin defects and allergies and a loss of the normal insulation around nerves in the brain and spinal cord. Most of these problems occur in miniature and toy poodles rather than those of standard size. Generally, the largest and smallest breeds tend to suffer the most genetic weaknesses.

Some other examples of problems created in breeding "un-wolfly" shapes and sizes of dogs include the bulldog, Chihuahua and others bred to have a small pelvis. Many of these animals require cesarean deliveries. Giant breeds such as Saint Bernards and Great Danes are known for their bone problems and their short lives. Breeds that have abnormally short noses and jaws (bulldogs, Pekingese, boxers and Boston terriers) generally suffer with breathing problems, and, as might be expected, dogs bred to have short legs (dachshunds and basset hounds) also tend to have deformed spines. Among cats, breeding for cats that are tailless (the Manx breed) has also led to litters with severe malformation of the urinary tract and genitals.

Environmental Influences on Birth Defects

Environmental poisons and stresses also contribute to congenital problems. Some of these hazards (mutagens) can cause a change in one or more genes that can be passed on to future generations. The result could be a sad legacy of genetic defects and diseases as well as spontaneous abortion, lowered disease resistance, decreased life span, infertility or unnatural behavior. Add unwise breeding practices to the mix, such as mating affected parents and their offspring, and the effects can be even worse.

Other hazards (teratogens) attack the embryo but are not passed on. Depending on the timing and the amount of exposure during pregnancy, such factors can cause deformed bodies, miscarriages, retarded growth, congenital tumors and various disabilities or abnormalities that surface after birth.

If you are planning to breed an animal, it is very wise to take special care to minimize certain risk factors suspected of damaging genes and/or fetuses. The following are the most important to avoid because they can pose a threat both before and during pregnancy.

- Radiation (the worst threat; use filtered water and avoid unnecessary diagnostic x-rays and radioisotopes)
- Lead, mercury and cadmium (see chapter 8)
- Chlorpromazine, phenobarbital and urethane (veterinary sedatives and anesthetics)
- The insecticides carbaryl, dichlorvos, dieldrin and lindane (some are banned, yet they persist in the environment and accumulate in animal fat, so emphasize diets with lean meats; also minimize use of any chemical insecticides)
- Aflaxtoxin (may be in moldy or spoiled foods)
- Fungicides (especially captan and griseofulvin)
- Anti-cancer drugs (not a good idea to breed an animal that has had cancer anyway)

In addition, do your best to protect your pet from the following:

Before breeding: the antibiotics Actinomycin D, erythromycin and streptomycin; the antiseptics hexachlorophene, mercury chloride and hydrogen peroxide; the drugs Butazolidin, EDTA, methylene blue and ethidium bromide; canine distemper (or the live vaccine); the herbicides 2,4-D and 2,4,5-T; chemical soil sterilants; formaldehyde (see chapter 8); and benzene (found in cigarette smoke and car exhaust; don't keep your pet in a garage).

During pregnancy: overheating (from being in a hot car or exercising in hot weather); lack of oxygen (from anesthesia, high altitude, anemia, air pollution or chemical exposure); traumatic injury; most veterinary antibiotics, corticosteroids and sedatives; aspirin; feline leukemia virus (or vaccine); microwave ovens; herbicides, especially paraquat and MCPA; many chemicals, especially complex organic hydrocarbons (follow advice in chapter 8); general underfeeding and malnourishment; insufficient levels of vitamins A, D or B complex, iron, magnesium, zinc, copper, iodine or manganese; excessive amounts of calcium, vitamin A, iodine or salt; certain poisonous plants (jimsonweed, locoweed, skunk cabbage and wild pea).

Some of these factors are known to cause reproductive problems only when given in high doses to experimental animals. For that reason they may not be an issue under ordinary exposures. However, their safety is questionable and it is best to err on the side of caution.

The harm caused by these agents can show up in everyday veterinary practice, not only in laboratory experiments. For instance, pups born of a mother given corticosteroid therapy during pregnancy have been born grossly swollen with fluid. Also, extreme leg and leg joint deformities occurred in an entire litter of cocker spaniel puppies born to a mother treated with the corticosteroid dexamethasone during the second half of pregnancy.

Now that we have a better understanding of the contributing causes behind congenital defects, let's look at some of the more common problems found in various breeds of dogs and cats.

COMMON BIRTH DEFECTS IN DOGS

The parts of the dog's body most frequently affected by congenital problems are the central nervous system, eyes, muscles and bones. For example, the German shepherd, collie, beagle, miniature poodle and keeshond can inherit epilepsy. Also, a variety of other nervous system disorders are sometimes passed on within certain breeds. These include paralysis of the front and back legs (Irish setter), a failure of muscle coordination (fox terrier), idiocy (German shorthaired pointer and English setter) and abnormal swelling of the brain (Chihuahua, cocker spaniel and English bulldog).

Congenital eye abnormalities, including cataracts, glaucoma and blindness, are found in *most* of the common breeds.

Hernia is a typical muscular problem. The basset hound, basenji, cairn terrier, Pekingese and Lhasa apso all have a high risk for inguinal hernias (the gut protrudes into the groin). Umbilical hernias (gut protrudes through the navel) are inherited defects in the cocker spaniel, bull terrier, collie, basenji, Airedale terrier, Pekingese, pointer and weimaraner.

Besides the bone-related problems such as those mentioned in very small, large or short-legged dogs, many canines suffer lameness from abnormal hip formation (dysplasia), probably the most common inherited defect among dogs (see "Hip Dysplasia" on page 280). It is seen in most purebreds, particularly cocker spaniels, Shetland sheep dogs, German shepherds and many large breeds.

For more specific information on particular breeds, see "Behavioral Patterns and Congenital Defects in Dogs" on page 124.

COMMON CONGENITAL PROBLEMS IN CATS

While there have been very few thorough studies of birth defects in cats, the most common problems occur in the nervous system, including the brain, spinal cord and skeletal tissues. (This is true of all domestic animals and humans.) In alphabetical order, these are the special congenital problems that affect cats.

Brachycephalic head (Peke face): Marked by an unusually short and wide head, the deformity is exemplified by long-haired Persians and newer strains of Burmese. Cats from these lines produce lethal birth defects involving the eyes, nasal tissue and jaws in nearly one out of four kittens. Also, a brachycephalic head is associated with an increased incidence of cleft palate.

Brain and skull problems: Cats that have an undersized cerebellum in the brain may have poor coordination, tremors, excessive tension in the limb muscles and slowed reflexes. Swelling of the brain (hydrocephalus) can be inherited in the Siamese. In some cats the roof of the skull does not close, causing abnormal expansion of the brain. In others the brain degenerates even before birth (a condition that's usually fatal).

Cancer of the ear: White-haired cats are the prime victims of this ailment because of repeated sunburn of their sensitive ears.

Cardiovascular defects: The main malformations include a narrowing of the aorta, the heart's main artery, or nonclosure of the aortic duct. Both conditions are common causes of heart murmurs. Cats may also have other kinds of heart and aorta malformations.

Cleft palate: In some Siamese a cleft palate seems to be hereditary, but it can also be caused by various drugs ingested during pregnancy.

Cryptorchidism: The phenomenon of undescended testicles is not unusual among male cats.

Deafness: Many blue-eyed white cats are deaf from birth and often have poor resistance to disease, reduced fertility and impaired night vision.

Eye and eyelid defects: The absence of the outer half of one or both upper lids (seen in Persians, Angoras and the domestic shorthair) is included here, along with an albino or a multicolored iris (which is sometimes associated with deafness on the same side, sensitivity to light and eye incoordination), degeneration of the retina (particularly in Siamese and Persians), strabismus (an inward rotation of one eye when the other is fixed on an object, common in Siamese) and nystagmus (involuntary movements of the eye).

Hair abnormalities: Some cats are born with (or bred for) hairlessness or curly, short, plushlike hair, such as the "Rex" mutant, which has missing or abnormal guard hairs.

Hair balls (frequent): It's well known that this is a chronic problem in longhairs.

Kidney missing: This abnormality occurs most often in males, and usually the right kidney is missing.

Limb defects: Kittens sometimes show missing or extra toes or legs at birth.

Mammary gland abnormalities: This occurs in the formation of the ducts that supply milk.

Spina bifida: The vertebrae fail to close normally around the spinal cord, leading to motor and sensory problems in areas fed by affected nerves. The Manx, in particular, suffers from this problem because it is associated with the gene for taillessness. Symptoms can also include a hopping gait and incontinence.

Tail defects: A missing tail is typical of the Manx but rare in others. Associated defects include spina bifida with hindquarter deformities and an abnormally small anus. Other cats can be born with a kinked tail.

Umbilical hernias: Part of the intestines or some fat protrudes through the navel in this commonplace defect. Hernias of the diaphragm are also frequent.

PREVENTING CONGENITAL PROBLEMS

You can't always help an animal that is born with a congenital problem. Sometimes surgery can correct a structural defect, and proper grooming, veterinary care and feeding can control certain other problems. But the very best treatment for congenital defects is prevention. That means:

Never breed unhealthy animals. Avoid breeding those pets who have obvious birth defects or behavior difficulties. Even though the animal may not have a specific genetic problem, its overall support system is under par for developing healthy offspring. Also, avoid acquiring such animals unless you are willing to provide them with the special care they need.

Don't breed or select animals with family health problems. If their close relatives have congenital defects or inheritable behavioral or physical troubles, stay away. The tables beginning on page 124 help alert you to particular problems that may plague the breed(s) you are considering. Try to check on the medical histories of both parents and what percentage of related puppies or kittens have had defects. It should be less than 5 percent.

Do not breed close relatives. Mating two animals of the same family (such as parents, siblings, aunts and uncles and grandparents) tends to "fix" latent defects into their offspring.

Don't select or breed inbred animals. Be particularly careful with breeds that are currently popular in your area, because it's likely they have been weakened by intensive inbreeding.

Favor breeds that best resemble canine or feline ancestors. Look for size, face shape, ear shape, color, coat length and texture, tail shape, and limb proportions that most closely match that of wolves, coyotes and wild cats. (Try to match at least four or five of these characteristics.) Canine examples include most of the retrievers, sled dog breeds, basenjis, shepherds, pointers and spitzs. Feline examples include most shorthairs, especially those with more natural colors such as tabbies, silvers and ancient breeds such as Korats and Abyssinians. If a given characteristic differs, consider the potential effect. A curly coat, for instance, will attract stickers. A pushed-in face will cause breathing problems. Long, floppy ears may harbor mites.

Occasionally, I have had the opportunity to examine and treat injured coyotes or foxes, and never have I found one with a foxtail in its ears or anywhere else on its body! Every inch of their bodies reflects the intelligence of millions of years of natural evolution and adaptation. I have been quite impressed with how perfectly their teeth fit together and with their fine hair coats, fastidious cleanliness, natural grace and high intelligence. (Don't try to adopt a truly wild animal: The place for them is in the wild, and they do not make good pets anyway.)

Protect fertile and litter-bearing females. If you plan to breed your female pet, avoid use of potentially damaging flea powders, cortisone, vaccinations, sedatives, anesthetics and x-rays, unless natural aids fail and circumstances demand this kind of medical treatment. Feed her an optimal diet (see chapter 5) and make sure she does not consume food additives, moldy foods, poisonous household chemicals or lawn grass or other plants treated with toxic herbicides, insecticides or fungicides. This rule applies before and during pregnancy and during lactation.

Also, see that she does not become overheated. Excess heat can retard fetal brain growth. Don't leave her locked in a hot car with the windows closed (a good piece of advice concerning any animal) or overexercise her in hot weather. Nor should you take her on an arduous trek into high country or transport her in the baggage compartment of an airplane, because the lack of oxygen at high altitudes can induce a variety of fetal abnormalities.

Selecting a Healthy Animal

The tables that follow will alert you to potential problems in various breeds and mixed breeds. But how can you tell if a *particular* animal is healthy? Here is a "checkup" list you can use to pinpoint any congenital defects present. It also helps assess the likelihood of chronic health problems to come.

What color is the coat? White animals, beautiful as they are, often fall victim to extra problems, such as skin cancers or deafness in white, blue-eyed cats. (Test for deafness by clapping your hands behind the animal's head.) Gray collies sometimes have a blood immune problem with increased susceptibility to infection.

Check the nose and jaws. Are they unusually long and pointed or unusually short and pushed in? Odd shapes here should act as a warning against trouble with teeth and gums, in addition to potential respiratory problems.

Are the eyes normal-looking? Are they both the same color? Be cautious about eye trouble if the eyes are unusually small or large compared to other canines or felines. Discharges from the eyes signal plugged tear ducts because tears and liquids would ordinarily be discharged through the nasal cavity.

Does the animal move normally? Or does it swing its hips from side to side as it walks—a warning sign of possible canine hip dysplasia? Are the legs a normal length, and are the front and back legs in the right proportion relative to each other?

Does the pigmentation over the nose look normal? If not, the animal may be subject to sunburn and skin cancer.

Observe the animal carefully for normal temperament. Be wary of animals that seem unusually aggressive, clinging, jealous, fearful, suspicious, hyperactive, noisy or unaware. Whether because of inheritance or environment, such problems may be difficult to live with and even harder to correct. If you want a playful or affectionate animal, choose the one that responds to your overtures. Roll a dog on its back and hold him there. If he fights to get up, he may be difficult to train and aggressive. A dog that keeps its tail low or acts submissive will be the most devoted and easiest to train.

Once you have the trust of the animal (and with the owner's assistance, if necessary), take a closer look for problem signs.

Is the coat attractive? Does it look and smell healthy and clean, or is it slightly greasy or thin? Are there reddish patches? Is the skin light pink or off-white in color, pliant and firm, or are some areas unusually thin, thick, dry, dark, red or crusty? Is the skin covered with fleas?

Does the animal breathe quietly and easily? Raspy, heavy sounds, especially after a little exertion, are not good signs.

Look inside the ears. Check for any signs of inflammation or dark, waxy discharge. This could signal a chronic tendency toward ear trouble.

Feel around the navel. You're looking for a lump, which could be a sign of a hernia.

Check the scrotum in an adult male for the presence of both testicles.

Are the upper and lower jaws the same size? Do the teeth fit together well? (This particularly applies to dogs.) Are the gums pale or inflamed? Is there a red line at the edge of the gums next to the teeth?

In spite of the many problems inappropriate breeding has caused, it is still possible to find a genetically healthy animal or one with only minor problems. If you don't plan to breed the animal and don't mind the extra work of caring for an animal with inherited problems, you can select from a wider variety. Although you cannot always foresee or control potential congenital problems, with just a bit of common sense you can actually do a great deal to minimize the risks. In the process, you will be doing a big favor not only for your own animals and yourself but also for those whose time is yet to come!

CHOOSING THE BEST PET FOR YOU

When choosing a dog or cat, pick a breed that suits your lifestyle and preferences. Both dogs and cats vary widely in their temperaments and their needs, often along breed lines. Every day humane societies must euthanize healthy animals turned in because their unhappy owners did not anticipate certain issues. For instance, a mild-mannered person would be unwise to select a large dog from a breed that tends to dominate the owner. Similarly, a family with toddlers in the house should choose a breed less likely to snap at children. Those who live in an apartment with no yard should pick an animal suited to smaller confines, such as the Korat cat.

It is also important to consider size variations when you are selecting a dog. Clusters of traits tend to go with size. Small dogs, for example, may be especially active and have a high demand for affection. Large dogs tend to be quieter and more patient with children. Dogs that are unusually large or unusually small tend to have the most genetic problems, especially structural ones. Larger and more active dogs require the most space and consume the most food, which involves economic and ecological considerations. For example, a 70 to 80 pound dog needs as many calories every day as an adult woman. So if you plan to feed your dog a natural diet, as recommended in this book, it will be easier to deal with a smaller dog. Many people find it too expensive or too much work to prepare food for a larger dog. Such dogs almost always end up on a diet of commercial food, with the accompanying lower level of health.

Behavioral Patterns and Congenital Defects in Dogs

Breed	Weight (lb.)	Physical Needs	Training	Companionship
Toy and Small Dogs				
Basenji	23	Should sleep indoors.	—	—
Beagle	20–35	Should sleep indoors.	More difficult.	Very active.
Boston terrier	15–25	Should sleep indoors.	—	Very affectionate, active, needs attention.
Brittany spaniel	25–40	Regular grooming. Should sleep indoors.	Easy. Submissive.	Patient with toddlers.
Chihuahua	2–6	Lots of exercise. Should sleep indoors. Sensitive to cold.	Difficult. Dominant. Nondestructive.	Very affectionate, active, needs attention. Not very playful. May snap at toddlers.
Cocker spaniel	20–30	Regular grooming. Should sleep indoors.	—	Very affectionate, but may snap at children.
Dachshund	15–25	Should sleep indoors.	Destructive (chews, digs).	—
Fox terrier	17	Regular grooming. Should sleep indoors.	Difficult. Dominant. Destructive (chews, digs).	Not so playful. May snap at toddlers. Very active.

Footnotes appear on page 136.

Watchdog and Aggression	Possible Congenital Defects*	Notes
Quiet.	Anemia. Hernias. Opaque cornea. Enteritis (diarrhea).	Clean, no odor. Doesn't bark. Natural size, shape and coat. Patient.
Barks excessively.	Cataracts, glaucoma and other eye problems. Epilepsy. Hemophilia. Cleft lip and palate. Spinal deformities. Short or missing tail. Skin allergies.	—
More likely to bark at intruders. Barks excessively.	Cataracts. Obstructed breathing.† Pituitary cysts.‡ Deformed spine, knees. Tumors. Excess or missing teeth. Hernias.	—
Less likely to bark at intruders. Nonaggressive.	—	Sweet, well-mannered. Good swimmer.
More likely to bark at intruders. Barks excessively.	Deformed spine, knees. Dislocated shoulder. Heart and breathing problems.† Hemophilia. Swelling of brain.	—
Less likely to bark at intruders.	Cataracts, gradual blindness, glaucoma and other eye problems. Kidney disease. Hemophilia. Cleft lip and palate. Misshaped jaw, tail. Deformed spine, knees. Dislocated shoulder. Swelling of the brain. Hernias.	—
Strongly defends territory.	Bladder stones. Pituitary cysts.‡ Deafness. Diabetes. Circulatory problems. Disk disease. Incomplete kidney. Cleft lip and palate. Malformed jaw, spine, limbs.	Long-haired dachshund more tranquil, barks less.
Barks excessively. Strongly defends territory. Aggressive.	Glaucoma. Deafness. Nervous and cardiovascular defects. Excess or missing teeth. Dislocated shoulder. Skin allergy. Muscular incoordination. Goiter.	Very excitable, may try to dominate owner.

(continued)

Behavioral Patterns and Congenital Defects in Dogs—Continued

Breed	Weight (lb.)	Physical Needs	Training	Companionship
Toy and Small Dogs—Continued				
Lhasa apso	10–15	Regular grooming. Should sleep indoors.	Dominant.	Very affectionate, needs attention. Not so playful.
Maltese	6	Regular grooming. Should sleep indoors. Sensitive to cold.	—	Very affectionate, needs attention. May snap at toddlers.
Pekingese	10–14	Regular grooming. Should sleep indoors.	Difficult. Nondestructive.	Very affectionate, but not so playful. May snap at toddlers.
Pomeranian	5	Regular grooming. Should sleep indoors.	Difficult.	Not so playful. May snap at toddlers.
Poodle (miniature)	12–25	Regular grooming. Should sleep indoors.	Easy.	Very affectionate, active, playful, needs attention.
Poodle (toy)	8–12	Regular grooming. Should sleep indoors.	—	Very affectionate, needs attention. May snap at toddlers.
Pug	16	Should sleep indoors. Sensitive to heat.	—	—
Schnauzer (miniature)	12–15	Regular grooming. Should sleep indoors.	Dominant.	Very affectionate, playful, active, needs attention. May snap at toddlers.
Scottish terrier	20	Regular grooming. Needs lots of exercise. Should sleep indoors.	Difficult. Dominant. Destructive (chews, digs).	May snap at toddlers. Very active.

Watchdog and Aggression	Possible Congenital Defects*	Notes
Barks excessively.	Inguinal hernias. Kidney defects.	Can be stubborn.
Barks excessively. Nonaggressive.	—	Less aggressive than most small dogs. Long-lived.
Barks excessively.	Eye abnormalities. Obstructed breathing.† Pituitary cysts.‡ Deformed spine. Hernia.	Classic apartment dog. Ancient breed.
Barks excessively.	Dislocated shoulder. Deformed knees. Collapsed trachea. Heart defects. Underdeveloped teeth.	Usually excitable but some are calm. Most natural size, shape and coat. Seasonal shedding. Related to spitz.
Barks excessively. Nonaggressive.	Gradual blindness, eye problems. Epilepsy, nerve and heart defects. Hemophilia. Bladder stones. Collapsed trachea, obstructed breathing.† Diabetes. Deformed spine, limbs. Dislocated shoulder.	—
Barks excessively.	Gradual blindness. Knee problems. Collapsed trachea. Heart defects. Muscle problems in lower rear legs.	More likely than other poodles to snap at children.
More likely to bark at intruders. Nonaggressive.	Male pseudohermaphroditism. Ingrown hairs in tissue.	Less aggressive, excitable and snappish than other small dogs.
More likely to bark at intruders. Barks excessively. Strongly defends territory. Aggressive.	Cataracts. Hemophilia.	—
More likely to bark at intruders. Strongly defends territory.	Nerve defects. Deafness. Bladder stones. Short limbs. Skin allergy. Tumors.	Needs regular, long walks. Barks less than many small dogs.

(continued)

Behavioral Patterns and Congenital Defects in Dogs—Continued

Breed	Weight (lb.)	Physical Needs	Training	Companionship
Toy and Small Dogs—Continued				
Shetland sheepdog	16	Should sleep indoors.	Easy. Submissive.	Very playful.
Shih Tzu	12	Regular grooming. Should sleep indoors.	—	Very affectionate, active. Needs attention.
Welsh corgi, Pembroke	27	Should sleep indoors.	Easy. Submissive. Nondestructive.	Very playful.
West Highland white terrier	16	Regular grooming. Needs lots of exercise. Should sleep indoors.	Difficult. Destructive (chews, digs).	Very affectionate, playful, active, needs attention. May snap at toddlers.
Yorkshire terrier	4–7	Regular grooming. Should sleep indoors. Sensitive to cold.	Difficult.	Very affectionate, active, playful, needs attention. May snap at toddlers.
Medium Dogs				
Airedale	50	Regular grooming. Needs lots of exercise. Should sleep indoors.	Dominant. Destructive (chews, digs).	Very playful, active.
Australian shepherd	40	May sleep outdoors in a doghouse.	Easy.	Very affectionate, playful, active, needs attention. Patient with toddlers.
Basset hound	40–55	Should sleep indoors.	Difficult. Submissive. Nondestructive.	Not so playful or affectionate. Patient with toddlers.
Dalmation	45	Should sleep indoors.	Dominant. Destructive (chews, digs).	May snap at toddlers. Needs attention.

Watchdog and Aggression	Possible Congenital Defects*	Notes
Barks excessively. Nonaggressive.	Eye and cardiovascular problems. Hemophilia. Nasal sunburn. Bladder cancer.	Seasonal shedding. Sometimes stubborn, suspicious of strangers.
Nonaggressive.	Cleft lip and palate. Kidney defects.	Less aggressive than many small dogs.
Strongly defends territory.	Bladder stones. Gradual blindness. Difficult births.	Good combination family pet/watchdog.
More likely to bark at intruders. Barks excessively. Strongly defends territory. Aggressive.	Skin allergies. Diseased jaw. Central nervous system problems. Inguinal hernias.	Very active, excitable and aggressive. Needs patio or yard.
More likely to bark at intruders. Barks excessively.	Knee problems. Displaced retina. Underdeveloped teeth. Birth problems.	Excitable.
More likely to bark at intruders. Strongly defends territory. Aggressive.	Small cerebellum. Trembling of hind quarters, nerve problems. Hernias.	Regular clipping customary. Needs affection.
Quiet. Nonaggressive.	Small eyes and other eye problems.	Benign watchdog. Energetic yet not high-strung.
Less likely to bark at intruders. Quiet. Nonaggressive.	Spinal deformities. Short limbs. Glaucoma. Hernias.	Mild. Descended from bloodhound.
—	Skin allergies. Deafness. Uric acid problems. Nerve system problems.	Can be melancholy if alone.

(continued)

Behavioral Patterns and Congenital Defects in Dogs—Continued

Breed	Weight (lb.)	Physical Needs	Training	Companionship
Medium Dogs—Continued				
English bulldog	50	Should sleep indoors.	Difficult. Nondestructive.	Not so playful or affectionate.
English springer spaniel	50	Regular grooming. Should sleep indoors.	Easy. Submissive. Sometimes destructive.	Very affectionate, playful, needs attention. Patient with toddlers.
Great spitz	40	Regular grooming. Should sleep indoors.	—	—
Keeshond	40	Regular grooming. May sleep outdoors in a doghouse.	Easy. Submissive. Nondestructive.	Patient with toddlers.
Norwegian elkhound	50	May sleep outdoors in a doghouse.	—	Not so affectionate. Patient with toddlers.
Poodle (standard)	35–50	Regular grooming. Should sleep indoors.	Easy. Submissive.	Very affectionate, playful, needs attention.
Samoyed	45–65	Regular grooming. May sleep outdoors in a doghouse.	Difficult. Dominant. Destructive (chews, digs).	Not so affectionate or playful. May snap at toddlers.
Siberian husky	35–60	Needs lots of exercise. May sleep outdoors in a doghouse.	Destructive (chews, digs).	Not so affectionate. May snap at toddlers. Very active.

Watchdog and Aggression	Possible Congenital Defects*	Notes
Less likely to bark at intruders. Quiet, nonaggressive.	Obstructed breathing.† Heart problems. Cleft lip and palate, excess or missing teeth. Birth, fertility problems. Pituitary cysts.‡ Deformed spine. Tumors. Swelling of brain.	—
—	Weakened skin. Hemophilia. Displaced retina. Some lines have abnormal aggression (attack people), so check lineage.	Playful family pet, safe with children, but can be destructive.
Less likely to bark at intruders. Strongly defends territory.	—	Natural size, shape and coat. Seasonal shedding. Considered ancestor of all breeds. Suspicious of strangers.
—	Epilepsy. Heart defects.	Natural size, shape and coat. Odorless. Seasonal shedding. Some lines may be more active, aggressive.
More likely to bark at intruders.	Gradual blindness. Tumors. Incomplete kidneys.	Natural size, shape and coat. Seasonal shedding.
More likely to bark at intruders. Strongly defends territory. Nonaggressive.	Cataracts and other eye problems. Bladder stones. Hemophilia. Skin allergies. Behavior problems.	Intelligent, good family dog. Can learn meaning of words.
Strongly defends territory. Aggressive.	Heart defects. Diabetes. Hemophilia.	Natural size, shape and coat. Seasonal shedding. Best watchdog of all the sled dog breeds. Odorless.
Less likely to bark at intruders. Strongly defends territory. Aggressive.	Different-colored irises.	Natural size, shape and coat. Seasonal shedding. More playful than other sled dogs. Hardy.

(continued)

Behavioral Patterns and Congenital Defects in Dogs—Continued

Breed	Weight (lb.)	Physical Needs	Training	Companionship
Large and Giant Dogs				
Afghan hound	60	Regular grooming and exercise. May sleep outdoors in a doghouse.	Difficult. Dominant. Destructive (chews, digs).	Not so affectionate or playful. May snap at toddlers.
Akita	85	Regular grooming. Needs lots of exercise. Should sleep indoors.	Easy. Nondestructive.	Not so affectionate or playful. Patient with toddlers. Calm.
Alaskan malamute	85	May sleep outdoors in a doghouse.	Can be destructive.	—
Bloodhound	90	May sleep outdoors in a doghouse.	Submissive. Nondestructive.	Not so affectionate or playful. Patient with toddlers. Calm.
Boxer	50–70	Needs lots of exercise. Should sleep indoors. Sensitive to cold.	Dominant.	Patient with toddlers.
Chesapeake Bay retriever	55–75	—	Easy. Submissive. Destructive (chews, digs).	Very affectionate, needs attention. Patient with toddlers. Calm.
Chow Chow	60	Regular grooming. May sleep outdoors in a doghouse.	Difficult. Dominant. Nondestructive.	Not so affectionate or playful. May snap at toddlers. Calm.
Collie	40–65	Regular grooming. Should sleep indoors. Sensitive to heat.	Easy. Submissive. Nondestructive.	Not so affectionate. Patient with toddlers. Calm.

Watchdog and Aggression	Possible Congenital Defects*	Notes
Less likely to bark at intruders. Strongly defends territory. Aggressive.	Cataracts. Malformed elbow. Decaying spinal cord.	Require good training. Hardy to weather.
More likely to bark at intruders. Strongly defends territory. Quiet. Aggressive.	—	Natural size, shape and coat. One of best watchdogs without dominating owner. Odorless.
Quiet.	Eye abnormalities. Hemophilia. Anemia with malformed bones. Dwarfism. Day blindness. Incomplete kidneys. Hemorrhaging.	Natural size, shape and coat. Clean, odorless. Does not bark. Okay in apartment with daily walks.
Less likely to bark at intruders. Quiet. Nonaggressive.	Susceptibility to distemper.	Very calm, quiet, polite. Excellent tracker.
Quiet. Strongly defends territory.	Cardiovascular defects. Obstructed breathing.† Extra teeth. Subject to rheumatism.	Short-lived. Good family dog/watchdog. Less destructive than most guard dogs.
—	—	Good family dog, swimmer.
Strongly defends territory. Nonaggressive.	—	Natural size, shape and coat. Seasonal shedding. Aggressive, but good guard dog with training. Loyal. Best with quiet owner.
Nonaggressive.	Retinal atrophy. Deafness. Epilepsy. Hemophilia. Hernia. Nasal sunburn. Bladder cancer. Eye problems. Cyclic neutropenia. Heart defects. Dwarfism.	Seasonal shedding. Good family pet, nonaggressive yet fairly good watch and guard dog.

(continued)

Behavioral Patterns and Congenital Defects in Dogs—Continued

Breed	Weight (lb.)	Physical Needs	Training	Companionship
Large and Giant Dogs—Continued				
Doberman pinscher	70	Needs lots of exercise. May sleep outdoors in a doghouse.	Easy.	—
German shepherd	60–85	Regular grooming. Needs lots of exercise. May sleep outdoors in a doghouse.	Easy. Dominant. Destructive (chews, digs).	Not so affectionate. Very playful.
German shorthaired pointer	45–70	Needs lots of exercise. May sleep outside in a doghouse.	Destructive (chews, digs).	Very playful, active. Patient with toddlers.
Golden retriever	55–75	Regular grooming.	Easy. Submissive. Nondestructive.	Very affectionate, playful, needs attention. Patient with toddlers.
Great Dane	100–150	Should sleep indoors.	—	Not so affectionate or playful. Patient with toddlers. Calm.
Irish setter	45–70	Needs lots of exercise. Should sleep indoors.	Difficult. Destructive (chews, digs).	Very affectionate, playful, active, needs attention.
Labrador retriever	55–75	May sleep outdoors in a doghouse.	Easy. Submissive. Nondestructive.	Very playful. Patient with toddlers.

Watchdog and Aggression	Possible Congenital Defects*	Notes
More likely to bark at intruders. Quiet. Strongly defends territory. Aggressive.	Incomplete kidneys. Spinal deformities. Heart degeneration. Bone problems. Liver problems. Eye problems.	Long-lived. One of best watchdogs, easiest to train.
More likely to bark at intruders. Strongly defends territory. Aggressive.	Cataracts. Epilepsy. Kidney and bladder disease. Heart defects. Cleft lip and palate. Behavior problems.	Natural size, shape and coat. One of best watch and guard dogs. Genetic lines vary a lot (check them out).
Less likely to bark at intruders. Nonaggressive.	Cataracts. Cardiovascular defects. Hernias. Behavior problems, idiocy. Cancer of connective tissue. Out-turned eye membrane. Swelling caused by obstructed lymphs. Decaying spinal cord. Skin cancer (melanoma).	Fine temperament, but can be destructive. Not for apartments.
Less likely to bark at intruders. Quiet. Nonaggressive.	Cataracts, gradual blindness. Generally a healthy, hardy dog.	One of best family dogs. Good swimmer.
Quiet. Strongly defends territory.	Heart defects. Bladder stones. Deformed spine. Out-turned eye membrane. Paralysis.	Bred as a guard dog. Size requires commitment to training.
Barks excessively. Nonaggressive.	Gradual blindness. Heart and nerve defects. Hemophilia. Paralysis of legs. Joint problems in forelegs. Degeneration of kidneys.	Very playful, lively. Long-lived.
Quiet. Nonaggressive.	Cataracts, gradual blindness. Bladder stones. Hemophilia.	Natural size, shape and coat. Good swimmer. Good family dog, safe with children. Hardy, healthy.

(continued)

Behavioral Patterns and Congenital Defects in Dogs—Continued

Breed	Weight (lb.)	Physical Needs	Training	Companionship
Large and Giant Dogs—Continued				
Newfoundland	140	Regular grooming. May sleep outdoors in a doghouse.	Submissive. Nondestructive.	Not so playful. Patient with toddlers. Calm.
Old English sheepdog	95	Regular grooming. May sleep outdoors in a doghouse.	Difficult.	Calm.
Rottweiler	110	May sleep outdoors in a doghouse.	Easy. Dominant. Nondestructive.	Not so affectionate or playful. Calm.
St. Bernard	100–200	Regular grooming. Needs lots of exercise. May sleep outdoors in a doghouse.	Difficult. Dominant. Nondestructive.	Not so affectionate or playful. Calm.
Vizsla	65	Should sleep indoors.	Easy. Submissive. Nondestructive.	Very playful. Patient with toddlers.
Weimaraner	75	Should sleep indoors.	Destructive (chews, digs).	—

SOURCE: "A Catalogue of Congenital and Hereditary Disorders of Dogs," in *Current Veterinary Therapy IX: Small Animal Practice*, ed. Robert Kirk, 1986, pp. 1281–1285.
*Miniature breeds: Tend to have collapsed tracheas, knee problems, difficult births and abnormal carbohydrate metabolism.

Watchdog and Aggression	Possible Congenital Defects*	Notes
Less likely to bark at intruders. Quiet, nonaggressive.	Out-turned eyelids. Heart defects.	Natural size, shape and coat. Seasonal shedding. Excellent temperament. Good swimmer. Quietest, least aggressive of large dogs.
Less likely to bark at intruders. Quiet. Nonaggressive.	Cataracts.	Much grooming required.
More likely to bark at intruders. Quiet. Strongly defends territory. Aggressive.	Diabetes.	One of best, calmest guard dogs and bodyguards, though may dominate owner.
Less likely to bark at intruders. Strongly defends territory.	Out-turned eye membrane. Missing eye lens. Hemophilia. Paralysis.	Calm, but may dominate owner, snap at children. Not for indoor life.
Less likely to bark at intruders. Quiet. Nonaggressive.	Hemophilia.	Good family dog, safe with children.
—	Nerve defects. Hemophilia. Hernias.	Moderate in most characteristics. Fairly lively, affectionate. Can be stubborn.

Giant breeds: Hip and elbow dysplasia (joints improperly joined, causing lameness) and bone cancer are common.
†Caused by small nostrils and overly long, soft palate, predisposing to collapse of larynx.
‡Can result in diabetes, genital atrophy and obesity.

Behavioral Patterns and Congenital Defects in Cats

Breed	Physical Needs	Companionship
Short-Haired Cats		
Abyssinian	Clean coat with a wet mitt or glove. Prefers outdoors.	Affectionate, likes attention. Cautious. Active, inquisitive. Bonds to one person. Can learn simple tricks.
American shorthair	Regular brushing. Prefers outdoors.	Affectionate, likes attention.
American wirehair	Regular brushing. Prefers outdoors.	Affectionate, likes attention.
Bombay	Clean coat with a wet mitt or glove. Prefers indoors.	Affectionate, likes attention. Sedate.
British shorthair	Likes indoors or outdoors. Adapts to cold.	Affectionate, likes attention.
Burmese and Malayans	Clean coat with a wet mitt or glove. Likes indoors or outdoors.	Affectionate, likes attention. Enjoys travel. Vocal, "talkative."
Egyptian Mau	Likes indoors.	Sedate.
European shorthair	Likes indoors or outdoors. Adapts to cold.	Active, inquisitive.
Exotic shorthair	Regular brushing. Likes indoors.	Affectionate, likes attention. Sedate.
Japanese bobtail	Regular brushing. Likes indoors or outdoors.	Affectionate, likes attention. Active, inquisitive.
Korat	Clean coat with a wet mitt or glove. Likes indoors.	Can learn simple tricks.

Footnotes appear on page 142.

Hunting and Aggression	Possible Congenital Defects*	Notes
—	—	Natural shape and coat. Needs special attention from owner (petting, playing) or becomes sad, may run away.
Good mouser.	Abnormal or short tail, indented nose, extra toes. Thin or obese. Eyelid defects. Deafness in white, blue-eyed cats.	Fur adapts to cold, wet, thorns. Needs occasional brushing after outdoor excursions. Accepts baths well if started young.
Good mouser. Aggressive with other cats.	Crooked tail.	Wiry coat a mutation. May dominate other cats.
—	Curly hair, abnormally short tail.	Tranquil, good indoors.
Good mouser.	—	Natural shape and coat. Fur adapts to cold, wet, thorns, etc. Large, strong.
Good mouser.	—	Natural shape and coat. Long-lived, healthy. Requires affection, quiet. Good indoors.
Good mouser.	—	Natural shape and coat. Okay indoors. Delicate to changes of weather.
Good mouser.	Deafness in blue-eyed, white cats.	Natural shape and coat. Long-lived. Resists cold. Strong, adapts to many environments.
Good mouser.	Short or abnormal tail.	Tranquil, good indoors (Persian-American shorthair cross).
Good mouser.	—	Loves fish.
Aggressive with other cats. Good mouser.	Tends to get respiratory infections.	Natural shape and coat. Dislikes street noise.

(continued)

Behavioral Patterns and Congenital Defects in Cats—Continued

Breed	Physical Needs	Companionship
Short-Haired Cats—Continued		
Manx	Regular brushing.	Active, inquisitive, playful.
Rex	Clean coat with a wet mitt or glove. Prefers indoors.	Sedate.
Russian blue	Regular brushing. Prefers indoors.	Affectionate, likes attention. Sedate.
Scottish fold	Regular brushing. Likes indoors or outdoors. Adapts to cold.	Affectionate, likes attention. Bonds to one person.
Siamese (also Colorpoint shorthairs, Oriental shorthairs)	Regular brushing. Likes indoors or outdoors.	Active, inquisitive. Bonds to one person. Enjoys travel. Accepts a leash. Vocal, "talkative."
Sphynx	Prefers indoors. Sensitive to cold.	Affectionate, likes attention. Sedate.
Long-Haired Cats		
Balinese and Javanese	Extra grooming to avoid hair balls. Likes indoors or outdoors.	Active, inquisitive. Bonds to one person. Vocal, "talkative."
Birman	Extra grooming to avoid hair balls.	Sedate.
Himalayan (Colorpoint longhair) and Kashmirs	Extra grooming to avoid hair balls.	Active, inquisitive. Bonds to one person.

Hunting and Aggression	Possible Congenital Defects*	Notes
Good mouser.	Taillessness compromises balance. Hopping gait. Incontinence. Stillbirths. Lack of undercoat. Small head. Spina bifida, hind limb and pelvic deformities, small anus.	Muscular, playful. Friendly to all. Likes to climb.
—	Kinked tail.	Likes indoors. Very inquisitive.
—	Obesity.	Natural shape and coat. Good indoors, likes quiet. Especially affectionate.
Good mouser.	Folded ears may harbor ear mites, impair hearing.	Content indoors with occasional escape. Resists cold weather.
Aggressive with other cats.	More susceptible to disease than other breeds. Nasal obstruction, chin malformation, cleft palate. Retinal degeneration. Weak legs.	Natural shape and coat. Long-lived. Sensitive, unpredictable. Jealous. Needs space. Can be walked on a leash.
—	A hairless mutation. Susceptible to catching colds. May have overly wrinkled skin.	Must live indoors in temperate climate.
Good mouser.	Weak hind legs. Can be sickly. Crossed eyes.	Affectionate, but mostly with one person. Similar to Siamese.
—	Crossed eyes, kinked tail.	Tranquil, devoted.
Good mouser.	Crossed eyes.	Adapts to indoors, but likes a lot of space. Affectionate, does not fight with other cats.

(continued)

Behavioral Patterns and Congenital Defects in Cats—Continued

Breed	Physical Needs	Companionship
Long-Haired Cats—Continued		
Maine coon cat	Extra grooming to avoid hair balls. Likes outdoors. Adapts to cold.	Affectionate, likes attention. Bonds to one person.
Persian/Longhair	Extra grooming to avoid hair balls. Prefers indoors.	Affectionate, likes attention. Sedate.
Ragdoll	Extra grooming to avoid hair balls. Prefers indoors.	Sedate.
Somali	Extra grooming to avoid hair balls. Prefers outdoors. Sensitive to cold.	Active, inquisitive. Somewhat standoffish.
Turkish Angora	Extra grooming to avoid hair balls. Prefers indoors.	Affectionate, likes attention. Bonds to one person. Sedate.

SOURCE: Siegal, Mordecai (ed.) and Gino Pugnetti, *Simon and Schuster's Guide to Cats* (New York: Simon and Schuster, 1983).
*All long-haired cats tend to get hair balls.

Hunting and Aggression	Possible Congenital Defects*	Notes
Good mouser.	Generally healthy, can withstand cold.	Natural shape and coat. Prefers a yard, but okay indoors. Likes fish. Muscular. Friendly, but bonds to one person.
Good mouser.	Must be brushed daily to avoid hair ball problems. Eyelid defects. Retinal degeneration. Peke face.	Tranquil, home-loving. Muscular. Sociable even to other cats. Affectionate. Classic indoor cat.
—	Crossed eyes, deformed tail.	Soft body, mild character. Requires quiet owner, best indoors.
Good mouser.	Excessive shyness.	A long-haired Abyssinian. Sometimes mistrustful. Needs some outdoor space.
—	Short tail.	Progenitors of Persian/Long-hairs. Easier to brush than Persian. Almost shorthaired in summer. Sweet, well-behaved. Best indoors.

CHAPTER TEN

EMOTIONAL CONNECTIONS AND YOUR PET'S HEALTH

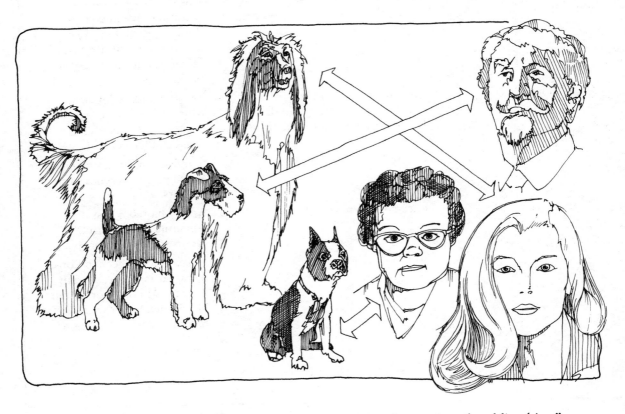

With the big hulk of a dog glaring at me suspiciously, I carefully examined the foul-smelling, hairless patches that oozed bloody discharges on his back, underside, legs and muzzle. As if to demonstrate just how bad it was, he jerked around and chewed violently on the base of his tail.

"Stop that, Bandy!" his owner yelled sharply. Calming down, he explained, "The biting and chewing only makes things worse, so I always make a point of scolding him."

"There are some particularly bad spots under his tail," the man's wife pointed out. Slowly, I started to raise the big dog's tail to take a look.

Hurling around, he snapped at me angrily, barely missing my hand. Pronouncing the exam complete, I sat down with the distraught couple to find out more about how this problem began.

"It happened pretty quickly," the woman began. "He had just a slight mange on his face when I got him as a puppy three years ago, but the real problem—chewing and licking all over himself—has gone on for about six months. The vet called it a flea allergy but didn't offer much for it. We ended up taking the dog to several vets, one of whom said it was 'hot spots.'" The woman described how the veterinarian shaved the areas and gave Bandy antibiotics and cortisone. But, she said, nothing really helped. Finally, the veterinarian told the couple that they would either have to put Bandy to sleep or do a bunch of expensive treatments that still might not work.

"Do you have any idea why it got bad six months ago? Anything special happen around that time?" I inquired.

"Well, all I can think of was that our baby was born a couple of months before it started. I didn't want Bandy to be around the baby— you know, worms and all that—and the dog was acting jealous because he wasn't 'Number One' anymore, so we started keeping him outside all the time. Maybe that affected him. I don't know. I've had itchy skin myself for years, and I've never been able to find out the cause."

As we went on to discuss the dog's irritability, the woman mentioned that she *preferred* an aggressive dog. That way she felt safer living in the country. Occasionally, the man would interject something. As he did, I sensed an underlying tension between the couple.

This case came to me soon after I first began to look at medicine in a new way, exploring a wide variety of factors that might affect an animal's health. It prompted me to pay closer attention to the emotional fac-

tors in pet illnesses. Through the years I have repeatedly observed several patterns that I first noticed in Bandy's case as well as some others. In summary, the patterns go like this.

- Pets may develop health problems soon after an upsetting change in the household, usually involving a loss of attention, relationship or territory.
- The health of a pet can be affected by recurrent feelings of tension, anxiety, depression, anger and other emotional upsets in the home.
- The owner's attitudes and expectations about the illness or disturbance can have a pronounced effect on the outcome.
- Pet illnesses often mirror those of the primary person with whom the pets are bonded.

I have noticed these connections particularly in pets with emotional and behavioral problems, but such patterns often seem to affect chronic physical problems as well.

By paying special attention to emotional issues in the home, it's possible to foster the kind of positive emotional climate that helps a pet maximize its ability to restore and maintain health.

PROBLEMS THAT START AFTER LOSSES

Many animals suffer a loss of attention and/or territory when a baby or a new pet arrives in the home. The same may occur when the family moves (perhaps to a small apartment or to an area with unfriendly neighboring pets). It can happen when someone dies or leaves the home, or when the owner takes a time-consuming job, goes on a long vacation or just loses interest. Or perhaps the house has just been redecorated and the animal is no longer welcome inside.

This loss may soon be followed by a decline in the pet's health. In cases like Bandy's (banished to the outside after the baby was born), boredom and frustration may combine with a pre-existing tendency for skin irritations and lead to excessive licking, scratching and chewing. This, in turn, may aggravate what was only a slight weakness, creating more inflammation and irritation. Before long, a vicious cycle is well underway, with the skin increasingly inflamed and itchy.

Quieter types of pets may react by becoming more lethargic and apathetic. This inactivity and disinterest, in turn, lowers the strength of the immune system, and the pet may become susceptible to an infectious disease.

In yet another scenario some pets may become stressed by territorial conflicts caused by a new animal's presence in the family or even in the neighborhood. If the disputes are not resolved, the constant stress can wreak havoc on the first animal's well-being, once more setting up fertile ground for germinating new health problems.

Problems like these may even be reinforced unintentionally by a well-meaning owner's reactions. Say your dog is feeling lonely because you went back to work and just don't have as much time for him as you used to. Before long, he develops a minor symptom—a cough—that worries you. Every time he coughs you rush over, pet him and murmur comforting words. (This sounds a little bit like dog training, doesn't it?) Pretty soon the dog gets the idea that every time he coughs he gets what he

wants—your loving attention. What incentive is there for him to get well and stop coughing?

Even if you were to scold the dog (as Bandy's owner did for scratching), he could perceive the scolding as a reinforcement of sorts. Even such negative attention, when attention is denied, is preferable to neglect.

Such scenarios are most likely to develop with symptoms such as coughing, limping or scratching that involve some action over which the animal has some control. Veterinarian Herbert Tanzer, author of *Your Pet Isn't Sick (He Just Wants You to Think So)*, has found that teaching owners to stop coddling pets in response to a symptom and to coddle them more at other times has resolved many irksome cases that seemed to have no physical cause.

What to do: Watch for any changes in your pet's psyche that might be because of new household schedules or a family crisis. Animals are individuals just as people are. Some require more attention, social bonding, territory and routine than others. Try to see altered situations at home from your animal's perspective and use your common sense in trying to make adjustments that will ease the situation. Perhaps you simply need to spend some special one-on-one "together" time with each animal; on the other hand, you might have to construct a solid fence to keep out intruding neighborhood dogs. Maybe one person's German shepherd needs daily walks, but just holding and petting a Siamese more often could be all that's required to calm her.

Sometimes the answer lies in confining a new pet to limited space until the "senior" pet accepts the newcomer. With animals that are particularly hostile or territorial toward other animals (especially cats), you might have to remain a one-pet family. However, with highly sociable animals, especially dogs who've just lost an animal companion, you might do well to get a new pet, particularly one of the opposite sex, from a breed noted for its friendly attitude. It could be as difficult as deciding that your animal needs a more suitable home than the one you are able to provide. But then, it could also be as easy as allowing Rover back on his favorite chair and protecting your new upholstery with a towel or blanket.

Resist the temptation to baby your pet or to fuss over him whenever he limps, coughs or scratches. Instead, pet him and play with him more at the times when he's behaving normally. And, of course, take him to the vet for a professional evaluation and give him whatever care he needs.

HUMAN EMOTIONS AND ANIMAL PSYCHES

The well-being of our pets is also affected by our feelings. Most dogs and cats form strong bonds with their owners, the people they depend on for food, shelter, safety and affection. That's why it's especially important for them to tune into our emotional cues. Except for perhaps a few brief verbal commands or names, pets rely completely on the emotional messages communicated by our posture, tone of voice, facial expressions and, well, just plain feelings in the air.

As a result of this connection, pets often seem to soak up angry, sad or fearful feelings from family members who are experiencing tension or conflict over issues that have nothing to do with the animal. Frequent arguments in the home are especially

stressful for a pet, who may react with irritability or fear. Emotional tensions in particular may affect health problems that have either a behavioral component (such as increased aggressiveness, destructiveness or extreme restlessness) or a nervous component (such as irritated skin, ears, bladder and the like). Just as a pet might react to losses (described above), an emotionally stressed animal with a predisposition to skin or bladder problems, for example, might scratch or urinate still more, further irritating the tissues and setting up the conditions for a vicious circle.

Other times, the owner's anxious emotions and expectations can aggravate a pet's existing health problem. Most commonly, an owner becomes upset on first noticing that a family pet is not feeling well. Deeply worried that the condition may worsen or even become fatal, the owners may be afraid of doing something wrong in treatment and losing their dear friend as a result. The animal senses this anxiety. Something must be wrong! The uncertainty only increases the pet's anxiety, which may already be heightened by the discomfort of illness. The animal may even begin to hide. Fearful and stressed, your pet may have a diminished capacity to heal.

Conversely, your calm, positive response to a pet's first symptoms relaxes and reassures the animal, helping to strengthen its immune response. All else being equal, I have observed time and time again that the animals likeliest to recover from chronic and difficult illnesses are those whose owners manage to be calm and maintain a positive outlook. While it may be difficult to find calm in the face of suffering, it's the best thing you can do for your animal.

Besides sending a danger signal to your pet, your anxiety could also hinder treatment. Clients have often told me that in acting from fear or a sense of urgency they made decisions that they later regretted. When animals get tumors or cancers their owners often feel under tremendous pressure to have the growths immediately removed, as though every passing hour were critical. But there is no evidence to support such urgency. In fact, the stress of the surgery can make the animal even more difficult to treat when using less drastic methods. Similarly, the intense scratching that accompanies skin allergies sometimes drives owners to get corticosteroids, which can undo several weeks of progress resulting from nutritional and homeopathic treatment. True healing of chronic disease requires, above all, patience. The desire for immediate relief is very seductive. That's the appeal of using strong drugs to control symptoms. But since they don't actually cure the underlying ailment, the illness recurs, gradually worsening over time or taking a different and more difficult form.

Over-anxiety can also push owners to jump from one veterinarian or treatment to the next, whether conventional or holistic. This can overwhelm and confuse your pet's body, never allowing any one method a chance to work. On the flip side, worry and discouragement can lead owners to give up on medical treatment without really trying.

One final way our psyches may impact our pet's health is something of a mystery. Veterinarians see many cases in which pets develop the same problems as their owners, seemingly beyond coincidence. This could owe to a common toxin or other agent in the environment. But it's also possible that the strong bond between some pets and people can create a kind of sympathetic resonance, akin to "catching" a yawn or the urge to scratch from someone nearby. Many experiments and anecdotes attest to a mysterious, seemingly extrasensory connection between animals and their owners. This could come into play.

What to do: First, don't worry about whether your emotions have affected your pet's health. Even if they may have, it was never intentional. In any case, the best thing from this point forward is to be as relaxed, confident and calm as you can. Whenever you are in an upset state, it is best not to engage in too much interaction with your pet or other family members. Taking a break can give you a fresh perspective. (For some useful tapes and books on coping with common emotional issues, see page 357.)

Don't let yourself be hurried into medical decisions. Give treatments a chance to work and make any changes purposefully and carefully, in cooperation with your veterinarian.

Finally, learn to have faith in the power of healing. Life always seeks to right itself—to close a wound, to lift up our spirits. Try also to accept the fact of death, for it is part of a larger cycle of eternal renewal. After the winters of our lives—all the disappointments, the lows, the losses—spring will always come again.

CHAPTER ELEVEN

NEIGHBORLY RELATIONS: RESPONSIBLE PET OWNERSHIP

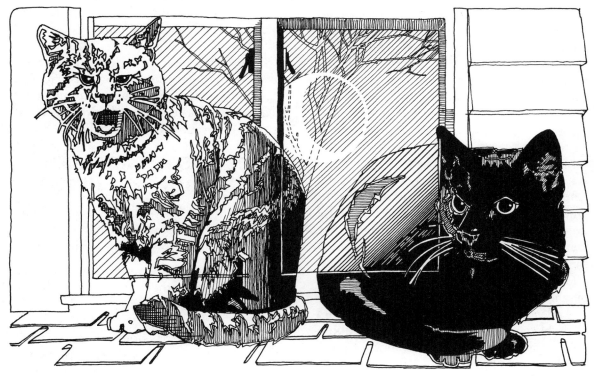

Living with animals can be a wonderful experience, especially if we choose to learn the valuable lessons animals teach through their natural enthusiasm, grace, resourcefulness, affection and forgiveness. In that same spirit, a kind person is very dear to an animal. But when it comes to living habits, the natural tendencies of people and animals often differ widely. To some of us, the joys of an animal's company are well worth the little extra mess or noise that may be part of the package. However, our neighbors may not be as tolerant of muddy pawprints on the car, loud barking in the early morning, dug-up flower beds or extra "watering" of the bushes.

That's why taking responsibility for the impact our dogs and cats have on the rest of

149

the community is one of the most important aspects of our ownership. Whether it's someone else's pet or our own, we all know the unpleasantness of dealing with animals that have not been well-taught or restrained. In fact, a nationwide survey revealed that the number-one citizen complaint made to city governments concerned "dog and other pet control problems."

I recall a neighborhood Doberman who used to bound into my front yard, relieve himself, then run up to my window and bark angrily at me as I sat in my own living room. And how many times have you walked through a parking lot when a big dog suddenly thrust its head through an open car window and barked ferociously, its huge jaws just inches from your face? I think of a veterinarian friend whose hand was painfully mauled by an aggressive dog. And I remember a town I used to live in where packs of roaming dogs used to chase down joggers and bicyclists as though they were prey. Think of the many songbirds that have fallen victim to prowling cats. Such situations often pit neighbor against neighbor, with pets caught in the middle.

And yet if animals could speak, they would probably complain about us humans—about being tied up or locked up too much, for example. Some might growl softly as they reflect on life with a rock 'n' roll fan addicted to top-volume stereo. Pets injured by cars might demand to know why we have to rush around so dangerously. And the millions of pets dropped off at animal shelters by their owners every year might tell how it feels to be abandoned. (Over half of these were given up because of unresolved behavioral problems.)

How can we, as caring and responsible pet owners, address the inevitable conflicts between animals and people? I say start by considering the viewpoints and needs of all concerned—both humans and animals. Often a pet problem results from conflicting views on how animals should behave. For example, a dog owner might think it's most natural, and therefore best, for his dog to roam freely; however, his neighbors think the dog should be confined. In other cases, the owner has definite ideas about how his pet should act—but the *animal's* ideas are different!

So first let's look at various ideas about how companion animals can best fit into human communities. Once we humans are clear on our basic standards, we can work out our differences with our pets.

WHAT IS APPROPRIATE BEHAVIOR FOR PETS?

Certain rules for pet behavior are pretty clear. That's because we apply the same standards to ourselves. We do not permit:

- Jumping on, biting, scratching, chasing, attacking or other aggression (except in defense to real threats).
- Excessive noise.
- Messes or destruction (especially inside the house or on someone else's property).
- Trespassing onto another's territory.

I list these because I've seen owners stand by as their dogs barked threateningly at harmless strangers or relieved themselves on a neighbor's lawn. To excuse such behavior by saying, "Well, dogs will be dogs," is not acceptable. Of course, we can't expect dogs to be just like us, but we *can* expect their owners to control them or at least clean up after them.

Numerous communities have laws that require dogs to be on a leash when not on their own property. But many pet owners resent such interference with their pets' freedom. Well-intended as this attitude toward animals' rights might be, it overlooks the very real problems created by large numbers of dogs and cats on the loose in an environment quite unlike a natural habitat. Completely dependent on humans, these animals exist in our communities in numbers far greater than a natural ecosystem could support. As a result, these animals endanger both the community and themselves in several ways.

- More than a million dogs and cats are killed by cars in the United States annually. Unconfined pets also *cause* thousands of car accidents every year when people swerve or brake to avoid hitting them.
- Every year at least a million people are bitten by dogs in the United States, making dog bites our second most commonly reported public health problem. A survey revealed that people in some areas of Pittsburgh feared being bitten by roaming packs of dogs as much as they feared being mugged. Dogs harass elderly people carrying groceries as well as young children with lunch bags.
- Free-roaming dogs kill or injure wildlife, livestock and other pets. I've treated my share of small dogs and cats chewed up by such packs. The owners of the attacking dogs usually have no idea what the family dog really does on an afternoon romp. Too many cats prowling through a neighborhood can also be a menace to birds, small wildlife and each other.

- Pets excrete a huge amount of body waste into the environment, much of it deposited in public places and on neighbors' lawns. These wastes can transmit harmful organisms to humans through sandbox play and gardening. They can also ruin a good lawn.
- Wandering pets may fall victim to poisons, sometimes intentionally placed. More often they fall victim to their scavenging instincts unavoidably merged with our toxic world—ingesting antifreeze, pesticides, decaying roadkills and bait for wildlife control.
- Others may be kidnapped. Every year in the United States hundreds of thousands of dogs and cats are nabbed and sold to research labs, where they may be subjected to painful experiments. Millions of other lost pets are impounded by animal control agencies. Usually, they are held for several days so that owners may claim them. But if the owner is used to a roaming pet's absences (especially cats), he may not check until it's too late and the animal has been euthanized.
- On the loose, unaltered pets freely follow their mating instincts. Competing males may engage in bloody and occasionally fatal fights. Multiplying far beyond the carrying capacity of either the natural ecosystem or our society, only about one in six of the millions of puppies and kittens born yearly in this country will find a home.

Government attempts to cope with animal control problems are a significant public expense, costing taxpayers many millions of dollars a year—in addition to untold private expenses for injuries, damaged property and protective measures.

Let's look at how to get our animals to understand and agree to some basic behaviors that will enable them to live successfully in the human community. The issues and the solutions differ a bit for dogs and cats, so let's take up each in turn. I'll start with dogs, who are much more apt to cause problems for our neighbors than cats are.

CONTROLLING YOUR DOG

Responsible care of a dog starts with confining him to your property at all times, unless he's under your direct control and supervision. This doesn't mean to just lock him in the house or garage or tie him up outside. Your neighbor's desire for privacy might be satisfied, but your dog's natural needs for attention and exercise would be frustrated. This plan might even backfire, because frustrated and unhappy pets are the ones most likely to develop behavioral problems such as destructiveness or excessive barking. (Some owners have their dogs "debarked"—an operation that removes the vocal cords and which I personally will not perform, since dogs can be taught not to bark excessively.)

Ideally, you should have a securely fenced yard to keep your dog from roaming when he's outdoors. If you tie him to a stake, the chain can tangle, limiting your pet's range and possibly endangering him. Barking and aggression are likely to result. If fencing is impractical, clip his leash to a metal ring that slides along a clothesline or suspended cable. This allows greater freedom of movement with less likelihood of tangling. Or you could construct a large pen. Some people install "Invisible Fence" or other electric

systems that train a dog to stay in its boundaries. However, aggressive dogs have been known to overstep the boundary in response to strong temptations. When your pet is in your yard, be sure to provide a snug shelter or install a pet door that allows him to go in and out of the house at will.

If you don't have a yard, choose one of the breeds that are relatively sedate or small and adapt well to a life spent largely indoors. But many dogs are more naturally active, exploratory and hardy and strongly desire to be outdoors. With such a dog you need to make a commitment to regular, vigorous walks and lots of attention. If that is not possible, the fairest thing may be for you to find your dog a new home that is more suited to his needs.

All dogs do best with daily walks—which are good for you, too! So you must be sure to teach your dog how to behave on an outing. This includes his walking on a leash without pulling you and without jumping on, barking at or chasing any humans or animals encountered on the way. If he is well behaved, you may be able to let your dog loose under your supervision in some areas. (Be sure to bring a scooper and a bag to clean up after him wherever you go.)

Make sure your dog always wears a current license and identification in case he should get loose. If he were to get lost and impounded, a license would be the key to his safe return. Always include a current phone number and address on the tag. People are more willing to help return a lost pet if the owner can be reached easily. A tagged animal also stands a better chance of receiving necessary medical care.

When you're home together, give your pup lots of affection. Most important, build a relationship together that allows you to leave him relaxed and comfortable when you must part. In fact, to have a wonderfully well-behaved dog, you need only to understand a few basic principles about what it takes for him to feel secure and to cooperate fully. From that foundation, you can teach your dog all he needs to know. While a comprehensive training program is beyond the scope of this book, I can present an overview. (For more information on specific issues, refer to "Recommended Reading and Tapes" on page 357.)

WHY WE NEED A WIDE-ANGLE VIEW OF CANINE CULTURE

It's essential to understand the deeper emotional makeup of your pet as a species. Of course, our pets have much in common with us emotionally (one reason we share our lives with them), but each sees the world through its own very different dog or cat senses. Unless we interact with them with these inborn traits in mind, we get limited results or even trigger behavior problems.

With our pets we share a need for affection and for rewarding interactions with other creatures and our environment. If a healthy diet is the foundation for your animal's physical health, a steady "diet" of positive interactions with you and with the world is essential for your pet's psychological health, and the key to a peaceful relationship for both of you. These emotional needs are just as continual and demanding as physical needs. We wouldn't consider letting our pets go unfed for several days at a

time, but an animal's desire for attention often goes unmet for that long.

Social needs are especially important for dogs. Just as some species need a particularly high level of protein in order to thrive, the dog must have a steady diet of happy social encounters. He also needs a clear, trustworthy leader in his immediate family. These two traits evolved strongly in wolves, enabling them to hunt and live together cooperatively, which enhanced their chances of survival. Dogs are not wolves, but they've inherited this need for social order from their ancestors.

Most dog owners have heard about the importance of playing the role of "alpha wolf" in the "pack" that now includes you, your dog and your family. The concept is that every pack of wolves or dogs must have one established leader that looks out after the whole group.

Unfortunately, this useful idea is sometimes misunderstood. The alpha wolf role is misinterpreted as a macho, tough guy in a heavy-handed boss/servant relationship. Few of us had this in mind when we decided to get a dog. We wanted a companion, not a slave. You don't have to dominate your dog (in fact, domination is both unnecessary and possibly even dangerous), but you do have to be a responsible leader.

If you neglect this role of leader or don't make it clear on a consistent basis, you're being unfair to your dog. That's because he will feel compelled to fill the leadership vacancy himself. Since he's a dog living in a human world, it is impossible for him to do this successfully. The normal behaviors of a dog doing his best to lead will get him in all kinds of serious trouble in our society. He may become aggressive to visitors, children, other dogs and even to you. He may bark excessively, run away, not come when called or be overprotective of food, toys or the family car. He may pull on the leash or jump on people.

If we try to correct these behaviors, the dog will get irritated with us because, for subordinates, we are acting way out of line. Then he tries to correct us, and we get more upset—which gets him more upset. Dogs have a strong desire for stability. So when we accidentally signal to a dog that he is to act as a leader, then later reprimand him for doing so, we can upset his mental stability and derail his predictability. Unfortunately, this situation exists in many caring households. Unless we understand the dog's point of view and adapt our efforts to it, things won't improve.

Eternal vigilance is the leader's primary responsibility. He must be concerned with every sound, every stimulus, every change in the environment. When it's clear that someone else is in charge, a dog is apt to go sleep in a corner. But if he's trying to take care of his pack, he notices everything. He'd like to react, to investigate, but he can do very little because he's confined.

Inadequate human leadership can make the family dog more vulnerable to "separation anxiety." This is a discomfort some dogs experience when left alone, and they show it by whining, barking, chewing, digging, pacing, escaping, and urinating and defecating in inappropriate places. The dog is not "getting even" for being left alone. He's just trying to relieve his internal anxiety about being left with the only activities available to him. They give him a temporary respite from tension but, unfortunately, they can easily become habits. Lack of exercise and stimulation, bad diet, poor health, breed characteristics and emotional changes in the family can all contribute to this type of anxiety as well, but a key factor often overlooked is that the dog is confused about leadership roles in the family.

BECOME A POSITIVE LEADER FOR YOUR DOG

So how do you become the good leader your dog needs? Wolf packs succeed best when their members are happy, healthy and in relative harmony with each other. If they were constantly squabbling over their rank, they'd be at a disadvantage for rounding up food. So, to maintain social stability, wolves use ongoing nonviolent signals to remind each other of their standing in the pack.

The need to train your dog provides a perfect context to mimic this repeated posturing and to make your leadership clear to your dog again and again. The idea is to convey to your dog that *he gets what he wants in life when he listens to you first.* You make this work by applying it dozens of times daily, in little ways.

First, make it fun for your dog to watch you for signals. Whenever he sustains eye contact with you, constantly reinforce him with treats, affection and whatever he loves to do (playing ball, going for a walk and so on). Associate it with a command like, "Rover, watch!" Make it fun, and soon the command itself will be enough to get your pet's attention. Once you can get his attention in this way, you're ready to proceed to other lessons.

Next, show the dog in lots of little ways that he must look to you first to get what he wants. If your pet wants to go outdoors, you tell him to wait. You walk out first. Then he gets to go out. If the dog wants to eat, first tell him to sit. When he sits, you feed him. If the animal wants affection, first tell him to lie down and have him stay for 30 seconds. Then you release him with a code word like "okay" and play together. Once the routine gets going, and your pet knows a few simple commands and learns that getting it right earns him lots of praise *plus* the thing he wants, he'll love it.

Every time you tell your dog what to do and he listens, it gently reinforces the idea that you're in charge, so he doesn't need to be concerned. It constantly signals to the dog that you're the leader, and it provides an ongoing supply of the attention he loves. Some dogs will accept this at once, others will put up a struggle about who's top dog. But consistent, daily, enjoyable reminders of your roles will lead to a more relaxed and confident pet.

Make praise and reward the cornerstone of your relationship. Simply by applying the central command to "Watch," you will soon be past the struggling stage in teaching your dog the basics. Learning itself will become an enjoyable game for him. Your pet will eagerly try to figure out what you want so he can do it!

MAKING LEARNING FUN

When you need to correct a misbehavior, always praise your dog as soon as he does the right thing. Show him, if necessary. For example, suppose your puppy jumps up on you when you come home. The limited approach is that you put your knee in his chest or pull down on his collar, saying "Off." With repetition, he'll learn to stop jumping up on you. But if you also praise the animal enthusiastically as soon as his front feet hit the ground, then give a treat, he will be even more interested in playing the learning game. He may jump up on you again, just to get the treat once more. Again, quickly correct the dog and praise him the instant he's back on the floor. After a few times, praise him even when he is "off," but hold back the treat. Tell him to "Sit." Show him how to do it if he doesn't know or is too excited, then give him the treat as soon as he even comes close to getting it right.

Now your dog is really eager to figure this thing out. As he keeps trying, you keep showing him which action has bad consequences and which action has good consequences. If your pet starts to think he's supposed to run up, jump on you and then sit, you'll have to modify the correction to get the "jump up" part out. Eventually the concept will click inside: "Maximum pleasure comes if I run up to my owner and sit." By the time the situation arises again, he may have forgotten how it works, but it will soon come back to him.

It takes many repetitions to teach a dog certain behaviors. That's why showing him what to do and rewarding him when he does it works so much better than merely correcting the pup for misbehavior. When a dog just gets a correction, he usually tries to figure it out for just a short while, and then he goes elsewhere. If he's forced to stay, he'll stop paying attention. Your dog will stick with you in learning if you make the instruction fun, so that every misbehavior becomes an enjoyable opportunity to learn what is expected. Not only will the pup get it right, but it will be ingrained.

Responses to certain commands are fairly

easy to teach once you get into the right mode: Watch, Sit, Stay, Down, Off (no jumping), Wait, Let's Go (walking on a loose leash), Gentle (no biting) and simple tricks like Roll Over.

For example, to teach a dog how to walk on a leash without pulling you, first teach him to place his primary attention on you (the "Watch" game described above). Put him on a leash. Using a pleasant tone, tell the dog, "Rover, watch!" Then say, "Let's go" or "Close" and start walking. Whenever he steps in front of you, focuses his attention elsewhere or pulls away on the leash, repeat the command "Stay close" or "Let's go." As soon as he moves toward you and slacks up on the leash, offer profuse praise and/or a treat. Head off again promptly. If he doesn't respond to the command, give a quick correction with the leash and change the direction you're walking to get his attention. Repeat these steps each time he pulls on the leash. He'll soon learn that a loose leash when walking is a great idea. It can take some high energy and quick reactions on your part to do this at first, but future years of relaxed walks with your dog are well worth it.

Similarly, you can use a reward to train your dog to come when called. Holding a treat that he loves in your hand, tell him, "Look, here's a treat!" While the pup is running to get it, tell him, "Come!" Reward him with the biscuit and plenty of praise. After several weeks of repetition, he'll associate the word "come" with good things, and you'll need to use the treat only occasionally to keep his interest up. Don't, however, be too eager to test out his understanding of "come" in challenging situations. It may take months of practice before he

knows "come" well enough to come when there are strong temptations close by (like another dog to investigate).

There are many resources available to help you with additional specifics of training certain behaviors. "Recommended Reading and Tapes" on page 357 contains several resources I recommend.

ADDITIONAL TIPS FOR TRAINING

Bearing in mind what I have already said, here are some related tips to help you get started or get a fresh start with the pet you already have. Most of these apply to cats as well as to dogs.

Remember that all animals learn by association. In attempting to understand the world around them, dogs build associations. Jumping on the couch is followed closely by a feeling of soft comfort, so an association is built between jumping on the couch and feeling good.

Your animal is constantly learning. The couch consistently rewards his jumping on it with softness and comfort, which encourages more jumping (unless you give another message even more consistently). If your dog runs through a screen door and gets slammed on the nose as it closes, he'll be less likely to try that again.

Be careful about what you teach your animal unintentionally. Our pets learn from all their interactions with us, not just the ones we think of as training. When your nervous dog barks fearfully at something and you pet him to calm him down, you have just unintentionally told him, "Good dog, that was a good response to that situation." Do you want your dog to respond that way all the time? If not, you must tell him so in some other way.

Teach your pet that you're worth learning from. At first your dog will listen to you because your voice is new and interesting. But if you don't capitalize on that initial interest and consistently reinforce his paying attention to you, don't be surprised if your dog starts to tune you out unless you raise your voice or take strong action.

Make it real. Take pleasure in your dog and your role as his teacher and leader. You can't fake it for long. Your dog provides an excellent excuse for you to be enthusiastic, silly, playful and creative. Using treats helps to pique a dog's interest in new things, but unless you link your praise and enthusiasm with this initial motivation, he'll end up responding to food but not to you.

Be clear about what you want and show him exactly what it takes to be a "good dog" in your eyes. You don't want your dog to rush up to visitors and bark at them, but what do you want him to do? A dog will find it much easier to learn "When the doorbell rings, I go and sit quietly on my bed" than the vague concept "I can do anything but rush up at people and bark too many times." The simpler and more consistent the association, the more likely it is to build. Doorbell-bed-sit is much easier than "Anything but. . . ."

Put a beginning and an end on your requests. Called a "release," this important dog training idea often gets neglected in practice. When you teach your dog to stay, watch or heel, teach him that your command continues till you say it's over with a word like "okay." This signals that he now may get up or look away or stop heeling. If you let a command end without a release, he

learns that you're in charge of when things start, but he can decide when they end.

Have high expectations of your dog, but be sure they're reasonable ones. Do expect your pet to listen to you the first time you make a request that he has learned thoroughly. Correct, don't punish, if he doesn't. But don't expect him to make judgment calls. If he's allowed on the couch at home, don't get mad at him if he jumps on the couch at your in-laws'.

Use gentle training aids. There are new halters for dogs that can be especially helpful for gaining control gently. We wouldn't think of trying to lead a horse around by the neck, but that's what we do with dogs.

Individualize your training to suit your dog's temperament. Breeds and individual dogs differ widely in their interest in and responses to training and handling. Is your dog a timid Sheltie or a gregarious Lab? Adapt the intensity and timing of your corrections and praise accordingly. Terriers require lightening-quick responses. Hounds welcome extra enthusiasm. Notice what kind of activity your dog especially loves, such as playing ball or going for a walk, and use that as a reward.

Use repeated cues to help get your point across. To praise your dog, speak in a varied and interesting voice, petting him and showing your affection. To discourage undesired behavior, give timely corrections with a leash and use a no-nonsense tone of voice.

Use proper timing. Always correct your dog *while* he is misbehaving, never after the fact, while he is partially behaving well. He will associate your correction or your praise with what he did a half-second ago, not with what he did or thought before that. For instance, if you scold him as he's taking his sweet time ambling over to you after you've called him, he won't know that you're unhappy about his slowness, he'll just think it's a bad idea to come at all.

Think of training your pet as an exercise in cross-cultural communication. We are a highly verbal species, but dogs are not. You are helping your pet understand the language of the dominant culture (human). To do so, you must try to become at least a little bilingual, taking the time to learn dog (or cat) culture. You may sometimes feel more comfortable interpreting your pet's behavior in human terms than in trying to grasp the perspective of another species. But it will be easier to get past that obstacle if you embrace the challenge of showing your pet how to fit into this world successfully.

Be patient with yourself. You're learning something new, too. Building a solid relationship with your pet is a great investment, and it does take plenty of time and energy. You may feel awkward as you ease into the task. It can be emotionally challenging at times to be firm, patient and clear, or to keep from venting your anger at your pet's mistakes.

Hold on to the deeper parts of your connection with your pet. Don't let your leader role be an obstacle to your companionship. You're not dominating or taking advantage of your dog; you're showing you care enough about him to learn a way to interact that makes his life happier and more successful.

PROBLEM BEHAVIORS IN DOGS: BARKING

Many canine problem behaviors—such as excessive barking, biting, destructiveness, chasing and other aggressive actions—are beyond simple training techniques. Here's where the whole-relationship, whole-environment approach outlined earlier in this chapter is really crucial. Sometimes a simple change will solve a problem. Bringing your dog inside at night may stop his barking. But often, undesirable behaviors are a normal canine response to a confusing environment. Are you giving mixed or unintended messages? Are your pet's important emotional needs being met? Deal with the problem head on as soon as you can. Otherwise, it can be a time bomb that explodes into serious consequences.

The noise that barking dogs inflict on neighbors' ears and nerves is one of the biggest complaints pet owners hear. Just as a considerate person will not play music at full volume or subject the sensitive ears of a pet to loud noise, a pet should not be allowed to make noise that bothers people. Constant barking can drive anyone mad.

If a dog is not well-trained and is barking from aggression or anxiety, it's hard to get him to stop. It's even more difficult as the intensity and emotion of the barking escalates. Remember, yelling at a barking dog is like barking back at him. You may stop him that way for the moment by intimidating him, but the barking problem will persist.

You probably want your dog to bark when visitors or possible intruders arrive on your property, and then to stop barking when assured that things are fine. Dogs can learn to do this, but you'll need to start the training for this early. When unusual noises occur or when strangers approach the house, you can praise your dog for giving two or three warning barks. However, he will also need to know a command like "Quiet," so when you tell him to stop barking, he understands what you expect. You can't wait until the problem situation arises to work on this if you expect results. You must lay the groundwork by setting up situations that allow your dog to learn "Bark" and "Quiet" under relaxed circumstances, not with the pressure both of you feel when a real visitor arrives. If your dog is accustomed to learning from you, this is not difficult. Even if he has already learned to bark non-stop, you can teach him to replace it with something better by commanding "Chew on your bone" or "Go find your toy." Only when he knows you're in charge is he likely to let you handle the situation. If he's barking because he thinks that's what you want, and he has learned a command for "that's enough," then he'll probably stop when you tell him to be quiet.

PREVENTING DOG BITES

Dog bites can be serious business. Every year a handful of Americans, mostly small children, are killed by family pets or neighbors' dogs. United States medical personnel treat at least a million dog-bite cases annually, ranging from nips on the ankle to mutilation requiring stitches or reconstructive surgery. It's true that vicious bites come mostly from guard dogs and roaming dog packs; however, the majority of dog bites come from animals known to their victims, dogs that have a reputation for being "nice." Your own child could be the victim of such a dog, perhaps even of your own pet.

There are many causes of canine aggression. Problems can often be traced to an inconsistent leadership or an overly emotional home. Other factors that can lead a dog to bite are: too little exercise, violent treatment,

teasing, failure to correct dogs that nip you in play, too much confinement, physical discomfort from aging or injury, poor breeding and minimal human contact during puppyhood (more likely for dogs from puppy mills). Also, chronic encephalitis underlies many canine behavior problems, including aggression. This condition is an inflammation of the central nervous system from vaccine reactions or auto-immune disease (see "Vaccinations" on page 321).

You should prevent your dog from endangering strangers by keeping it inside or secured behind a fence, or else under your control on a leash. If your dog is left alone in a yard with a fence that a neighbor child can reach through, talk to local parents, urging them to make sure their children understand possible dangers. (If necessary, put up a warning sign.)

Watch for subtle warning signs of a problem and take them very seriously. Many people mistakenly deny that their dog poses a potential danger, either because they see it as an insult to the dog or themselves or because they don't know how to solve the problem. Their dog might have actually snarled or bit at someone, but they make excuses—he was startled or had his tail stepped on, for example. Such aggressive reactions tend to get worse, not better, especially in older pets. Don't wait to react. Think how you'd feel if you ignored the problem and a child's face were bitten.

Play it safe. The guidelines that follow should reduce the risk of dog bites from your own dog as well as someone else's. Make sure your children understand and follow them.

First, learn these tips on how to avoid provoking a dog.

Don't disturb a dog while it's eating or sleeping. If your leadership with your own dog is clear, you should be able to take his food. But if there is any doubt, don't try.

Do not intrude upon the private territory of a restrained or confined dog. Neutral territory, like a park, is usually much safer for any interaction.

Never tease a dog by dangling food or toys over its head. A playful nip can easily get out of control.

Stop hugging or holding a pet that wants to be free. He may feel he has to fight (bite) to get away.

Teach children to avoid stray dogs completely. Also, it's dangerous to pet a strange dog walking with its owner, unless you ask the owner if it's safe. The dog might be a watchdog trained to attack.

Do not scream and wave your hands around dogs. Children who do this when scared or excited can unintentionally provoke aggressive dogs.

Once you know how to avoid provoking a dog, it's also helpful to know how to mollify a dog that approaches you in a threatening manner. You can tell from a dog's body language whether he means serious business or just wants to engage in some rough-and-tumble play.

A friendly dog avoids direct eye contact, looks to the side, perhaps exposes his throat and even grins. He keeps his ears flat, tail tucked down and body low. If his head is lower than his tail, but he is crouching, pouncing or thrusting about, he's probably just playing and is not a threat.

Be on the lookout for signs of a potentially dangerous dog: ears raised up and forward, teeth bared in a snarl and hair raised on the shoulders and rump. Even more threatening signs: becoming stiff-legged, raising a front leg, urinating, growling, staring you in the eye and slowly waving a high, arched tail.

An animal that bites out of fear may give mixed messages, so read the whole animal carefully and avoid threatening any dog that acts wary of you. Unfortunately, some dogs attack without any of these warning signs. Some Shar-peis, pit bulls and chows are especially notorious in this way, endangering even experienced animal handlers.

If a dog runs at you, stay calm. Turn partially sideways and speak in a soothing voice. Keep your head slightly lowered and your hands down. This conveys peaceable intentions. Do not face the dog head on or stare it in the eye. Do not turn and run unless you are certain of reaching safety. The dog tends to see a running creature as escaping prey. Some veterinarians and animal handlers confound threatening animals they must approach by whistling softly or calling in a friendly tone.

If a dog chases you on your bike, slow down and speak soothingly. Get off your bike if you can, on the side away from the dog. Walk at an unhurried pace, without turning your back to the dog.

If a dog should bite you, stay calm. A scream may provoke the attacker further. Try to put an object (like a purse, newspaper, book or jacket) near his mouth that will give him something besides you to bite. Wash the wound with soap and water. Call your doctor for advice. Report the incident right away to the public health department and establish the dog's identity if you can.

When two dogs fight, get out of the way.

If you feel safe at a distance or behind a barrier, the best way to break up a fight is to turn a hose on both dogs.

CONTROLLING AND TRAINING CATS

There's general agreement that dogs should not be allowed to wander (it's the law in many cities). But the attitude toward cats is somewhat different, leading some people to keep their cats indoors and others to let them out. Here are some of the main things to consider in making your decision.

Cats cause less harm to people or property outdoors. They mostly endanger themselves, each other (from accidents, dogs, cat fights, transmission of feline leukemia virus) and small wildlife. Most people welcome their natural tendency to kill mice, rats and gophers.

If allowed outdoors, cats can't be confined by a fence and most cannot be walked on a leash. Unlike dogs, cats resist training. They come "as is." Their natural behavior is pretty much what you get.

They use gardens and children's sandboxes as litter boxes. This can be a considerable nuisance and even a public health problem. A cat afflicted with toxoplasmosis can pose a risk to pregnant women gardeners, who may become infected with the organism via buried feces (see below).

Indoor life generally suits cats better than dogs. That's because cats are less active, less social, normally sleep more and take readily to using a litter box. Some cats actually seem to prefer living indoors.

Many people who live in apartments, in congested urban areas, near busy roads or in areas frequented by packs of dogs or coyotes keep their cats inside as a safety measure. With proper care many cats live indoors contentedly, especially the more home-loving breeds—Korats, Persian longhairs, Bombays, Angoras and ragdolls. Be sure to offer an indoor cat plenty of attention, toys and a nice shelf by a sunny screened window. If you're away a lot, consider getting a second cat as company for the first. Persian longhairs, Himalayans and Kashmirs tend to be most sociable and are least apt to fight with other cats.

Some cats have an instinctive love of the outdoors. As a group, outdoor cats are hardier, better hunters and more active. These include shorthairs, Abyssinians, Somalis and Maine coon cats. While they can adapt to indoor life, especially with a good window spot or screened porch, they really prefer an occasional romp in a garden. If you live in a fairly safe neighborhood (low traffic, no aggressive animals on the loose, no neighbor houses full of sickly cats), I feel it's often wise to allow a cat some freedom. This choice may mean a shorter life (there is always the risk of injuries from traffic or from other animals), but it may be a more satisfying one for the cat.

If it seems too dangerous to let your cat roam outdoors, there are a couple of safer ways to give your cat a taste of nature. The first is to build a fully enclosed pen (called a cattery), which could be constructed to connect with a window that opens onto your backyard. (Avoid the use of preservative-treated wood, which can make cats sick.) The other option, which works for a few cats (especially the Siamese-type breeds), is to take your cat for an occasional walk on a leash and harness.

If you do allow your cat to wander outside at times, here are some guidelines.

Spay or neuter your cat. This will reduce fights and spraying and address the pet overpopulation problem as well.

Confine your cat at any sign of disease. It's especially important to keep your cat indoors and separate from other cats if it has a contagious disease.

Teach your cat to come when called. Repeat her name often when you are playing together or feeding her. Ring a bell or whistle just before feeding her dinner. Call her frequently, offering a tidbit of her favorite food. Praise her and give her lots of affection when she responds. Soon she will associate pleasant things with coming when she's called, and she may begin to associate the bell or whistle with feeding time.

Be sure your cat is wearing a collar and identification tag with your name and phone number on it. Soft leather or nylon collars are the most comfortable. To avoid the danger that she'll get her collar caught on something, fit your cat with the special quick-release type that automatically opens with sufficient pressure on the collar. Attach a bell to the collar to warn birds.

It is safest for your cat to keep her in after the evening feeding. Cats are more apt to get into fights or get hit by cars at night.

Invite your neighbors to let you know if your cat is causing problems for them. If you get such reports, take responsibility for your cat's behavior and do what's needed to rectify the situation.

Be prepared to break up occasional cat fights. If you catch two felines staring each other down, a loud clap of the hands will usually cause one or both to back off. If the fur is already flying, splash water on the combatants.

Regardless of whether you let your cat outdoors or keep it inside, you need to teach it to accept a carrier. A few days before your cat's first visit to the veterinarian, place an open carrier out in the house. Encourage the cat to view it as a fun place to explore. To entice him further, place a tidbit inside. Without this familiarity, you could have a battle on your hands trying to shove a resistant cat into a cage on your way out the door to the vet's.

CAT BEHAVIOR PROBLEMS

What's called good behavior in a cat varies greatly from household to household. If you allow your cat to sleep on your neck, wake you up at 4:00 A.M. for breakfast and walk on the countertops, that's pretty much your business. It won't affect your neighbors.

However, it could take its toll on you and your home. Most cat behavior problems veterinarians see involve inappropriate urination and defecation (for example, spraying or not using the litter box). Others involve aggression, usually toward other cats, but sometimes even to the owner, excessive fearfulness or fussiness and scratching furniture. Let's look at some of these.

Begin by bearing in mind how life looks from your cat's point of view. Like humans and dogs, most cats enjoy affection and attention, but their primary focus in life really revolves around having a comfortable, safe environment with food and a sunny place to sleep. Cats want to secure these things for themselves, and since you're the source of food, that means you, too.

In nature most cats are loners and must fend for themselves in adult life. They must keep constant tabs on their world and make sure other cats don't intrude on their hunting range, which can only provide limited support of carnivores. They spend much of their lives watching and waiting, dozing, but keeping an eye out for passing prey (or predators). Cats need to know their territory well and all that's going on there. They like predictability. And they like cleanliness (smells are dead giveaways to prey).

Some of the most troublesome cat problems can be resolved if you take on a feline attitude. For example, when cats urinate and defecate outside the litter box, they are usually unhappy about something in the environment. It's a cat's way of expressing agitation, not a personal message to you. Inappropriate elimination often means the litter box is not clean enough or the particular litter that's used is not to their liking. Some longhaired cats get upset because the dirty litter gets in their fur. Sometimes the cat is just reacting to a change of litter box location, which is best done in a gradual manner. Certain cats just seem to want a more vertical surface, a problem that may be solved by propping a second litter box on its side, inside the main horizontal one. One of my clients has solved this problem by setting up a piece of plexiglass at one side of the litter box (any rigid washable material would do). She then drapes a small terrycloth towel over it, which her cat seems to prefer, and washes it frequently.

If your cat is spraying (the way cats mark territory), it can mean that he is disturbed by recent adjustments in his life and surroundings—a new person in the household, a more anxious attitude from you because of stress, or a move to a new home. A very common cause of agitation can be the presence of a new cat, even if it's just in the neighborhood. Inappropriate elimination may also signal chronic health problems such as allergies.

Many other problems are a matter of proper training, and you can apply similar principles to those discussed for dogs. If you don't want your cat to jump on your counter, scratch your couch, get on your lap when you're at a table or a desk, bat at you when she's hungry or wake you early in the morning, you can usually head off these problems if you nip them in the bud. It's best to decide on your limits from the beginning, then enforce them consistently. Say "No" and gently but firmly push her away, shove her off or put her out for a while. Never yell at, scold or strike your cat; it will frighten her and she will avoid you or your touch. If a situation seems to require serious discouragement, try a spray bottle. Draping plastic over a couch or chair leg for a time will reduce its appeal, especially if you place a scratching post nearby.

Act when she first starts the behavior, and, if you're consistent, the behavior will not build. If you let things slide, it can be very difficult to retrain a cat out of a bad habit. Unlike dogs, cats don't get as involved with you and your enthusiasm and praise, which makes cats much less interested in the training game.

It also helps to remember that both cats

and dogs are gamblers. Research shows that if they are positively rewarded for a behavior as few as 1 time in 20 tries, they may continue the behavior. They're willing to gamble on the reward despite the long odds. This is what you're up against in trying to get a cat to change its behavior. If you don't want kitty on the counter, but every once in a while when she gets up there she finds food, that jackpot will motivate her to try again at least another 15 or 20 times. On the other hand, negative consequences (being pushed away, told "No," squirted, finding an uncomfortable piece of plastic) often have to be much more consistent to condition an animal.

Because of this, your training efforts are even better spent in making sure your animal is never "rewarded" for undesirable behaviors. Keep food off the countertop. Don't pick your cat up to remove her from the counter, admonishing her sweetly and scratching her affectionately in the process. Avoid the temptation to say "Yes" now and then when you really should say "No."

Another effective technique is to channel your animal's behavior into a rewarding direction. Give her a treat whenever she earns it. Or consistently greet her with affection when she jumps on your lap in appropriate times and places, like when you're stretched out in your easy chair in the evening. Provide her with an appealing scratching post (see below) and some toys for pouncing. Most cats behave much better if you create suitable outlets for their energy.

Sometimes a cat trains itself into a bad habit and the "untraining" job falls to you. Be ready to call on any tool available to you—psychology and physiology included—

to get the job done. One common problem that can take months to untrain is the cat who wakes her owner early in the morning to be fed. If you respond, the cat is likely to waken you earlier and earlier. The next thing you know, it's happening in the middle of the night.

You can thwart this problem early on if you start a new habit of feeding your cat later in the morning and you stick to it. However, her body clock is still used to the early habit, and even if you stop feeding your cat until later, she'll be restless and anxious from hunger. To reverse the trend, you'll have to move the feeding time, gradually later and later, over a period of weeks or even months until you reach the time that works best for you.

SCRATCHING AND BITING: WHAT TO DO

A common training problem with cats is teaching them not to scratch your carpets, drapes and furniture. The best solution is to "reward" your cat for appropriate behavior by providing a scratching post that beats anything else. Pet stores carry scratching posts or you can order an excellent one by mail (see "Other Useful Pet Supplies" on page 354). The best ones are covered in natural sisal rope, which many cats enjoy scratching. Rub a little powdered catnip into it occasionally to make it irresistible.

To make your own post, nail an untreated 4 × 4 (2 to 3 feet tall) to a base of ½-inch plywood about 16 inches square. Then wrap the post with sisal rope or a piece of carpeting turned inside out to expose the rough side (posts with soft coverings are not sufficiently attractive to most cats). For maximum stability, lean the post up against the corner of a room or tilt it on its side. Make sure the post is secure. If it falls over and frightens your kitty even once, it may be enough to make her avoid the post altogether.

If your cat needs instructions on the use of a scratching post, simply lay it sideways and place her on top of the post. Scratch the post yourself with one hand and use the other to firmly stroke her neck and back (that will stimulate the urge to scratch). Don't try to push your cat's feet against the post, as cats will resist force. If your pet is still inclined to scratch at the furniture or drapes at times, move the drapes or the chair slightly and put the post in that spot. Move the post gradually and put the furniture back when the cat is actually using the post instead. You may need to cover a corner of the couch or roll up the drapes temporarily until your cat makes the transition. It's often good to position the scratching post near the spot where your cat sleeps, since many cats like to stretch and scratch on waking from a nap.

Declawing your cat is *not* a suitable solution to scratching problems. It is a painful and difficult operation that many veterinarians refuse to do. In fact, it's the equivalent of removing the first joint of all your fingers. It can impair a cat's balance, weaken it (from muscular disuse) and cause a cat to feel nervous and defenseless. The resulting stress can lower your pet's immunity to disease and make it more likely to be a biter.

It *is* helpful to trim your cat's claws. Because they are shaped like a scythe, their very tip is the part that does the most dam-age. A cat will slide that curved tip behind a loop of upholstery fabric and pull its foot straight back—snapping the loop. If the cat makes a practice of this, your sofa will soon look like it needs a shave.

The nail tip is also the part that so easily punctures the skin. It can be removed with ordinary nail clippers. (Be sure to clip only the very tip, or you'll hurt the cat.) Wait until your cat is relaxed, perhaps taking a nap in your lap. To extend a claw for clipping, press your index finger on the bottom of her foot while pressing with your thumb just behind the base of the nail at the top of the foot. Press *gently*. The claw will slide from its sheath so that you can get at it with the clippers you're holding in your other hand. You may get to cut only two or three claws in a single sitting, but you can try again later.

Here's another piece of advice about claws. Never let a cat or kitten scratch your bare hands—even in play. If you do, the animal will think it's okay to bite and scratch you and won't understand that he can hurt you. So when playing games like "pounce on the prey," use a toy or a piece of cord. Save your hands for stroking and holding.

If your cat has developed a habit of clawing or biting at you, you can break it fairly easily by consistently following a method described by Anitra Frazier in her book *The New Natural Cat*. If the claws are in you, relax and calmly disengage them by first pushing the feet a bit forward. To get out of a bite grip, relax and press your arm or hand *toward* the teeth (which confuses the cat). Then put the cat away from you with a gentle but firm message of disapproval and disappointment. To underline the message, ignore her for several minutes. Don't even look at her. A few repetitions are usually all that is needed for a cat to learn that if she wants to play with you, it's not acceptable to claw and bite. Thereafter, she will respect your wishes.

To avoid more serious contact with cat teeth and claws, which are quite sharp, never try to hold on to a cat that wants to be free (unless you are trained in handling cats properly). Teach children this point, too. If you must restrain a cat to give it medicine, wrap it firmly in a towel or blanket. To transport it, use an animal carrier. (I know of more than one serious accident caused by a frightened cat bounding loose in a moving car.)

A few cats have a more deep-seated problem with aggression. I'm talking about cats that are completely, violently intolerant of all other cats, even their own adult offspring. And once in a while, I've treated cats that are pretty nasty to their owners, too. Over the years I've come to the conclusion that many of these problems are more rooted in the constitutional makeup of certain cats than in situations.

Chronic disease can also play a role in such behavior problems. In many cases, careful, individualized homeopathic treatment has helped. Cats that are unusually timid or aloof for no apparent reason have also responded to this treatment.

GOOD SANITATION: A BASIC NECESSITY

Sanitation is an important issue for both dogs and cats; it's right at the top of the initial training agenda.

For puppies, the most painless house-breaking takes advantage of two things, a pup's natural cleanliness and the regularity of his bowels. Well-socialized pups go outside of their own den to soil. It's not reasonable to expect a young puppy to understand that your whole house is his den.

When mistakes are made in the house, a pup has usually run into another room (outside the den to him) to go. So set your pup up for success. For his first few weeks, confine him to a crate or very small room in the house at all times that you're not directly involved in playing with or watching him. Feed him on a regular schedule and take him outside a few minutes after each meal and nap. When you put him outside to relieve himself, go with him to make sure that he goes. Praise him when he does. Afterward, let him run around a bit indoors. Then put him back in his crate or room to sleep. Gradually, expand the size of the area you call his den—include uncarpeted areas first, just in case he makes a mistake. If he does, don't scare him and don't punish him, just take him outside. Then back up your training a day or two and shrink the size of the area he can roam in until he's doing well again.

If you have to work all day, you may need to have someone else come in to let him out, or else train him to use papers when he's young and then switch to outside only as he becomes able to hold his bowels longer. Don't expect a young pup to be able to go more than four to six hours at most without a pit stop. Do still keep him confined to a small area while you're gone. For a young pup this space should be at least the size of a large dog's kennel and no bigger than a very small kitchen.

Animals instinctively seek to relieve

themselves away from their own living area, which is why the neighbor's yard is often a favorite bathroom. You can wean a dog away from this habit and save a major part of your own lawn, too, by teaching him to use just a certain portion of your yard, such as behind the garage or near certain shrubs. Place some of his stool there and take him to that spot when it's time for him to answer nature's call. When he uses the spot, praise him enthusiastically. Placing some kind of low border around the area can help to make its limits clear to him and to friends and family.

When you're walking your dog on stormy days or in cold weather, you naturally want him to do his business A.S.A.P. Some people choose to put command words like "hurry up" with the act of defecating or urinating. This may sound funny, but it can be very useful. On cold or rainy days, this command can actually encourage your dog to go.

To discourage defecation in certain areas of the yard or garden, promptly remove droppings from areas you don't want the dog to soil. If necessary, spray those areas with a dog-repelling deodorant made with natural ingredients like citron, lemon oil, eucalyptol, geranium oil, capsicum and oil of lavender.

Dispose of accumulated pet wastes regularly. Though I don't recommend composting them because temperatures may not be high enough (140°F) to kill harmful organisms, you might consider using a small mechanism made especially for dog and cat wastes, known as the Doggie Dooley. Buried in the ground, it works like a small septic tank (see page 354).

Both the danger of spreading disease and simple common decency dictate that you clean up any solid wastes your dog may deposit on someone's lawn or in public places. Various types of scoop gadgets make it convenient to pick up and dispose of droppings. Though it may not be the most pleasing chore in the world, it certainly won't be any better for the person down the street. If you think of animal wastes in the same category as human wastes, it makes your responsibility for cleanup much clearer.

For cats it's usually a simpler matter. Just provide a full, clean box of litter. Cats prefer litter of a sandy, granular type. Keep it clean and keep it in the same place. Too much odor or too much change could put your cat off. Keep a clean litter box in your yard as well as in your house, and the cat will have something else to use besides Mrs. Jones's flower bed. Keep the boxes out of reach of toddlers and clean them regularly. Wash your hands well afterward because cat feces can carry potentially harmful organisms. (This is a good practice to follow after a dog cleanup, too.)

UNDERSTANDING AND PREVENTING ANIMAL / HUMAN DISEASES

A vital aspect of responsible pet ownership is working to prevent the spread of disease from pets to humans. Many public health authorities see these diseases as a serious problem. The most effective measure is prevention—through careful sanitation practices, avoiding bites and scratches and keeping your pet healthy. Reasonable precautions will minimize the spread of disease.

Most diseases picked up from cats and dogs fall into three groups depending on their means of transmission (through feces or urine, skin and hair contact or bites and scratches) and, therefore, their means of control. Let's consider each group individually.

DISEASES TRANSMITTED IN WASTES

Roundworms *(Toxocara canis, Toxocara cati):* The infectious form of these worms are their eggs, which incubate for several weeks in the ground where an animal has defecated. If a child plays there and puts his dirty hands in his mouth, he can swallow the eggs and become infected. Thus, migrating animal roundworms are most often seen in toddlers. The disease is only rarely fatal. More commonly it is mild and long-lasting.

When children swallow these common parasites carried by dogs and cats, the parasites often migrate through the body tissues and cause damage, including liver enlargement and fever. These symptoms may last as long as a year. In some children the larvae may enter the eye and cause inflammation. This is serious business, since surgeons have been known to mistake the eye lesions for early cancer and unnecessarily remove an eye.

Hookworms *(Cutaneous larva migrans):* These parasites are similar to roundworms, but they enter the body differently. Infectious larvae of the cat and dog hookworm directly penetrate the skin where it comes in contact with feces-contaminated soil or sand. Though the parasites try their best, they are not really suited to living in people and eventually die after moving several inches under the skin. The inflammation is called creeping eruption and eventually ends after several weeks or months. In the United States it is most often seen in the South.

Leptospirosis: Swimming in or otherwise coming in contact with water contaminated with animal urine is the way this serious bacterial disease is usually acquired. Many animals can carry it, particularly rats. Pets can catch it by drinking contaminated surface water (or licking it off their fur) or by eating food on which rats have urinated. In humans the disease is similar to flu, with fever, headache, chills, tiredness, vomiting and muscular aches. In addition, the eyes and the membranes covering the brain and spinal cord can be inflamed. In some cases the liver and the kidneys are damaged. Few die from this condition, but it can make you miserably sick for two or three weeks.

Tapeworms *(Dipylidium caninum):* Pets can pick up the common tapeworm by biting at and swallowing fleas or eating gophers, which can carry the infectious form. Children can get tapeworms either by ingesting fleas while nuzzling the pet's fur or being licked on the mouth by an animal with a flea on its tongue. Human infestation is rare, however, compared with infestations of other types of tapeworms we can get from eating undercooked infected beef or pork.

Toxoplasmosis: Many people are exposed to this infectious disease through ordinary activity and develop a natural resistance to it. On rare occasions, however, it has killed adults. More often, it causes birth deformities in children born to women infected for the first time during pregnancy, before they have developed immunity. It can be picked up by contact with feces from an infected cat or with contaminated soil. Also, the disease can come from eating raw or undercooked meat. Because the fetus of a pregnant woman can be very vulnerable, this problem is covered in detail under "Toxoplasmosis" on page 315.

PREVENTION OF DISEASES TRANSMITTED IN WASTES

Besides cleaning up your pet's droppings, there are a few simple precautions you should take and should teach your children.

- Wash your hands after contact with soil where an animal may have relieved itself.
- Avoid going barefoot in areas where an animal may have relieved itself, particularly in warm climates, where hookworms flourish.
- Remind children to wash their hands before eating and not to put their hands in their mouths while playing with animals or on potentially contaminated grounds. Teach them all other precautions as well.
- If your dog has gone swimming or wading in a pond or creek that could be harboring leptospirosis, give it a bath.

DISEASES FROM SKIN AND HAIR CONTACT

Fleas: Though fleas prefer feasting on pets, they will make a meal of people if the opportunity appears. Flea infestation is often at its worst in a house that was formerly occupied by an animal and then left vacant. Many young fleas, recently hatched, will be eager to eat.

Ringworm (*Microsporum canis*): Caused by a fungus that eats skin and hair, ringworm often shows up in humans as circular, scaly, red areas. As the organism grows, it spreads outward in a circle much as a ripple forms when a stone is dropped into a pond. In dogs, affected areas tend to be hairless, thickened, scabby and irritated. They are typically disk-shaped and about an inch or more in diameter. But most ringworm transmitted by pets comes from cats, who tend to show very few observable symptoms (dogs can also carry the spores without showing visible signs). An infected cat may have hairless gray areas without inflammation or scabbing. Generally, the animal doesn't itch either.

Children are more susceptible to ringworm than adults, though humans can get it at any age. The disease is on the rise and is now the most common fungal disease reported.

Rocky Mountain spotted fever (*Rickettsia rickettsii*): While usually not fatal to humans (it is commonly treated with antibiotics), this infectious disease can still make a person mighty sick. Starting suddenly with fever, headache, chills and reddening of the eyes, it may last several weeks. In the eastern and central United States the responsible organisms are carried by the dog tick (*Dermacentor variabilis*). In the West they are borne by the wood tick (*Dermacentor andersoni*). Incidence of the disease has risen sharply in North America in recent times.

The most common means of contracting spotted fever is from a direct bite by an infected tick. Pets can readily transport these infected ticks into a house or yard, where people can later be bitten. (All the tick's young will carry the infection, too.) It also is possible to become infected while pulling a tick off your animal if the tick's body is crushed or its feces are released. So it's safest to wear gloves when you remove ticks.

Scabies *(Sarcoptic mange):* In dogs this form of mange is less common than the demodectic ("red") mange. However, it does occur in both dogs and cats and causes itching, irritation and thickening of the skin. People can be infected by contact—usually from holding an afflicted animal close. The result is intense itching, especially at night, and in those areas that were most in contact with the animal (like the inside of the arm, the waist, chest, hands and wrists). Though the animal mange mite can live in human skin, it cannot reproduce there. So eventually the problem ends on its own, if reinfection does not occur. Note that we humans have our own brand of scabies mites, which can cause us prolonged aggravation.

PREVENTION OF DISEASES FROM SKIN AND HAIR CONTACT

A healthy animal is less likely to harbor parasites like fleas, ringworm and mange mites. Therefore, proper nutrition and overall care are important preventive measures for both of you. In addition, frequent grooming and inspection, along with herbal repellents, will catch most of these problems early. Be especially attentive when your animal has been in contact with other pets or is under stress from disease, emotional upset or a stay in a kennel.

Nuzzling and hugging animals can be great fun, but if you like to do a lot of this, you take your chances whether your animal may carry these diseases. Wash your hands after prolonged contact. Minimize contact with animals that may have ringworm. Also, since stray hairs can carry active ringworm spores, too, keep the house clear of hairs if your animal is infected (or keep your pet outside until the problem is cured). Avoid or minimize bodily contact with an animal with mange and do not let it sleep on your bedding, clothes or towels.

DISEASES CAUSED BY BITES AND SCRATCHES

Cat scratch fever: After being scratched by a cat, some people develop a fever, malaise and enlarged lymph nodes near the area of the scratch or bite. These symptoms usually occur one to two weeks after the injury. The condition is not serious or fatal, but it is uncomfortable and may be followed by complications. Nobody knows what causes it. A cat bite infected with the bacteria *Pasteurella multocida* looks similar and should be differentiated from cat scratch fever by your doctor.

Rabies: Everyone has heard of this disease and of its high fatality rate (essentially 100 percent once the clinical signs appear). Caused by a virus transmitted through the saliva of a biting animal, it travels from the bite area to the brain in a matter of days or weeks. There it causes severe tissue inflammation that has symptoms such as convulsions, hysteria and frothing at the mouth. The most common sources of human exposure are skunks, foxes, raccoons, bats and dogs, though theoretically almost any warm-blooded creature can acquire the disease and transmit it.

The animal with clinical signs of rabies shows peculiar or erratic behavior. For instance, a wild animal may approach humans or be sluggish and unable to dodge a speeding car. A dog may show evidence of a personality change—acting friendlier than usual or hiding in dark places. Eventually, a staggering, glazed-eyed, aggressive condition may develop—the stereotype of the rabid dog.

PREVENTION OF DISEASES CAUSED BY BITES AND SCRATCHES

The best way to prevent cat scratch fever is to be cautious when handling cats, as suggested earlier. However, cats are not always predictable and might turn on you suddenly when frightened or ill. After a scratch or bite, encourage the wound to bleed for a minute or two to help flush it out. Then wash the wound well with soap and water and soak it in a hot Epsom salts solution. Alternate the hot soak with a soak in some cold tap (not ice) water, going back and forth several times to stimulate blood flow and immune response. Do your final soak in the cool water.

Stray dogs or wild animals should never be handled unless you have special training or equipment to do so safely. If you see a dog or wild animal with symptoms resembling rabies, get away from it and phone an animal control agency or the police as soon as possible. One complication is that a dog can transmit rabies through a bite (or saliva-contaminated scratch) three days *before* any clinical signs appear. So if you're bitten by any stray or wild animal, get help, and try to follow the animal to learn where it lives so it can be caught and tested. If necessary, you might try to catch a small creature like a bat or a skunk, using a bucket, tub or dog carrier. If you must kill it, don't injure the head. It is needed for diagnosis. The testing procedure begins by putting a live animal in quarantine for ten days, during which time it is observed by a veterinarian. If rabies symptoms develop, the animal is killed and the brain sent to a lab for verification.

If you are bitten by an animal that's a stranger to you or by one you suspect might be rabid, follow the same procedure as for cat scratches and bites. Also, report to your doctor as soon as possible. Your chances of getting rabies are really very low. About 35,000 Americans require rabies postexposure treatment annually. Only about 30 percent of untreated people bitten by animals known to be rabid actually get the disease. Dog bites account for less than 5 percent of the rabies cases in North America.

THE PET POPULATION PROBLEM

Finally, one of the most important ways to be a responsible pet owner is to ensure that your animal does not add to the burgeoning pet overpopulation problem.

Spaying your female pet will keep packs of males from invading your property every time she comes into heat and will keep her in better health as well. The chance of her getting breast cancer is reduced and you won't have to worry about pyometritis (an infected uterus).

Neutering a male will reduce his desire to roam and fight, which your neighbors will appreciate. Moreover, that one simple procedure in a cat will spare you years of trying to remove the offensive odor of tomcat urine from your house.

Why do people allow their pets to breed when there are already too many being born? They believe:

◆ Their children should witness the process.
◆ They can find homes for the litter, or

they assume the local humane society will do the job.

- ◆ A spay or neuter operation is expensive, painful and holds possible adverse health effects.
- ◆ Neutering a pet is unnatural and takes away a pet's true self.
- ◆ It's easy and fun to make a little extra cash selling purebred offspring.

Yet when you consider the vast suffering that befalls unwanted, homeless dogs and cats, these reasons have little merit. For example, it is surely more important to teach children responsibility to animals in general than it is to bring more surplus pets into the world as "an experience" for the children. Humane societies cannot find homes for most of the animals they receive. And even if the owner can find homes for the animals he breeds, how many pets will be kept? And how many offspring will *they* produce? If she and her descendants are allowed to breed freely, one female dog can be the source of thousands of animals in just five or six years. Cats are even more prolific. And assuming you are able to find good, responsible owners for each puppy or kitten, consider that these people might otherwise have adopted animals that were destroyed for want of homes.

Anyone who can afford to provide decent care for a pet can also afford a spay or neuter operation. Many towns and cities have low-cost clinics. Ask your local humane society for information about these. The operation is painless, performed under anesthesia by skilled veterinarians and involves very little risk. It not only prevents unwanted births and discourages straying and fighting among the animals, but it prevents health problems like cancers of the reproductive organs, stress and complications from breeding, and abscesses and injuries from mating. Contrary to popular belief, neutered pets do not automatically get fat. Because they may be less active, they may burn less energy. So the solution is just to feed less.

If you are extremely conscientious, the old-fashioned methods of animal birth control, the door and the leash, may work for a female dog. Lock her up securely inside your house during the two- to three-week period of her heat. Be prepared for the fact that male dogs for miles around are likely to gather on your doorstep.

Confinement does not work for cats. They come into heat more often than dogs, they can be very vocal and they are very persistent in trying to get out. They almost inevitably succeed at some point. You should also know that an unspayed female cat prevented from mating will often develop hormonal imbalances from complications caused by not completing the reproductive cycle.

The idea that keeping pets intact reproductively is best because it's "more natural" is very short-sighted. We don't live in a natural world. These are not animals out in the woods hunting for their food and being hunted, falling victim to disease and hardship, living as an integral part of a balanced ecosystem and being governed by a complex interplay of hormones, social systems and territories that regulate their breeding. These are descendants of wild animals living in close company with us and with thousands of other animals in an entirely unnatural and overpopulated environment. A male wolf in the wild is exposed to the scent of females in heat only a few weeks out of the year. An intact male dog is bombarded by the same scent much more frequently. That's a long way from being natural or fair.

As for the profit incentive behind breeding pets, not only do such ventures often yield little financial return, but repeated breeding can cost you money if the female's health breaks down. Most "puppy mills," which add 2.5 million puppies to the glut of dogs born annually in this country, are actually small home businesses run by amateurs whose ignorance and carelessness in breeding is a direct cause of much of the rise in congenital and health problems in many breeds. Surely there must be a better way to earn a buck.

I can understand and appreciate people's desire to see their pets bear young. But, un-like most people, I have had direct exposure to the scope and everyday reality of the pet overpopulation problem. I worked for several years at a humane society clinic associated with an animal shelter, where I saw firsthand the tragic results of uncontrolled breeding. The sheer numbers are staggering. Estimates are that 5 to 12 million animals are euthanized each year in U.S. shelters. The reality—in flesh and blood and not just as abstract statistics—is devastating. Each one looks at you, and each is capable of much love and potential. And most never leave that shelter alive. When every pet owner takes responsibility for pet overpopulation, we'll see an end to the suffering it causes. It's best for society and best for the animals.

CHAPTER TWELVE

LIFESTYLES: TIPS FOR SPECIAL SITUATIONS

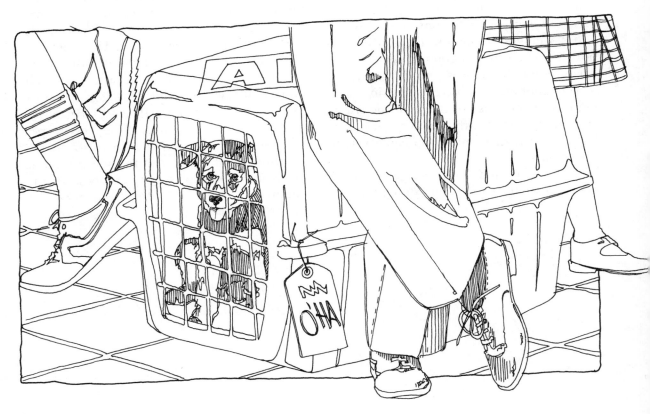

Every now and then you read the true-life story of a remarkable pet. Perhaps it's about a cat that survives without food or water for a month after being trapped accidentally in a transcontinental delivery truck. Or it tells of the family dog that gets lost during a cross-country move and somehow tracks down its owners hundreds of miles away.

Such stories of resourcefulness and devotion are both inspiring and amazing.

But all too often such incidents end badly. Everyday life poses special challenges for pets and their owners. For example, there is the emotional stress of travel and moving, the ease with which an animal can get lost in our busy cities, the dangers common household gadgets hold for our four-footed housemates. With a little planning we can make the going smoother for all involved.

VACATIONS AND TRAVEL

For many of us, travel is part of day-to-day living. Sometimes it's just an overnight business or a weekend fun trip; sometimes it's a month-long vacation. Whether your four-legged friend travels with you or stays at home, you need to give some thought to your pet's special needs at such times.

If you and your pet have a close bond, the animal could grieve during an absence that lasts several days or more, unaware that you plan to return soon. A long absence can sometimes lead to such an emotional upset—particularly for a dog—that your pet remains depressed for weeks after your return. In fact, it could spell the beginning of the end for a weak animal.

A deeply concerned owner wrote me this letter.

My dog, Lassie, will soon be 18. We've had family troubles including several deaths in these last two years, and now my husband and I are planning a ten-day cruise which we believe is necessary for our own health. But we will have to leave Lassie in a kennel. I read in a book that if you leave an old dog in a kennel, it might not last until you return. This has troubled us terribly, as Lassie is so accustomed to our care. Do you have any suggestions on how to care for our wonderful mutt, who has served us so well?

I sympathize with their plight. Not only would Lassie miss her human companions at a kennel, but she would be confined in a strange and perhaps uncomfortable run or cage, surrounded by barking and whining animals that might disturb her rest. She might not accept the unfamiliar food offered her, and, while in that stressed and weakened state, she could be susceptible to such diseases as "kennel cough," a contagious respiratory ailment (common where groups of dogs are housed). Even some younger animals do poorly during kennel stays. On the other hand, people do need to get away sometimes, and they can't always take a pet along.

Though it would not be my first choice, many an animal may be successfully placed in a kennel, if it is responsibly run and if the stay is not too long. You should definitely check out the facility in person before committing your animal to it. Look for such things as the degree of privacy provided (each animal should have a place to rest quietly), the sanitation, the noise level and the availability of sunlight, exercise space, fresh air, water, decent food and medical care, should the need arise.

If your animal is weak, if you plan a long absence or if you simply want to provide a better alternative, try in-home care. Ask a veterinarian, breeder or pet store owner to recommend a professional pet-sitter who will stop by once or twice a day to feed, groom, pet and exercise your animal and bring in the mail and water the plants, too. In our area this service presently costs $6 to $8 per visit. I have had very good luck with this alternative. If you can't get any leads from professionals, you might seek out teenagers who want a summer job, students in an animal health technician program or humane society volunteers.

A close friend, neighbor or relative who already knows and likes the animal might even take pleasure in providing the care you want for your pet while you're away. In such cases it might also work out for a friendly and well-behaved dog to stay at the sitter's residence. In contrast to dogs, cats are generally less stressed by being left alone, as long as they're on their own turf.

Here are some pointers on how to make the whole process go smoother.

Introduce the sitter to your pet before you leave. Professional pet-sitters like to meet the pet before you leave and make sure they understand its routine. Do what you can to encourage your pet to be friendly with this new person. You could even arrange for the sitter to spend some time with your animal—perhaps going for a walk, playing or holding it quietly for a while. Such preparations alleviate much of the stress and concern for the owner and are particularly good for an old or easily excitable pet.

Make certain the sitter you hire can and will provide adequate food, water, exercise and attention. Leave money and necessary instructions for taking the animal to the vet in case of an illness or an emergency. Provide phone numbers where you or a close relative can be reached during your trip. If you usually feed your pet a natural food diet, try to prepare some meals in advance and freeze them for the sitter's convenience.

Add anti-stress supplements to your pet's diet. If your pet tends to be excitable or seems likely to be upset at your absence, you can help him cope with emotional stress through nutrition. Starting about a week before the trip, add a complete B-complex tablet (including vitamins B_2, B_6 and pantothenic acid at the level of 5 to 15 milligrams, depending on the pet's size) and/or a liberal amount of nutritional yeast to the food. Also, give one to two grams of vitamin C, particularly after any stressful period. If possible, space the vitamin C dosage throughout the day. The sitter should feed the vitamins while you're gone, and you should continue to give the supplements for about a week after your return unless your animal seems fine.

Pay the sitter adequately. The fee or barter should be sufficient to convey a sense of your animal's value to you.

When you say good-bye to your pet, do so with a calm demeanor and untroubled mind. Since animals readily pick up people's feelings, you might start things off on the wrong note if you are nervous or upset when you leave. It may even help to look the animal in the eye and visualize a happy reunion scene. Once you are gone, don't cause yourself needless worry and anxiety. You did what you could.

Occasional absences, if thoughtfully handled, should not be a problem. However, some animals do develop physical or psychological ailments after being passed around from one temporary home to another. An owner with wanderlust or other out-of-town pursuits that cannot include a pet should consider placing her dog or cat in a permanent and supportive home where the pet will be better off.

TIPS FOR TRAVEL

What about taking a pet along on a vacation?

People find that many dogs and some cats (primarily the Siamese and Siamese-related breeds) can be excellent traveling companions if they are basically well-behaved and psychologically and physically healthy. However, certain precautions and considerations are basic.

Make sure your pet is wearing a current I.D. Should you get parted, you need some way for the finder to reach you. Many pet shops sell waterproof identification "barrel" tags in which you can enclose a small piece of paper that says "If lost, please call—collect." Give the phone number of a friend or relative who is willing to take messages, or else provide the number of the place where you are staying.

On long road trips, give your pet daily exercise. For traveling dogs, at least half an hour of a vigorous game of fetch or a jog with you is important. If you like to let your dog run loose, do so only in a safe and appropriate area and, even then, only if the dog is well-trained to return on command.

Cats should be kept in a harness attached to a leash. Car rides and strange places are more upsetting to a cat than to a dog, and felines might bolt. Once your cat has relaxed into the journey, and if he will come when called, you might let the animal off the leash under your supervision—but be cautious! For an added measure of safety, free the cat *before* feeding time, so hunger will provide an additional incentive for a prompt return.

Never leave a pet in a sealed car on a hot day. Heat can build up very fast in a closed car, which acts like a solar oven, causing an animal to go into heat prostration. This may lead to serious brain injury and even death. See "Handling Emergencies and Giving First Aid" on page 337 for first-aid treatment should this problem ever occur.

Take familiar items with you. A basket or piece of bedding from home can make any animal feel safer and more at ease. You could also take favorite toys to give your pet something to do.

Use commercial pet health foods for convenience, if necessary. But add vitamin C and vitamin B complex (as suggested above) to help traveling animals deal with stress.

Anticipate nature's calls. For a cat a litter box is basic gear for a road trip. Take a dog on a short stroll on a leash at least twice a day. Carry disposable bags and a scooper to use in public parks, cities, motel properties and beaches.

Prepare for health problems that are common to most travelers. *Constipation* can plague traveling pets. It can be caused by lack of exercise or water, infrequent stops or anxiety about strange new territories. Temporary constipation is not a serious problem and will usually clear up before long. For a dog you can prepare a useful preventive with figs, prunes and raisins as well as fresh berries or other fruits in season. Bran or psyllium husks are also helpful.

Nausea grips some animals when they ride in a car or plane, and they will either vomit or salivate excessively. The B-complex supplementation mentioned above will help prevent nausea. Also, encourage your pet to lie down on the floor of the car as a preventive. If motion sickness does occur, give your dog some peppermint tea or peppermint capsules to help settle her stomach (not so well tolerated by cats). An alternative to using peppermint tea is a formula made from the 38 flower preparations discovered by Dr. Edward Bach (see chapter 14 for more information). Mix together Aspen, Elm, Scleranthus and Vervain and give two drops of this formula every two hours to relieve the emotional upset and subsequent nausea.

Occasionally, it is wise to fast a susceptible pet the day before departure or on the first day of the trip. For an animal going by public transit in a carrier, a 24-hour fast before the trip will generally prevent it from eliminating during the journey.

Aconitum napellus 30C is very useful for minimizing fear and upset before traveling. Give one pellet of this homeopathic remedy an hour before leaving home; give another pellet just a few minutes before actually leaving the house. This usually is enough for most animals and most trips. If nervousness returns, give your pet another dose (one pellet) during the trip itself. Rarely will this remedy be needed more than three or four times; in fact, most animals travel well with just the two doses given before leaving home. This medicine is very safe to use and often functions better than a tranquilizer. (See page 354 for sources of this medicine.)

Eye irritation may occur in a dog that likes to ride with its head out the window, testing all the interesting scents it passes. Sometimes dust and debris enter the dog's eyes at high speeds, scratching the cornea and irritating sensitive membranes. For a minor irritation, I suggest washing the eyes out with this mild salt (saline) solution quite similar to tears: Add a level ¼ teaspoon of sea salt to one cup of pure water and stir. Keep the solution at room temperature; pour a small amount into a cup or dish and apply it by dripping it from a saturated cotton ball into the eye or by using a glass or plastic dropper. Administer the liquid until it runs out of the eye to flush out irritating substances.

For more serious irritations, use a cup of the same saline solution to which you add only five drops of tincture (or alcoholic extract) of the herb *Euphrasia officinalis* or eyebright. Use this solution in the eye four times a day.

If your pet has a serious corneal injury, the animal will keep its eye shut most of the time. In such a case seek veterinary help. (See also "Corneal Ulcers" on page 268.)

Do not take an unhealthy pet on an airline. If you do take a pet on a flight, make sure that the animal won't be exposed to extreme temperatures or possible suffocation. If your pet is small enough to stand up and turn around in a 20″ long × 13″ wide × 9″ high container, most of the major airlines will allow you to carry it on. Otherwise, it will have to be shipped in the cargo compartment, in a sturdy plastic kennel with metal doors. Try to determine if the cargo compartment is temperature controlled. If not, avoid layovers exceeding one hour and avoid flights in or out of any city with expected temperatures outside the range of 45° to 80°F. Reservations for cargo space are usually required. Animals may also be shipped, unaccompanied, by air freight. This service costs extra.

You will also need to get certification of your pet's health from a veterinarian. This is required for public transportation, interstate shipment and foreign travel. I do not advise taking your pet if your destination is a country that has a lengthy required quarantine time or any special health hazards. Check on the destination country's requirements before making your plans.

Respect motel and campground properties. You and your pet are much more apt to be welcome if you assure the owners that you will:

◆ Never leave a dog alone in a motel room while you go out for an extended period (which may lead to barking and chewing). If you must leave, confine the pet instead in your car, parked in the shade with the window slightly open to prevent heat buildup. A cat can be kept in a car or carrier in your absence.

◆ Have a bag and scooper with you and clean up any messes, inside or out.

◆ Only bring a neutered or spayed pet. This discourages wandering and territory-marking.

◆ Keep the pet on a leash at all times, so it doesn't charge through tender flower beds or bother other guests.

These guidelines help make you welcome with your pet when visiting at people's homes, too.

PETS ON THE MOVE

Besides our round-trip vacations, every year many Americans make a significant one-way trip —moving to a new residence. This means an awful lot of animals have to pull up their roots, dealing once more with the stress of getting used to and claiming a new territory as well as adjusting to new neighborhood challenges.

These relocations can easily disorient animals, so they run off, get lost and can't find their way back. So make sure your pet is under your control at all times while the move is in progress. During the hustle and bustle of packing and unpacking, confine the animal to a quiet room, perhaps the bathroom, laundry room or (for dogs only) a securely fenced yard. During this time provide your pet with some familiar items

for reassurance, such as its bed, some toys or a favorite rug.

Some unlucky pets are simply left behind when their owners move. This usually means slow and painful starvation, illness, bewilderment or (if they're lucky) a quicker death by euthanasia in an animal shelter. Others may be foisted off onto a reluctant new owner, in which case the animal can be neglected, eventually destroyed or given to someone else. Pets forced to switch owners too many times can develop insecure personalities and behavior problems that make them undesirable to anyone.

For the same psychological reasons, a high turnover of family members (through such events as divorce, marriage, birth, death and children leaving home) can also be stressful to an animal's sense of security. As much as possible, try to give your pet some special attention during times of change or upheaval.

Unfortunately, even the most loving owners sometimes find they cannot keep a pet because of housing problems, allergies, animal incompatibility or other situations that make dealing with animal care an impossibility. If so, follow the Humane Society guidelines (below) to help find your pet a good home. These guidelines also apply to placing a litter of puppies or kittens.

FINDING A NEW HOME

Begin your search for a good adoptive owner by advertising through the local paper and posting notices. Run newspaper ads several times to ensure wide coverage. List the animal's qualities (such as "Loves kids, healthy, quiet, house-trained and affectionate") and state simply that it needs a home. Post photocopied notices (preferably with an appealing picture of the animal) where responsible people might see them—in community centers, health food stores, doctors' and veterinarians' offices, churches, senior citizen centers and employee lunchrooms.

If you advertise that you're giving away a pet "for free," you might attract people who would neglect or mistreat it or sell it to a lab. Unfortunately, such things do happen to pets given away indiscriminately.

When someone calls to express interest, take your pet to *their* home so you can check the new place out for yourself. This may ease the transition for your pet also. Ask yourself the following questions.

- Does the house have a safe, fenced yard of adequate size?
- Is there a dangerous highway nearby?
- Will the pet be left alone too much?
- Does the interested party appreciate the basics of responsible pet ownership?
- Does anyone in the family oppose the adoption?
- Is the potential owner apt to move around a lot?
- What happened to any former pets? (Beware of people who have gone through a series of pets that were lost, hit by cars or given away; this will likely be the fate of yours as well.)

If you find it difficult to ask these kinds of questions, remember that a responsible pet-owner-to-be will appreciate your concern for your animal.

Though it may be difficult and even sad to place your old friend in a new home, you will feel best in the long run if you take the time and care to do the job well. Some time later you may return to find everyone pleased with the new relationship.

LOST PETS

The danger of losing a pet is not limited to moves and vacations. The possibility is ever present By tagging your pet with proper I.D. and licenses and keeping it under your supervision, you greatly reduce its chances of being lost or stolen. However, despite the most thoughtful precautions, animals sometimes still get lost. Here's what to do if your pet is missing.

Visit your local animal shelter. Go in person every day for a week or more after the disappearance. Most such organizations try to find you, but if a pet is unlicensed or not carrying identification, locating an owner is almost impossible. In any case, the burden of responsibility is really yours. Visit all appropriate kennels, asking to see any quarantine, isolation, holding and receiving rooms. Call out your pet's name as you go. Giving kennels or shelters a brief description over the phone is inadequate, since only you know your pet for sure and there may be many animals there.

While at the shelters, be sure to fill out a lost pet report, providing photos, if possible, as well as noting any unique markings. Also, check out reports of found pets. To prevent possible euthanasia, people who find lost pets often keep them at their homes and just file reports with the humane society. I once reunited a dog with its grateful owner this way. Frightened by fireworks, the dog had jumped into the wrong pickup truck during a Fourth of July celebration. When this same truck accidentally rear-ended me on the way home, the driver was

LOST

Date:_____

This area:_____

HAVE YOU SEEN OUR PET?

(dog or cat)	(breed)	(colors)
(sex)	(age)	(collar)

(special I.D. or comments)_____

DON'T WAIT—WE
MISS OUR PET

PLEASE CALL: (name and address)
_____

(phone)_____

PHOTO

---

astonished to find a dog in the back of his pickup. I filed a "found pet" report and, fortunately, was able to make contact with the owner, who never would have traced this same path with his own inquiries.

Check with local police. This is particularly important if you have reason to suspect your animal was stolen.

Place an ad in a local daily paper. Put it in the lost-and-found section. Give a description of the animal, note the area where you last saw it and, if possible, offer a reward.

Post notices in the area where the pet was lost. The form above is a good model.

Most photos will reproduce adequately on a good copier. Post the notices on telephone poles, at laundromats and on grocery store bulletin boards. Ask around. Ask the mailperson, children and housewives in the area if they have seen your animal; they are the people in the community who are usually most aware of strays.

HAZARDS IN THE HOME

Often, animals are unable to understand and avoid certain dangers unique to their human environment. It's hard to anticipate all the unexpected things a pet can get into, and we needn't worry excessively about them, but here are a few basic concerns.

- Cats can sometimes die from the complications of swallowing yarn, string or rubber bands. Because their barbed tongues make it difficult to spit objects out, they may be unable to stop the process once it starts. So offer them a ball of yarn for play only when you're there to supervise.

- Be on the lookout for ways your pet could ingest the many poisonous materials found in most homes. This ingestion could occur unintentionally (through skin or paws) or out of curiosity (through chewing or swallowing). Most homes contain numerous poisonous substances from toxic houseplants, antifreeze, insecticides and drugs to caustic cleansers and mothballs (beware of letting a cat sleep in a closet or drawer full of these little buggers—rather, debuggers). The challenge for you is like the one parents of toddlers face. See chapter 8 for more detailed coverage of dangerous substances.

- Make a habit of glancing in your car, oven, refrigerator or any drawer, cabinet or closet before closing it. Your curious cat may have jumped inside when you weren't looking. Such oversights can be fatal.

- Take care that your animal does not chew on electric cords. Don't confine a puppy or kitten in a room with an exposed cord. Reprimand it firmly if you catch the animal chewing on or playing with one.

- Also make sure that your pet doesn't chew up and swallow inedible objects like newspapers, books, plastic toys or bags and other such things. A rawhide bone makes a good substitute chewing toy.

- If you have toddlers, make sure they don't handle a small animal too roughly, because that endangers both parties. Also, the child may unintentionally cause a great stress for an animal by making a loud noise near its sensitive ears.

- If a child is responsible for taking care of a pet, make sure the job gets done the same way you would do it, every day. Don't let the animal become the victim of a learning experience in "natural consequences." Teach your child the necessity of sticking to any responsibility he or she has assumed for an animal.

- If you live in an upper-floor apartment, screen your windows. Despite their agility, cats can and do fall out of windows and off balconies.

By taking these precautions and by adopting an overall attitude of watchfulness and consideration, modern life need not hold undue peril or stress for your animal or for you; instead, it can provide unique opportunities for adventure and enjoyment.

CHAPTER THIRTEEN

SAYING GOOD-BYE: COPING WITH A PET'S DEATH

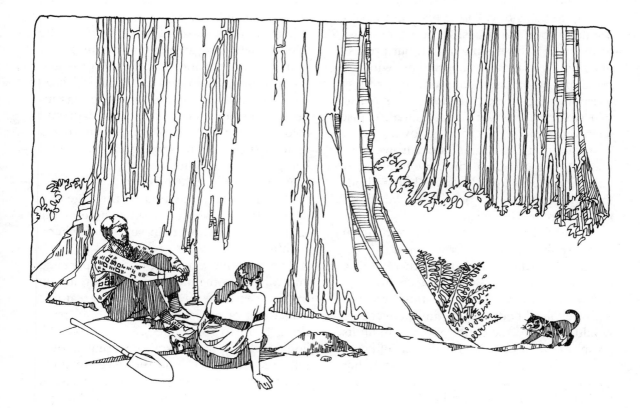

The evening wore on, the music from the radio drifting out and enveloping us all. And with each moment my wife and I could see that the small black kitten she held in her lap was edging ever closer to death. Only a week before we had adopted it from the animal shelter clinic where I had twice saved its life—first from the ravages of parasites and then from the institutional procedures

that required unadopted strays to be put to sleep after a certain period.

But now further postponing seemed impossible. I had done what I knew how to do and yet Miracle, as we'd dubbed her because of her heroic though brief rebound, was surely on her way out.

The signs were clear. Her small body grew steadily weaker and more limp and her legs began to stiffen. Her eyes stared, dilated and motionless, fixed upon some awesome eternity. Occasionally, she waved her head in small convulsions and feebly licked the inside of her mouth.

We had already discussed the possibilities. We could have struggled to save her all the way up to the end, violating her dignity with needles, tubes and drugs. Or to spare her—or maybe ourselves—the drawn-out process of dying, we could have injected her with the standard euthanasia solution, a painless passport to a quick end. Yet somehow, in that situation and with that animal, it just seemed right to let her go in her own way.

Without having to talk about it, we both knew it would be best this way. Looking at her, we realized how little we knew about the mystery of death or of life. We didn't know who or what a cat was, really.

We didn't know where she had come from or where she would go. Yet we knew that beneath our surface differences, there was a oneness, a bond uniting all living creatures.

And we knew that soon this graceful, highly evolved body and its tiny, perfect eyes would return to the earth, never to fulfill its promises. We thought of how we would miss her innocence, her playful grace, her courage—and a wave of sadness swept over us. Yet, what must be must be. And it was all right to be as it was.

Finally, the broadcaster announced the arrival of Sunday morning, and shortly after 1:00 A.M., we turned out the lights and placed Miracle near us on the bed. Her breathing grew weaker and faster. It would soon be over.

Gently and slowly, the darkness began to lower us into that unknown into which we all go each night. Through the growing silence came a few sounds—long, low half-groans, half-meows. We reached over and felt Miracle's temperature. It was dropping.

We placed her into her sleeping box atop some warm bottles covered with cloth and settled back into bed. Once, in the middle of the night, we awoke to hear another of the strange sounds, this one deeper, longer, with an air of finality.

The sunlight was streaming through the window when we awoke that morning, full of a fresh appreciation for the gift of living. We got up and looked in Miracle's box, knowing what we would find. She was indeed gone now. Her body was rigid and cold. Her eyes and mouth were open, frozen as if in surrender to some great force that had passed through her.

We found the right place to bury her, beneath a towering redwood on the edge of a nearby forest. We dug a small hole at the foot of the tree and then simply sat there, silently.

The redwood was magnificent, sparkling and waving in the morning light, surging up from the earth to the sky. Into this great tree something of our small friend would pass. From form to form, life would go on. We laid her body in the soil, covering it over with the tree's roots and the sweet-smelling forest loam. As we tamped down the last of it, we heard a small rustling in the bushes. We turned to see.

It was a cat, watching.

Mostly, we think of death as something to be feared, to be put out of mind and avoided at all costs. Yet in the end it comes to all organisms. It will come to your animal, and one day it will surely come to you and me.

But as the passing of Miracle and of others we have known has taught us, death need not be feared. In fact, being fully with it and letting its significance speak to you can make such an experience a thing of beauty. It can remind us, if we have forgotten to notice, just how mysterious and wondrous life truly is.

That is why it saddens me when I see and hear from so many people who are deeply burdened and upset at the anticipation or the memory of a pet's death. Their grief is real—often as great as that felt at the loss of a human friend or relative. But often, because they are unwilling or unable to face their feelings and thus learn from these emotions, people shut themselves off not only from the pain of death but also from its beauty and meaning.

A pet's death can be a complex thing. All sorts of emotions can arise, including sadness, anger, depression, disappointment and fear. With people for whom the relationship is especially important—such as a single person, a childless couple or an only child for whom the animal has been a "best friend"— the grief may be that much greater. And, too, if the death was sudden and unexpected or if it seemed preventable (as in an accident), the feelings of loss and disappointment can be particularly intense.

Often a death brings with it memories of past unresolved losses, regrets about things done and not done, a resurfacing of a loneliness that the relationship may have covered over and, perhaps deepest of all, the fear of your own death, of the idea of becoming nothing. But viewed positively, facing these emotions can provide real opportunities for learning and flowering.

In addition to those psychological hurts common to losing either a human or an animal friend, a pet's death brings its own unique challenges. For one thing, the euthanasia option can burden you with a difficult decision. Another problem is that it is

not socially acceptable to mourn openly over the death of an animal, although the grief may be just as real as if you had lost any other family member. It may be hard to find a sympathetic listener to help you work through the experience. And even sympathetic employers are unlikely to allow absence from work for mourning a faithful cat or dog.

In fact, it *is* socially acceptable to replace the lost pet with a new one immediately after death. However, if a woman were to remarry the day after her husband's funeral, eyebrows would raise. Simply replacing your last pet with a new one will not heal the grief you feel. Only time and insight can do that. And parents who rush out to buy a new pet for their bereaved child before he has really said good-bye to the one he just lost should realize that the unspoken message can be: "Life is cheap; relationships are disposable."

HANDLING GRIEF

Above all else, you need to know how to cope with the grief and other emotions that may surface before, during or after the death. If you can do that, any choices or actions required of you will come much more easily.

Lynne De Spelder, a friend who teaches, counsels and writes on the subject of death and dying, emphasizes that coping with the loss of a pet is much the same as coping with the death of a human friend: "It's really important to *handle* the grief. Research shows the costs of mismanaged grief can be great, illness among survivors, for example. Hiding from grief makes it worse."

How can you handle it? Start with the most important thing: Give yourself permission to grieve. Lynne observed, "Women often deal with grief better than men simply because they are allowed to cry. Also, it's good to find someone who'll listen. If your spouse won't, find someone who will. If anyone makes light of your grief, it's probably his own fear of emotion."

Suppose your crying and sadness seem to go on too long? That's a signal that you are dwelling too much in your thoughts and memories. Lynne and other grief counselors encourage people suffering from loss to discover and engage in nurturing activities—such as yoga, hiking, music or sports—that help people to let go of the past lovingly and open themselves to the goodness of the present.

When you must help a child cope with the loss you all feel, it's important to understand your own feelings first. You must be honest and open about what happened. But don't try to console the child with an instant replacement or with explanations that can be misinterpreted or taken too literally, such as "he went away" or "she was taken to Doggie Heaven." If the child wants to see the dead body before burial, understand that it is a natural curiosity and should be allowed, provided you are emotionally stable about it yourself.

Talk with the child and make sure he is not harboring misunderstandings. Don't let him blame himself or even you for the death. If you had the animal put to sleep because it was clear that a painful death was inevitable, make sure the child understands.

MAKING A CHOICE

If your pet is suffering and you are forced to consider euthanasia, familiarity with the procedure and its alternatives is a great help.

Euthanasia: The idea of "putting an animal out of its misery" has long been accepted as a humane option, even though we humans rarely accept it as a choice for ourselves.

Technically speaking, veterinarians perform euthanasia in their office or sometimes as a house call by injecting an overdose of a barbiturate anesthetic into a vein or the heart. The animal loses consciousness within a few seconds, slumps over, and the vital functions cease soon after. It is considered painless. However, if the animal is agitated (perhaps by its upset owner), that can make it harder for the doctor to do the job properly.

Personally, I've always found the whole process rather uncomfortable, and I think most veterinarians feel the same. Mercy killing can make sense, however, in cases where the animal is in great and prolonged pain and the death would be slow but inevitable.

It's unwise to make a hasty decision for euthanasia in a moment of anguish. Wait until you clearly and rationally understand the animal's chances of survival and can weigh the alternatives. Otherwise, you may be burdened with doubts and regrets forever, wondering if your pet might have made it, given more time.

If you do choose euthanasia, give two drops of Dr. Bach's stress-relieving rescue formula (see page 205) every one to two hours for several doses before seeing the vet to make the experience less traumatic for your pet. If your animal is very frightened, reacting to everything that is different or that seems threatening, change to a dose of *Aconitum napellus* 30C (one to two pellets) by mouth. This homeopathic remedy often works wonders by alleviating fear in such situations.

Hospital care: When your animal is so ill that you are considering hospitalizing it, ask your veterinarian for a realistic opinion of its chances of recovery. Special care often pulls an animal through a serious crisis, enabling it to live a few more years. However, some conditions, such as cancer or major heart or kidney degeneration, allow for little or no hope of recovery. Heroic efforts to prolong a pet's life might involve extensive care and expense as well as drawn-out suffering for the animal, only to prove futile in the end.

The cost of emergency treatment for an animal in a crisis can, of course, vary considerably. However, the typical cost is over $100 in the first few hours, and it can go up to several hundred dollars after just a few days of intensive care. Compared with human care in a similar situation, it's a real bargain. But because veterinary hospitals are usually small and privately owned, animal care is less intensive than in a human hospital, where a whole team of personnel and sophisticated equipment may be continuously used on the patient. A trained veterinary staff, however, can come close to this in quality of treatment.

Certainly there's a place for extensive medical care in some situations. However, in many cases it is obvious that the animal can't survive and that heroic measures are not really appropriate. When this occurs, the veterinarian can administer fluids and drugs that allow the animal to rest quietly. As soon as it becomes apparent that death is near, most doctors put the animal to sleep (with the owner's prior permission).

With other conditions—hind leg paralysis, for example—an animal might live for some years longer, but the permanent handicap requires a great deal of attention from the owner. Depending on the total picture and the specific condition, euthanasia might be best, in view of the long-term outcome.

Home care: Sometimes there is no real hope for a cure, and death appears to be relatively close, but with little pain. That's when it can make sense to consider a home death. If the family is prepared to handle the death of a pet, both in terms of time and emotional clarity, the experience can be positive for all involved, including the dying animal. Unless the pet has been heavily treated with drugs (such as chemotherapy for cancer), death from many serious conditions can be comparatively free of excessive discomfort. Of course, some conditions, such as accumulation of fluid in the chest or heart failure, can cause a lot of suffering and may warrant euthanasia after a certain point.

Here is a general guideline: If your pet seems reasonably comfortable and peaceful, you may wish to allow the process to unfold naturally. If the animal is restless, crying or has great difficulty in breathing or has convulsions, euthanasia is the recommended response.

In terms of physical care, don't feed a dying animal; just give it water or vegetable juices. Provide a warm, comfortable, quiet place to rest. Occasionally, your pet may need your help to go outside or to the litter box to eliminate. The dying animal may welcome the gentle and calm presence of those it loves, but do protect your pet from too much noise, activity or disturbance.

There are some homeopathic remedies that will assist the dying process. I hasten to add that these medicines will not *make* your pet die, the way a euthanasia solution injection will. Their role is to assist the dying process *if it is already under way.* If your pet is not ready to die, the remedy will either have no effect or perhaps even seem to improve the situation for a few days (temporarily).

All these homeopathic medicines are used the same way—give one pellet every two hours as needed for relief of symptoms. If there is no change for the better after a maximum of three doses, then the remedy is not appropriate to the situation. In this case choose one of the other ones or simply use Dr. Bach's stress-relieving rescue formula instead. Once some relief is seen, no more medicine is needed.

These are the three chief remedies to consider using.

- *Arsenicum album* 30C is the major remedy needed in handling 95 percent of dying animals. The indications are restlessness, fear, discomfort, extreme weakness, increased thirst and coldness. Not all these elements need to be present at the same time for this medicine to be appropriate. However, look for restlessness or weakness coupled with a low body temperature.
- *Pulsatilla* 30C is appropriate for the animal that is whimpering, complaining or wanting to be held. This remedy is also useful for the stage right before death when breathing becomes loud and labored.
- *Tarentula cubensis* 30C is most suitable for severe pain with tossing about, crying and intense restlessness. The restlessness and discomfort are greater than

when *Arsenicum album* is indicated. But the animal shows less fear.

When I discuss these remedies and their indications—such as restlessness, pain and so forth, I do not mean to imply that these states always occur. Nor do I mean that you should not just consider euthanasia. There are times, however, when it is really wonderful to know of these medicines and the relief that they can give.

How can you tell that the dying process is underway? When the end is very near, the animal will grow quite weak. The body temperature will drop. (The feet and ears will feel cold, along with the gums and tongue.) If you take the temperature with a rectal thermometer, usually death is near when the temperature drops below 100°F.

Often, breathing slows and the animal seems to go into a prolonged sleep or unconscious state. However, right at the moment of dying, breathing may be spasmodic and gasping. The pupils may dilate, and the animal may stretch out or perhaps pass urine. This final dying process generally lasts for only a few minutes. Rarely is it prolonged for more than an hour.

In some cases, of course, an animal dies so suddenly that you have no need to make such choices. But regardless of how the process occurs, I hope that when the time comes, your parting will be a peaceful one.

During the span of years you spent together, there were probably ups and downs. Through it all you both learned, loved and did the best you knew how. When you think of the past, let it be with gratitude for the beautiful times you had together. When you think of the future, let it be with faith that life will again bring such beauty your way.

CHAPTER FOURTEEN

HOLISTIC AND ALTERNATIVE THERAPIES

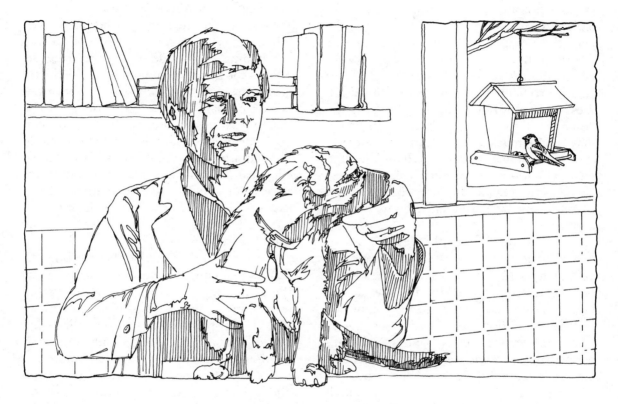

My dog has arthritis. Can you tell me what vitamin or mineral will help him?"

Many people who seek an alternative natural or drugless therapy for a sick animal are surprised that we don't handle health problems as though there were one simple pill or fix-it treatment good for all cases diagnosed as arthritis or asthma or

kidney trouble. I wish they would realize that the natural or holistic method of treatment is not the substitution of a vitamin for an antibiotic or a mineral for a hormone or an herb for a painkiller.

The truth is that health problems are rarely caused by just one factor. Ailments usually arise from a broad spectrum of

189

physical, emotional and mental influences. So, to respond effectively, we must take all these realms into account. We need to look at the whole picture of an illness and find therapies that will work with—not against—the whole body in the healing process. To me, this holistic approach to medicine is the path to a true cure.

In the practice of holistic medicine, we recognize that disease or illness affects the whole animal, so to understand and treat a health problem in its entirety, we must address all levels of the body and the spirit. We don't want to use a method of treatment that might mask a symptom or control a certain physiological process. If we did that, we might suppress an underlying weakness at the same time, and that weakness would be sure to surface eventually in one form or another.

Let's illustrate this with "Jesse," who is typical of so many dogs today, with chronically itchy and inflamed skin. Jesse's economy-brand commercial food is low in certain nutrients essential to healthy skin and nerves. In addition, her body is struggling to throw off excess toxins contained in this poor-quality fare and pollutants inhaled during frequent rides in a pickup truck on smoggy freeways. As a result, her skin is overly sensitive and reactive to fleas, which are abundant both in her quarters and in her coat, primarily because Jesse's owner, Tom, rarely grooms her, and he only vacuums the house about once a month.

Jesse is left alone in the backyard every work day, which also encourages her to bite and scratch herself out of sheer boredom. Between the fleas, the oversensitivity and the boredom, she often scratches rather violently.

To compound matters, Jesse's endocrine system doesn't function well. That's because her thyroid gland is sluggish from a buildup of poisons and from lack of stimulation from regular exercise. This fosters a greasy-looking and inflamed skin. All told, her problems are persistent and severe.

Jesse's owner finally takes her to the veterinarian, who prescribes cortisone to stop her itching. As a side effect, the drug depresses the dog's adrenal glands. The doctor also gives her an artificial thyroid hormone to compensate for her weak thyroid. Unfortunately, it discourages the thyroid's natural hormone production, which weakens the gland further. The vet urges Tom to use chemical flea powders, and they add to the toxic load. Finally, the vet suggests a more expensive kibble, higher in protein and fat—but still chock-full of preservatives and other chemical additives.

Now if the nutritional and environmental factors that contribute to the disease remain the same, but Jesse is given these well-intended but stopgap measures, you can see that the problem may be "controlled" but not solved. As the months and years pass, the dog's accumulated toxicity and poor nutrition, plus the boredom, weakened glands and lack of exercise will eventually lead to a more serious breakdown, this time involving more critical organs. This "new" disease is now treated with new drugs. And on it goes.

Instead of building up Jesse's health, this conventional treatment merely covers up her problems, allowing them to get even worse. And when that happens, the "new" disease is never even seen as an outgrowth of the original condition.

THE LIMITATIONS OF A CONVENTIONAL APPROACH

Like all veterinarians, I learned the conventional approach of diagnosis and treatment in school, and I practiced that philosophy for years. It has certainly produced some remarkable successes, particularly with acute infections and trauma. Yet, when we approach health problems from this perspective, our thinking tends to get so specialized and materialistic that we lose sight of larger patterns and processes. Instead, drugs and surgery claim our attention, often to the exclusion of a broader health-building and prevention program.

As a result, the major effect of contemporary medicine is to control and counteract symptoms and disturbances. The body's innate ability to heal itself when given the right support is almost ignored. Instead of strengthening the patient, such methods merely compensate for the body's weaknesses.

In our eagerness for quick and easy solutions, we seize on a certain drug (or vitamin) that may just cover up symptoms without addressing underlying causes. Unfortunately, some modern drugs are very good at this. The various forms of synthetic cortisone, for example, are powerful enough to stop a wide variety of symptoms in their tracks, but inside, the disturbance continues unseen.

When taking medical histories, my associates and I frequently observe that animals vigorously treated with such drugs (apparently successfully) go on to develop another condition within a few weeks or months. Usually, it is more serious. For example, a dog with a skin problem like Jesse's, continually suppressed with cortisone as hers was, may later develop calcification of the spine, pancreatitis or kidney failure. Often, a cat with a chronically inflamed bladder that is treated with drugs will eventually show a deeper problem like kidney failure, arthritis or leukemia.

Although most people tend to regard the new conditions as separate from the prior ones, I suggest they are related. The suppressed disorder has simply gone on to create more serious inroads in the body, now involving internal and more critical organs.

PROBLEMS DRUGS CAUSE

One problem associated with dependence on powerful drugs is the production of side effects or even iatrogenic (doctor-caused) diseases. Although iatrogenic disturbances are taken seriously in human medicine, veterinary researchers have barely studied them. I'm convinced, however, that they are also common in animal medicine. I have seen many pets improve considerably when prolonged drug treatment is simply stopped.

Some examples of drug-related complications are loss of appetite or diarrhea (from the use of oral antibiotics), and skin rashes, convulsions, hysteria or hearing loss (from the use of tranquilizers or antibiotics). If symptoms appear right after therapy begins, they are probably related to the drug.

Even in situations where drugs are not called for, they are sometimes used to appease the client and to justify the expense of the office call. For example, antibiotics are often prescribed to treat viral diseases, though we know antibiotics are only effective against bacteria, not viruses. But don't put all the blame on the doctor. Many people insist on a shot or some pills to take home, and if one doctor won't comply, they search for another who will. Unfortunately, we have been sold a bill of goods about the necessity for these drugs. I question that assumption, both on the basis of my own success and that of many other people who use more natural methods that work *with* the body's healing forces.

Why have we come to rely so heavily on drugs, surgery and the like? I think a lot of it boils down to several culturally shared attitudes most of us hold—doctor and client alike.

One of these is our insistence on a "quick fix." We avoid change in our lives and habits. We just want to eliminate anything unpleasant at once, even if we suspect that the measures we take will not be a permanent solution.

If we do undertake a change of habits or lifestyle, it's often only to adapt ourselves to a problem we assume we can't change. For example, we learn to avoid certain foods that cause allergic reactions. Yet, by taking the time and care to understand and treat the disorder, we might be able to do away with it altogether. In fact, some in-depth holistic approaches have actually enabled patients to recover from food allergies.

DIVERGENT VIEWS IN MEDICINE

An even more fundamental stumbling block is the materialistic view that has long dominated our Western science. While virtually all cultures and systems of healing in the history of the world, including ours, have recognized the presence of a unifying life force, Western scientists no longer do. The Chinese call this life force *chi*, the Polynesians *mana*, the Sioux *wakonda*, the Hindus *prana* and so on.

In our own history of Western medicine and philosophy, it was called the *vital force*. But as modern science was forming, a philosophical divergence arose between the *vitalists*, who asserted the existence of such a force that animated and governed physical organisms, and the *materialists* who denied it and said that all life could be explained in terms of chemical and physical processes.

Understandably, this turning point in the history of science explains why most of us today look almost exclusively to physical explanations for disease. We look first for germs, parasites, genetic defects or just plain wear and tear from old age. In addition, our bias is to focus our research money on those physical factors that best tie in with marketable solutions, such as a new drug, rather than those that would require a change of lifestyle or a cleanup of the environment.

So, although doctors may pay some lip service to avoiding emotional stress or may notice how often patients get sick after suffering a psychological upset, the usual "fix" for a health problem involves drugs or surgery. Even psychiatrists rely largely on drugs that suppress emotional states.

THE RE-EMERGENCE OF HOLISTIC THERAPIES

Today, however, many practitioners and laypeople alike feel limited by the materialistic approach. They are exploring and revitalizing a number of holistic therapies for humans and for animals that acknowledge and respect a vital force that governs living organisms.

Most practitioners with a holistic perspective, including myself, take the view that symptoms represent the action of the individual's life force. In creating symptoms, the life force is doing its best to throw off the disturbance by means of diarrhea, vomiting, coughing, sneezing, pus formation and the like. So, we try to work with the action of the symptoms, gently helping the body in its attempt to restore harmony.

We also consider emotional and mental factors in health, carefully observing fluctuations at these levels and often advising changes that will promote greater internal harmony. This is not to deny the importance of physical factors. Certainly, there are virulent microorganisms and environmental assaults of all kinds to consider. But individuals who are exposed equally to these factors vary tremendously in their resistance.

Have you ever noticed how there can be several animals in the same household, eating the same diet and exposed to the same environment, yet one of them seems to have all the fleas or to pick up every infectious disease that comes along? As I see it, the most important factor in susceptibility to disease of any sort is the strength of the individual's defense system—not just the physical responses immunologists describe but also the total state of the animal or person. This encompasses mental and emotional qualities as well as the subtle fields of energy of the life force.

The holistic perspective also casts a differ-

ent light on the process of diagnosis. Partly because of our culture's mechanistic attitude, we often view health problems as distinct, separate diseases that we must label correctly using interpretations of extensive and costly lab tests. These test results give us the illusion of certainty, tempting researchers to seek the one factor behind a given disease—the unknown virus, the missing enzyme, the damaged gene.

Holistic therapies tend not to seek single causes or cures, but to understand and treat disorder in the whole individual. Holistically minded practitioners do not divide diseases into separate components so much as they try to see how various disturbances in a person or animal are linked together.

SUPPORT FROM MODERN PHYSICS

Developments in modern physics support the holistic and vitalist views. When the materialist doctrine became dominant, physicists held the now-outdated Newtonian idea that the world is ultimately composed of minute particles, such as electrons, photons and neutrons. Modern physicists searched for ever smaller particles, hoping to find the one basic building block from which the rest are formed, but they never found it. Instead, they concluded that particles are merely concentrations of energy that come and go as aspects of a larger whole. In effect, it is an illusion to try to analyze things as though they are separate entities or parts, for all things are part of a whole.

This fundamental breakthrough of understanding in physics makes it clear that the fragmented approach to scientific knowledge, medicine included, is erroneous at its very root. We must look at problems as they relate to the whole, and not to the divisions of artificial labels and definitions.

HOW TO PUT HOLISTIC THERAPIES INTO PRACTICE

All right, this theory makes good sense to you, but how can it help your sick pets?

In many simple conditions all an animal really needs to get well is a supportive environment, some commonsense care and a little time. Nature does the job, either with us or in spite of us. But if recurrent or chronic disease or weakness afflicts your animal, a return to health will most likely require major lifestyle changes, plus specific therapeutic measures.

Start with the diet. Is it fresh and natural, or is it highly processed and of inferior quality? Will it keep a pet healthy? Next, consider the environment. Is it peaceful and wholesome or stressful and polluted? Is there adequate sunlight, fresh air and good water? Does the animal have a comfortable, secure and quiet place to rest? Is the sanitation good? Does your pet receive regular and proper grooming and exercise?

Now think of relationships. Does your cat or dog have plenty of friendly, happy companionship, either with people or with other animals? Or is it often neglected, bored and frustrated? What are your mental attitudes toward the animal's problems? Are you supportive and positive? Or do you broadcast anxiety, worry and fear? How is the animal expected to behave? Is it forced to be a guard dog, for instance, when its personality rebels at this task? Is there any animal or person in its environment that is a threat to your pet's well-being or wishes it harm? Had the animal lost someone or something dear when the ailment began?

Granted, it's not always easy to unravel the problem or to change some circumstances. If in doubt, start with the natural feeding program outlined in chapter 4, make sure your pet gets regular affection, exercise and grooming, and then see what problems (if any) remain. If a wholesome physical and emotional environment is not enough to restore health, the problem may be more deep-seated, involving a disturbance to the vital force. In that case, several drugless, holistic therapies can effectively help to rebalance the body's energies and stimulate healing.

It would require many volumes to detail all of the therapies that might help your pet. Let's look instead at the general philosophy and methods of some holistic therapies that veterinarians and others commonly use to heal animals. Then I'll describe in greater detail the approach I favor—homeopathic medicine.

Most of these holistic therapies overlap to some extent in their methods and their medicines. Their practitioners often advise a combination of methods. For example, herbal medicine and dietary changes are often used along with acupuncture. In the discussions that follow, I will suggest which methods will work best together.

NATUROPATHY

Defined by a medical dictionary as a "drugless system of therapy by the use of physical forces, such as air, light, water, heat, massage and the like," naturopathy is a comprehensive approach that emphasizes supporting the whole body's physical attempts to eliminate disease. Naturopaths believe the major physical cause of disease is an excessive buildup of toxic materials, often from improper eating and lack of exercise. They say these toxic materials clog the usual avenues of waste disposal.

Naturopaths employ a number of techniques to clean out the body, including some used by various cultures throughout recorded history. One is fasting, a way to rest the digestive system and allow the body to do some internal housecleaning. Patients who are fasting, plus other naturopathic patients, are often advised to drink a lot of pure water or juices to flush out the kidneys, and to take enemas or colonic irrigations to clean out the lower intestines.

Hot and cold treatments may be used to stimulate the circulation or encourage sweating. They may include baths, saunas, packs, compresses, steaming and the like. Other naturopathic methods include exercise, sunbathing, good hygiene and various massage and brushing techniques. Besides the cleansing processes, patients are put on supportive programs of good nutrition (often emphasizing raw organic foods and juices), specific food combining (to aid digestion) and judicious use of specific food supplements, vitamins, minerals and herbs.

Some of these methods are difficult to apply to animals, but others lend themselves easily—particularly fasting, exercise, good nutrition, sunbathing and grooming (a form of massage). I encourage their use in many cases.

Donald Ogden, D.V.M., who made extensive and successful use of naturopathic methods for years in animal medicine, reported that nine out of ten patients he treated for skin irritation recovered within two weeks. He attributed his success to bathing the animal thoroughly, then fasting it for seven days on vegetable broths and then for seven additional days on vegetable solids and soups. He advised breaking the fast with raw meat and raw or steamed leafy vegetables, followed by a balanced natural foods diet.

Dr. Ogden also found that quiet rest and fasts of three to ten days (until the pet's temperature is normal and symptoms disappear) are very beneficial for many conditions including: obesity, rheumatism and arthritis, constipation, chronic cardiac insufficiency, bronchial diseases, heart worm, kidney and bladder stones, gastritis, kidney disease, pyorrhea, diabetes, liver disorders (unless cirrhosis has developed), open sores and the fever stage of distemper.

However, he advised against fasting an animal with a wasting disease such as cancer, advanced uremia, tuberculosis, prolonged malnutrition, hookworm disease or distemper.

Naturopathic medicine works well in combination with other holistic approaches, such as herbal medicine, chiropractic and other manual therapies, acupuncture and Chinese medicine and homeopathic medicine.

HERBOLOGY

Herbalists use many of the same methods as naturopaths. Their main emphasis, however, is upon the use of specific herbal leaves, roots and flowers to assist healing. Basic to folk medicine in every culture since ancient times, herbology is probably the most fundamental system of specific remedies. When ill, wild animals have used herbs instinctively for eons.

In fact, many of our modern pharmaceutical drugs are actually compounds originally isolated from herbs and considered to be their active elements. For instance, digitalis derives from foxglove, atropine from belladonna (deadly nightshade), caffeine from coffee, theophylline from tea, arecoline from the areca (betel) nut and reserpine (used for high blood pressure) from *Rauwolfia serpentina*.

Herbalists contend that the pharmaceutical derivatives and the whole plants from which they come are not the same, however. The strength of herbs lies in the unique and complex properties of the original natural substance. Again, the whole is more than the sum of (or one of) its parts.

As compared with their pharmaceutical counterparts, herbs exhibit a slower and deeper action. They assist the healing process by helping the body to eliminate and detoxify, thus taking care of the problem that's causing the symptoms. For instance, they may stimulate physiological processes like the emptying of the bowels or urination. In addition, herbs can serve as tonics and builders that strengthen tissues in specific parts of the body (or the whole body, depending on the herb in question). They can also be highly nutritious, containing large amounts of various vitamins and minerals and other nutrients. And there are some herbal practitioners who believe that plant medicines, particularly those found locally, bring the healing energy of the environment to the user.

Herbal remedies have been used successfully throughout the centuries to treat many illnesses in animals. In recent years Juliette de Bairacli-Levy has popularized their use for this purpose through her detailed writings (which also emphasize the importance of natural diet and fasting). She reports good results in using herbs to treat dogs with worms, fleas, skin problems, mange, distemper, kidney and bladder trouble, arthritis, anemia, diabetes, leptospirosis, obesity, wounds and fractures, constipation, diarrhea, jaundice, heart disorders, warts and cataracts.

De Bairacli-Levy recommends using the freshly gathered herb whenever possible and replacing dried herbs yearly. I concur with this advice. In chapter 15 I will describe the standard methods of preparing infusions, decoctions and tinctures from herbs. In the "Quick Reference" section on page 221, I suggest specific herbs for various illnesses.

Besides the difficulty of finding fresh herbs, one disadvantage of using internal herbal therapy for animals is that the remedies are usually administered in sizable quantities at frequent intervals over long periods of time (weeks to months). Since they rarely taste good, you need to give them to your pet in capsules or disguised in food. As every animal lover knows, it's not easy to force medication down a pet's throat over a long period.

For that reason and others, I prefer to emphasize homeopathic medications, which taste good and are given less often. Many of these are also derived from plants. Another related system I use with animals is the 38 flower preparations discovered by Dr. Edward Bach. Both are described later.

However, I have seen the power of well-chosen herbs as well and recognize their value. I find them most useful for external treatments on animals (as in flea powders and rinses, mite control, skin problems and wounds) or for minor upsets (such as diarrhea, indigestion and the like) that do not require prolonged treatment.

Herbal medicine works well with naturopathy, chiropractic and other manual therapies, acupuncture and Chinese medicine and, *limited to only the milder herbs*, homeopathic medicine.

CHIROPRACTIC AND OTHER MANUAL THERAPIES

Since the time of Hippocrates, manipulative therapies have been in use throughout the world. Some, like chiropractic and osteopathy which were both founded in the nineteenth century, hold that disease conditions result from misaligned or abnormal bodily structures (especially in the spine) that interfere with the normal flow of life force, nerve impulses and blood circulation.

Chiropractic has become the largest drugless healing profession in this country. I first became interested in the potential this therapy holds for animals when a local chiropractor told me that many different conditions in pets (including epilepsy) have been helped by chiropractic.

Later I met a veterinarian who, with the help of a trained chiropractor and vitamin supplementation, was getting amazing results in one of his canine patients. The dog was afflicted with "wobbler syndrome," an inherited condition in which the neck vertebrae put pressure on the spinal cord and make walking difficult. Before treatment the poor dog could go only about three steps without falling over; after adjustment it could run all over and even jump fences! Also, some clients have reported to me that their dogs were helped by chiropractic adjustments when paralyzed by disk problems.

The original theory of chiropractic holds that subtle vertebral misalignments can block the essential flow of nerve energy passing through the spinal column. This irregularity, known as a subluxation, puts excessive pressure on the spinal nerves, thus interfering with various body functions. Treatment consists of careful manipulation of the vertebrae to restore correct alignment and full working order. To achieve this specialized skill, practitioners usually undergo at least four years of medical training.

A broader way to understand how manipulative therapies may work is to view the body and mind as a whole. Disturbances in any one part of the body reflect and affect the whole system. In fact, a number of advocates of diagnostic and manipulative therapy methods focus on certain parts of the body with the understanding that these parts reflect or represent the whole body. For instance, an iridologist "reads" disturbances in various organs by a careful examination of the iris of the eye. Practitioners of reflexology pinpoint and treat disturbances throughout the body by manual pressure on certain points of the feet and hands. Some acupuncturists diagnose and treat problems solely at points on the ear, which is said to reflect the whole body. I met one veterinary acupuncturist who treats only the ear to manage health problems successfully in horses, even lameness!

In the same way, body/mind disturbances may be reflected in the spinal column, associated with irregular muscular tensions and vertebral displacements. If so, they should respond to corrective spinal manipulation.

Regardless of why and how it works, chiropractic manipulation is a real boon for many animal patients. For example, a *Prevention* magazine reader wrote me to describe her 18-year-old cat's amazing response to chiropractic therapy. For over 12 years, her cat had been having severe attacks of vomiting, loss of appetite and intense itching of the face and shoulders. The poor cat licked and scratched until its skin was bloody. The owner consulted several different veterinarians, but their drug therapy offered only temporary help, at best.

By chance, this woman mentioned the situation to her chiropractor and he offered to try to help. Just one adjustment brought startling results: The cat stopped vomiting and began eating well. In all, four adjustments were done and the cat remained symptom-free.

Another case that was reported in a veterinary publication concerned a silky terrier diagnosed by his veterinarian as having a "protruding disk" with pain and loss of function. X-rays revealed calcium deposits in the area and a misaligned vertebral joint. Surgery was rejected because of the high cost. After two weeks of unproductive drug therapy and confinement, chiropractic treatment was suggested. Though the owner had to carry his pet into the office, within a couple of minutes after the adjustment, the dog walked out painlessly. The improvement was lasting. The chiropractor said he had also treated other animals successfully. In one case he had restored a cat's sight after relieving pressure on the spinal cord.

The use of chiropractic and allied techniques in treating animals has been slow to develop because only licensed veterinarians are legally allowed to charge for it, and they are not taught such methods in their medical education. Nevertheless, supporters from both professions have come together to share information. Postgraduate training in chiropractic has recently become available to veterinarians.

Chiropractic works well with herbal medicine, naturopathic medicine, acupuncture and oriental medicine and homeopathic medicine.

ACUPUNCTURE AND ORIENTAL MEDICINE

Perhaps the most significant impact made on the veterinary profession by a traditional, holistic approach is the use of acupuncture and other aspects of oriental medicine. The basic theory behind this ancient and comprehensive system is that the fundamental energy fields (*chi*) that comprise the body (as well as all aspects of the universe) manifest as two poles, *yin* and *yang*. They're reminiscent of the positive and negative electrical charges described by physics.

Yin is seen as disruptive, disturbing, expanded and negative, and yang as constructive, focusing, contracted and positive. Your state of health depends on the proper balance between these two, which are really two sides of the same coin. A skilled therapist can correct any excesses or deficiencies by manipulating certain critical acupoints along the body's meridians (channels through which the energy flows). The flow of energy cannot be simply blocked or suppressed; it must be redirected. This may be done by using needles (acupuncture), finger pressure (acupressure or shiatsu), burning the herb mugwort near the point (moxibustion) or, in modern times, electrical stimulation (electroacupuncture), injection of various solutions (aquapuncture), the use of ultrasound (sonapuncture), lasers and the implantation of small gold beads.

The American Veterinary Medical Association has taken an interest in acupuncture and has encouraged scientific documentation of its results. According to Dr. Allen Schoen of Sherman, Connecticut, who introduced acupuncture to the well-known Animal Medical Center of New York City, the kinds of conditions that acupuncture can best help include:

◆ Musculoskeletal problems, such as arthritis, slipped disk and hip dysplasia (dislocation)
◆ Skin diseases and allergic dermatitis
◆ Chronic gastrointestinal diseases, such as chronic diarrhea or vomiting, equine colic and prolapsed rectum
◆ Neurological problems, such as epilepsy and some types of paralysis
◆ A variety of other problems such as chronic pain syndrome, breeding problems, respiratory arrest and coma

Dr. Schoen notes that acupuncture, like other alternative healing methods, may take time and repetition to produce results. He asks new clients to commit themselves to at least eight treatments in chronic cases. "If someone has six treatments without seeing any results, and stops, that doesn't mean that acupuncture doesn't work. It can take a while to stimulate the body to heal itself," he emphasizes.

Like any system of medicine, however, acupuncture has its "miracles." Dr. Sheldon Altman of Burbank, California, an active teacher, writer and practitioner of veterinary acupuncture, tells of a Doberman suffering from panosteitis (a painful bone disease). After only one treatment the dog walked out pain-free after six months of limping. The pain did not return.

Ihor Basko, D.V.M., who practices in Hawaii, has also told me about some marvelous results, especially with spinal disk problems, arthritis, canine hip dysplasia, skin allergies, kidney disorders and metabolic imbalances. He has been able to reduce the use of conventional drugs dramatically since learning acupuncture. Dr. Basko described acupuncture's effectiveness as amazing in some cases of uremia (a toxic kidney condition).

Even advanced canine distemper and feline leukemia (diseases for which modern veterinary methods can do little) have yielded to this holistic approach. And when animals treated with acupuncture finally reach their end, death is usually more peaceful, with less suffering than we usually see.

Of course, such a holistic approach can also work to *prevent* disease, much like a "tune-up" for the body. In fact, the ancient Chinese, who developed the system over thousands of years of practice and observation, emphasized prevention above all else. They resorted to acupuncture or herbs only when the preferred methods (meditation, exercise, massage) were insufficient. Most contemporary acupuncturists emphasize a total approach to health and include advice on the use of food, herbs and the like in their methods.

Acupuncture and Chinese medicine, like homeopathy, is a complete system that stands on its own. For that reason it is best not to combine it with homeopathy; the two can interfere with each other. Some practitioners use acupuncture along with naturopathic and manipulative therapies, but that is best determined by an experienced practitioner.

HOMEOPATHY

We now come to my own particular love, the science of homeopathy. In my search for effective holistic therapies, I started out using nutrition and herbs. I still do, along with naturopathic methods. But, by themselves, they didn't always seem sufficient to me. So I kept my eyes and ears open for a system that might be more effective. Here and there I kept hearing praise for homeopathy, so I finally decided to examine it for myself. That decision was a turning point that expanded my horizons to embrace a medical approach of unique elegance, order and effectiveness.

Homeopathy is practiced on both humans and animals in most parts of the world. To my way of thinking, it deserves far more attention than it now receives in this country. The contributions of homeopathy to our general understanding of health and disease have been enormous. Because of its many virtues, I hope it will become a prominent medical art of the future.

The real beauty of the homeopathic system lies in the simplicity of its basic principles, combined with richly researched detail to guide the practitioner in choosing the most suitable remedy. *The Science of Homeopathy*, by George Vithoulkas, is an important modern discussion of the principles involved and is invaluable for those interested in *any* form of holistic therapy.

Conventional medicine seems to be a composite of various hypotheses and changing fads, but homeopathy was founded on one basic unifying principle, "Like is cured by like" (*Similia similibus curentur*), recognized by Hippocrates and many others. It has remained the foundation of homeopathy ever since the early 1800s when the German physician Samuel Hahnemann originated the system.

Hahnemann noted certain similarities between symptoms produced by some diseases and by the drugs most useful in their treatment. From that relationship, he formed this theory: A disease can be cured by careful use of a medicine that produces similar symptoms when given to a healthy person. Called the Law of Similars, its beauty is that the treatment provided goes with rather than against the body's own efforts to regain health.

A good practitioner can read a whole set of signals flashed by a disease. Rather than prescribe one medication for a headache, another for an upset stomach and a third for depression, the homeopathic doctor will provide a single remedy for the whole set of symptoms in the patient. The one medication chosen can produce all three symptoms if given repeatedly to healthy individuals.

By contrast, conventional drugs are generally used either to take the place of normal body processes (hormonal drugs), inhibit body responses (painkillers, anti-inflammatory drugs, antihistamines) or weaken or kill bacteria or cancer cells (antibiotics, chemotherapy, radiation therapy). Therefore, they are frequently used in combinations to treat different conditions in the same patient, like arthritis, pyorrhea and migraine headaches—each requiring its specific medicine. This increases the chance of side effects

How Homeopathic Medications Are Prepared

Most homeopathic preparations can be purchased in a specific strength. For example, if treatment for nausea requires *Ipecac* 3X, you simply purchase the medicine at that strength.

The number following the name of the remedy indicates how many times the original substance has been processed.

For example, 1X indicates that one drop of medication has been added to nine drops of alcohol and subjected to energetic shaking. The medication is now at $\frac{1}{10}$ of its original concentration. If you add one drop of this 1X mixture to nine drops of alcohol, the solution would be labeled 2X, at $\frac{1}{100}$th of its original strength.

Thus: $1X = \frac{1}{10}$ concentration; $2X = \frac{1}{100}$; $3X = \frac{1}{1,000}$ and so on. These same numerical indications of remedy potency also apply to powders, which are diluted with powdered milk sugar.

In rare instances the "Quick Reference" section directs you to dilute certain medications on your own. For example, you may be asked to dilute echinacea by adding ten drops of the tincture to one cup of water.

Simply follow the directions in the "Quick Reference" section as you would a recipe.

---

because the interaction of medicines is often unpredictable.

Homeopaths, on the other hand, consider that the patient has only *one* disease, which can create many symptoms and idiosyncratic characteristics. Therefore, only one remedy is administered at a time—the one found to be the best catalyst for the body's total defense response. This minimizes the use of medicines and also gives attention to all of the symptoms of illness at the same time.

The specially prepared remedies used in homeopathy contain minute doses of herbs, minerals or animal products such as bee venom and cuttlefish ink. These substances are diluted and repeatedly agitated numerous times, so that only minuscule amounts actually enter a patient's body. Sometimes the mixture is so diluted that skeptics wonder how the substance could have enough strength left to do any good. But many homeopaths (myself included) believe what Hahnemann originally said: The specially prepared medicine carries a healing energy derived from the original material.

I can testify from my own experience of more than 17 years that, regardless of the reasons, homeopathic remedies do work—and very, very well. When I am able to recognize the unique symptom picture clearly—taking into account the mental, emotional and physical levels—and match it to the right remedy, I can be certain the patient will respond.

Here's a simplified example of how homeopathy works.

We know that a bee's sting will cause a certain typical reaction, including swelling, fluid accumulation (causing a bump), redness of the skin, pain and soreness. Typically, all of this is made worse by the application of heat or pressure. Some sensitive individuals also experience mental symptoms such as apathy, stupor and listlessness, or the opposite—whining and tearfulness. If a homeopathically prepared dilute solution of bee venom is given to a person with these symptoms, *even if the symptoms are caused by something other than a bee sting,* the condition will begin to improve.

The essential requirement is a very close similarity between the remedy and the pattern of the disease. And because the active ingredient is given in such dilute form, it does not cause unwanted physical side effects. So we have the advantage of a treatment method that stimulates and accelerates natural healing forces without causing side effects.

To know what conditions a remedy can cure, it is first tested by a group of human volunteers who take the substance in a diluted form for several days or weeks. Each day they note their individual changes—mental, emotional and physical—in a diary. Combining this detailed information with that of the cases it has cured and any poisonings it has accidentally caused, homeopaths develop a characteristic "symptom picture" of each substance. Eventually, the treatment is added to a *Materia Medica*, a reference that catalogs the effects of hundreds of medicines.

Let me tell you about a few cases where animals were treated successfully using homeopathy.

When I was first learning homeopathy, I encountered Misty, a cat suffering with septicemia (a rare, postsurgical reaction involving bacterial spread in the bloodstream and a general breakdown of the blood-clotting mechanism) following a routine spay. She was in pitiable condition, with a high fever and vomiting. Dark blood leaked from her

back, her underbelly, legs, feet, mouth and vagina. I also detected bleeding under the skin (dark blue swellings under the eyelids and ears). Though antibiotics might help, I was not sure they would act quickly enough in this crisis situation. She seemed to get worse even as I examined her!

As a temporary measure I decided to administer fluids under her skin to help counter her moderate dehydration. In the process I immediately noticed that she was very sensitive to pain, far more than I would expect. She could hardly bear being touched at all. At this point I recognized the similarity between Misty's condition and the provings of the remedy *Arnica* (from the herb leopard's bane). Among the characteristics of *Arnica* are fever, hemorrhage, black and blue spots under the skin from bleeding, septic conditions, hypersensitivity to pain and an aversion to touch!

I immediately gave Misty a tablet of *Arnica* and repeated it every few hours. Later in the day she was much improved. By the next morning her temperature had dropped and she was no longer bleeding. Misty was obviously calmer—eating for the first time since she became ill. Within 48 hours the only evidence of what had so recently been a life-threatening condition were a few dry scabs where the hemorrhage had been, and Misty was discharged. She remained in good health. I was quite impressed that such results had occurred without any need to use antibiotics or other drugs.

I'm often amazed at how rapidly homeopathic medications can work. In acute problems they usually restore health much faster than drugs do, and I have used them to treat a gamut of acute problems from severe infections like parvovirus or distemper to gunshot wounds, bites, punctures and abscesses. But they also excel in treating many chronic conditions, which are the bulk of my practice—allergies, auto-immune diseases, hyperthyroidism, urinary disorders, appetite problems, behavioral abnormalities, paralysis, skin problems, gum disease and so on. In short, they are useful in treating the whole gamut of animal disease.

A recent case that comes to mind, for instance, involved an older cat whose lab tests confirmed feline infectious peritonitis—a terminal condition not curable with drugs. His symptoms included repeated vomiting, diarrhea, loss of appetite and swelling of the abdomen. Over several days my client and I gradually changed the cat's diet to a home-prepared one and increased his vitality through the use of vitamins and thymus gland supplements. I then recognized an appropriate homeopathic remedy, which, for this particular fellow, was *Arsenicum album*, or white oxide of arsenic. (Don't let this alarm you. The amount of arsenic in a homeopathic remedy is less than you'd find in the food you eat, when it appears as a trace mineral.)

So I gave him one dose, which was followed by a short aggravation of symptoms for a couple of days and then a continued improvement for a long period. Two months later the vomiting began to recur, and I gave one more dose. He quickly returned to normal health and has remained stable ever since. On top of it all, his personality improved, so that he is now considerably calmer and steadier, and his weight increased from 6 to 11 pounds!

Homeopathic remedies can even be used to treat personality problems. For instance, one client's cat had spontaneously developed a drastic personality change for the worse. Where she had once been friendly, she was now irritable, resistant to being held and generally stand-offish. Homeopathic treatment with *Nux vomica* restored her normal affectionate self.

In another example, a dog did a Jeckyl-Hyde transformation not long after getting a rabies shot. Formerly happy and friendly, he became suspicious, aggressive and "barky." Worse yet, he began biting people—hard! Fortunately, with one dose of a remedy called *Stramonium* (thorn apple), I was able to restore this dog to its normal, happy self. This remedy is used for disturbances of the brain when the above symptoms of suspicion, aggressive behavior and biting are present. (It's used in people who are mentally disturbed and who, believe it or not, exhibit this same behavior!) Unfortunately, we see these behavior disorders coming on after rabies vaccination much too often. Apparently, the vaccine causes a low-grade inflammation of the brain in some animals.

Homeopathic remedies should not be combined with acupuncture or oriental medicine, as they are too similar in their action and interfere with each other. Homeopathic remedies are, however, compatible with naturopathic and nutritional therapies as well as chiropractic and other manipulative therapies. Some mild herbs can be used with homeopathy, but tinctures of herbs, especially large doses and herbs that affect the nervous system, should be avoided.

TISSUE SALTS

I sometimes recommend tissue salts instead of homeopathic preparations. A system of therapy using these salts was devised by Wilhelm Heinrich Schuessler in the nineteenth century. Schuessler, a medical doctor, physiological chemist and physicist, based his treatment on the fact that the human body is composed of billions of cells that contain a perfect balance of water, organic substances and inorganic compounds. While the inorganic substances are present only in very small quantities, they are vital to living tissue—helping cells build or heal.

Tissue salts are prepared homeopathically. That is, they are divided into 12 separate salts—each serving to stimulate the body in a certain way. They are usually known by their abbreviated names, as follows:

1. *Calcarea fluorica* (Calc. fluor. or calcium fluoride). Preserves the ability of elastic tissue to contract.
2. *Calcarea phosphorica* (Calc. phos. or calcium phosphate). Used for rickets and to aid growth and development, digestion, circulation and general recovery.
3. *Calcarea sulphurica* (Calc. sulph. or calcium sulphate). Purifies blood of nonfunctional organic matter.
4. *Ferrum phosphoricum* (Ferr. phos. or iron phosphate). Carries oxygen into the bloodstream and to all parts of the body. Good for inflammation, pain or fever.
5. *Kali muriaticum* (Kali mur. or potassium chloride). Helpful in sluggish conditions.
6. *Kali phosphoricum* (Kali phos. or potassium phosphate). A nerve nutrient.
7. *Kali sulphuricum* (Kali sulph. or potassium sulphate). Often used where

there is a sticky, yellow discharge from the skin or mucous membrane.
8. *Magnesia phosphorica* (Mag. phos. or magnesium phosphate). Known as the antispasmodic tissue salt, its main function is to treat the nervous system and muscle cramps.
9. *Natrum muriaticum* (Nat. mur. or sodium chloride). Often called the water-distributing tissue salt, it controls the ebb and flow of body fluids. Excessive wetness or dryness in any part of the body can indicate a deficiency of this tissue salt.
10. *Natrum phosphoricum* (Nat. phos. or sodium phosphate). An acid neutralizer that is important for the proper functioning of the digestive tract.
11. *Natrum sulphuricum* (Nat. sulph. or sodium sulphate). Removes excess water from the fluids that bathe tissue cells. A tonic to the liver.
12. *Silicea* (quartz or silicon dioxide). A cleanser capable of breaking up accumulations of pus, as in the case of abscesses or sties. Helps to eliminate foreign material such as plant stickers or splinters.

The chief advantage of tissue salts, and the reason I mention them here, is their availability. Whereas homeopathic remedies must often be ordered by mail from a homeopathic pharmacy, tissue salts are sold in many health food stores (usually in the 6X potency). Both *Natrum muriaticum* and *Silicea* are often needed in treatment of severe chronic disease in animals.

Tissue salts will combine well with herbal medicine, chiropractic and other manipulative therapies. Some practitioners use them as an adjunct to other therapies such as acupuncture and Chinese medicine, even allopathic drugs. However, tissue salts are prepared in the manner of homeopathic remedies and best results will follow from using them with the same guidelines as given under the section on homeopathic medicine above. They are not to be used with other homeopathic medicines.

FLOWER ESSENCES

In addition to homeopathic remedies, I also use something similar—the flower preparations of Dr. Bach—to treat both behavioral and physical problems. Though these dilute infusions of flowers and tree buds are said to act primarily upon the mental state, a psychological improvement often brings a physical one as well. These extracts are given orally several times a day, often for several weeks.

One case in which I used a flower essence involved a dog, Jamie, that had a host of distressing symptoms. These included a loss of appetite, lack of energy, unusual behavior, vomiting, collapse, fever, a moist coat, a tense abdomen and enlarged spleen. In addition, laboratory tests showed that she was anemic, with abnormally shaped red blood cells, an above-normal number of white blood cells, elevated liver enzymes (showing liver damage), elevated cholesterol and bile pigments, high blood sugar and so on. The x-rays taken were normal.

All these were threatening symptoms and seemed to indicate a serious physical disturbance. Yet previous treatment with a synthetic cortisone preparation, antibiotics and vitamin B_{12} injections had no effect on Jamie.

Because I knew the family was under stress, I suspected that emotional disturbance was playing an important role. Accordingly, I prescribed one of the flower essences, *Larch*, to be given four times a day for a week. For the first few hours after starting the treatment, Jamie's symptoms became exaggerated, but she was markedly better by the next day. After a week her symptoms were gone and didn't return. In addition, her personality improved. For the first time she became playful and outgoing with the other animals in the family. This change has persisted even though the original treatment was only for a few weeks.

I've also found the flower preparations discovered by Dr. Bach useful in treating some conditions that develop shortly after a traumatic or upsetting experience. For instance, a woman brought in a cat a couple of weeks after it had been violently shaken by a large dog. The cat was uncomfortable, irritable and constipated and had a fever, weight loss, fluid accumulation in the lungs and a painful abdomen. His most severe injury was a displaced vertebra in the lower back, which I could feel was out of place. It hurt the cat very much when I touched it.

I prescribed the flower essence *Star of Bethlehem* (indicated for fright after trauma) in a dosage of two drops every two hours. Three days later, the cat's owner called to say that her pet was quite recovered. The drops had noticeably relaxed him. After a couple of days' treatment, he began stretching by hooking his claws in a piece of firewood and pulling from side to side. Apparently, the stretching corrected the back problem. Soon it was difficult to medicate the cat—he was too busy leaping tall fences in a single bound!

The 38 flower preparations discovered by Dr. Edward Bach are compatible with any other system of treatment. They are mild in their effect and cannot cause problems even when "overused."

As you can see, some pretty remarkable things can happen when we adopt a new view of the wholeness of the body and mind, and treat from there. The success of the holistic therapies described in this chapter depends on the skill of the practitioner, the strength and will of the patient, the degree of support in the environment, the appropriateness of the selected method and the cooperation of the owner in applying and following through with treatments.

This brief survey is meant to introduce you to the numerous exciting approaches that can help to relieve the suffering of animals. And if we are but willing to extend our mental horizons, how much more is possible?

CHAPTER FIFTEEN

HOW TO CARE FOR A SICK ANIMAL

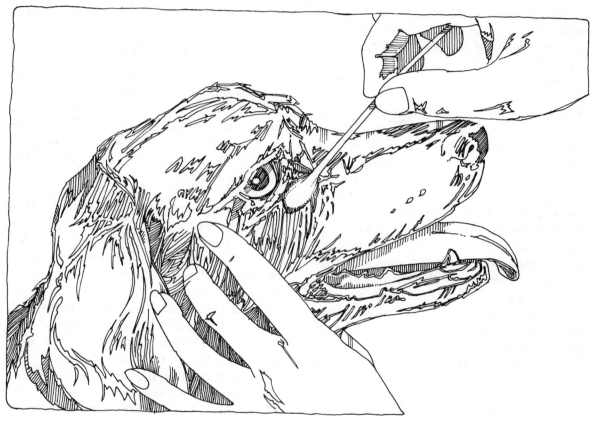

If your animal gets sick, there are several advantages to caring for it at home, if your family situation allows for seeing to the animal's needs. First, home is familiar and safe, free of the stress a pet is likely to feel trying to recuperate in a busy veterinary hospital filled with unfamiliar animals and people. Second, if you have the time, you can provide some really useful nursing care at home.

Fasting, special nutrition or meticulous cleaning might not be provided in a hospital, either because these things take too much time or because the philosophy of disease treatment is different. Third, at home you are in charge; alternative or natural forms of treatment can be used without conflict.

On the other hand, a veterinarian is a skilled professional. Years of training and experience enable him to assess the seriousness of a condition and use the proper diagnostic techniques. For conditions that are either very messy to take care of (like severe vomiting and diarrhea) or life-threatening (such as a car accident or severe infection), the veterinary hospital offers support that is impossible to provide at home, including such treatments as anti-shock therapy, intravenous fluids or surgery.

Both at home and in the hospital, your pet can recover faster and more completely if you utilize the general health care principles in this book (good nutrition and supplements, exercise, a supportive relationship and so on) and some of the nursing care methods in this chapter. If, however, you are giving your animal a prescription drug recommended by your veterinarian, do *not* use the homeopathic remedies suggested in the Quick Reference section of alphabetical entries at the end of this book, since they tend to work against each other. You can, however, use some of the herbal recommendations, particularly those that are suggested for external use or those whose primary purpose is to help rebuild the tissues.

A seriously ill animal has certain basic needs. When wild animals are sick or injured, they go off by themselves to rest in a secure, peaceful place and to allow nature to heal the condition. We need to provide our pets with a comparable opportunity. Most sick animals want to be quiet, safe and warm and to have access to fresh air and sunlight. Also, they often will fast instinctively. The loss of appetite seen in many diseases, especially acute infectious ones, is part of the healing response rather than a symptom to be forcibly overridden.

So provide comfortable bedding in a cozy spot that is free of drafts, disturbances and loud noise, where your dog or cat can rest peacefully and feel protected. Keep the area clean, changing the blankets or towels as necessary. If your pet desires it, allow some access to fresh air and sunlight (but don't impose it).

FASTING

Generally, it's good to encourage fasting the first day or two of an illness, especially if there is a fever. A good rule of thumb is to fast your pet until its temperature returns to normal—one to two days, or as long as four to five, if necessary, provided that the animal is in reasonably healthy condition to start with.

Fasting is one of the oldest and most natural methods of healing. Normally, the body constantly eliminates waste products, along with any tainted or toxic materials that were consumed. Fasting greatly reduces the body's usual assimilation and elimination load, allowing it to break down and expel older wastes that may have accumulated in the liver and fatty tissues. The body also gets a chance to unload the products of inflammation, tumors and abscesses. Once the body has cleansed itself, the overworked glands, organs and cells have a chance to repair and restore themselves.

Dogs and cats have been fasted for many days with excellent results and amazing recoveries. Of course, you should not attempt a long fast without professional guidance. See the section on naturopathy in chapter 14 for conditions that generally benefit from fasting as well as for those for which fasting should not be used.

The following program is a good basic

guideline for fasting your animal. It can be used during illnesses, but it also can help your pet switch from its old eating habits to a new natural foods diet.

The break-in period: Begin by easing the animal into the fast for one to two days. Feed it a lighter, simpler diet that includes a moderate or small amount of lean meat or tofu (if feeding a dog), along with some vegetables and cooked oatmeal. (Of course, if your animal is suddenly ill and loses its appetite, this step is not necessary or appropriate.)

Use vegetables considered beneficial to the kidneys and the liver, organs that will play major roles during the fast. They include broccoli, kale, cauliflower, cabbage, beets and turnips (with tops), dandelion greens, squash, spinach, corn, potatoes, cucumbers, parsley, carrots and tomatoes. Serve these foods either raw and finely grated (which is preferable) or lightly steamed.

The liquid fast: Next, proceed with the main part of the fast, a liquid diet. In acute problems, continue the fast until the temperature is normal (less than 101.5°F) and the animal is well on its way to recovery. In more chronic or degenerative conditions, the length of the fast may vary from about three to seven days—until there is substantial improvement and a hearty appetite returns. If you begin reintroducing solids and your animal doesn't seem hungry for them, stay with the liquid fast a little longer.

During this period, offer plenty of the following:

- ◆ *Water:* Use a pure source, such as bottled, spring, filtered or distilled water. Do *not* use tap water, which may contain chlorine, fluorine and other unwholesome chemicals.

- ◆ *Vegetable juices:* Use fresh juices only. Don't use juice more than 48 hours old. If you can't give your pet fresh juice, offer chopped or grated raw vegetables (especially greens and juicy ones blended with pure water and strained through a sieve). If you can't come up with either of these alternatives, feed water and the broth recipe that follows.

- ◆ *Vegetable broth:* Using the vegetables listed for the break-in period, make a soup stock by chopping and then simmering them 20 to 30 minutes. You may add a small amount of meat or a bone to flavor the stock, but no spices or salt. Pour off the liquid for the animal and save the solids for a soup or casserole for yourself.

If your animal is young or run-down and seems to need a little extra energy, you can occasionally offer it a teaspoon or so of honey.

If you notice your pet having strained or constipated bowel movements early in the liquid fast stage, you can help get things going by slowly (over one to two minutes) administering an enema (see the instructions under "Special Care" on page 211). Though an enema is seldom needed during a short fast if your pet is in fairly good shape, the animal with a chronic disease or an acute infection will benefit from several enemas during the longer fast.

Breaking the fast: When it's time to end the fast, give your pet a simple diet for several days. This transition diet should last two to three days for every seven days the animal was on liquids. Offer water, juice, broth and a moderate amount of raw or steamed vegetables (the same group used before) plus a little raw milk or plain yogurt. After this period, begin adding other natural foods, starting with oatmeal or flaked barley cereal (cooked), milk, honey and figs or prunes. Then, after a day or two, offer some raw lean meat (or tofu or cottage cheese), some other grains or dairy products and some nutritional yeast until you have worked into the standard natural diet with supplements.

It is very important that you break the animal out of the fast gradually and that you avoid any temptation to feed commercial foods or highly processed tidbits at this point, or else you may undo the beneficial effects of the fast and cause serious digestive upsets by overtaxing the system before it has fully reestablished peristalsis, the contractions that aid in digestion.

Carried out properly, a fast of this sort can be a great boon for your animal's health. I hope that you understand the spirit of the fasting instructions and do not misinterpret them. I am *not* saying that you can just put a sick dog on the back porch with no food and a little water to drink! I am not suggesting neglect by any means, but rather an attitude of support, which includes doing the right things at the right time. Though outwardly the two approaches may appear similar, your inner intent and concern is the decisive factor that makes the difference. If you are not sure what to do or how long to keep the fast going, then consult with a holistically oriented veterinarian before proceeding.

IF YOUR PET WON'T EAT

Sometimes an animal (usually a cat) starts fasting on its own but does not regain its appetite at the end of the fast. This can happen as a result of stomach upset, inflammation of the digestive organs or as a reaction to toxic chemicals in the body or the environment (from pollution or kidney failure, for example). Fasting becomes a problem if there is rapid weight loss and developing weakness that robs the body of the energy to heal. So it may be necessary to force-feed (put food in the animal's mouth) to keep a pet alive or to get it started eating again.

Before you do this, however, you may want to try tempting the animal into eating on its own by offering a tasty food that has a strong aroma, such as freshly broiled chicken or turkey.

If you must force-feed, try this healthful mixture.

PET PUREE

⅔ cup raw chicken or turkey (may contain giblets)

⅓ cup half-and-half or whole milk

400 milligrams calcium (or ⅔ teaspoon bonemeal or ¼ teaspoon eggshell powder)

Cat or dog vitamins, as recommended on the label for one day

Puree all the ingredients in a food processor. Adjust the liquid as needed to make a thick, smooth paste. If you only have a blender, thin the food down and prevent strain on the motor by using short bursts rather than a long run. Refrigerate extras up to 3 days; throw it out if it begins to smell sour.

Feed ½ to 1 cup a day to a small animal, proportionately more to larger ones. The easiest method is finger-feeding. Using one hand, pry the mouth open (as described below in the directions for giving medications). Scoop up a gob of this food paste on a finger and wipe it on the roof of your animal's mouth, behind the front teeth. Most pets will swallow it rather than spit it out. Allow plenty of time for swallowing before offering the next bit. If this doesn't work, you can thin the mix further and use a turkey baster or a plastic syringe without the needle (ask your veterinarian for one) to administer it. Give small amounts every few hours, rather than forcing the whole daily feeding down in one or two doses.

Caution: You may need to wrap your pet (especially cats) in a towel before the feeding to avoid getting scratched in the process.

SPECIAL CARE

Depending on the animal's condition and symptoms, you may also need to provide other kinds of nursing care.

Enemas: Animals can benefit from the use of enemas in some conditions, particularly in fasting, constipation, bowel irritation caused by bone fragments or the presence of toxic material (like garbage or spoiled food in the digestive tract), dehydration or excessive vomiting.

Use pure water that is warm but not hot (test it on your wrist)—only about two tablespoons for a cat and up to a pint for a large dog. (Even a small amount of fluid will stimulate the bowel to empty itself.) Add a few drops of freshly squeezed lemon juice to the water and administer the solution with a plastic or rubber syringe (or enema bag and nozzle with larger animals) over a two- to three-minute period.

Here's how: First, lubricate the end of the syringe with vegetable oil and, while someone else calmly and gently holds the animal while it stands on the ground or in a tub, insert the nozzle carefully into the rectum. With gentle, consistent pressure against the anus (so the fluid does not leak out), slowly fill the colon. If the solution does not flow in readily, it's probably because the syringe is up against a fecal mass, in which case you'll need to pull back on the nozzle or syringe and adjust the angle a bit. A bowel movement is usually stimulated within just a few minutes.

Administer an enema in this fashion once or twice a day for a couple of days. That's usually enough.

Dehydrated animals may simply retain the fluid. I have seen this many times. What happens is that the colon absorbs the fluid, which the body desperately needs. Thus, enemas are an excellent way to administer fluid therapy at home! Give them about every four hours under these circumstances, or until fluid is no longer retained.

If your animal has been vomiting a lot and can't keep water in its stomach, an enema can introduce fluid as well as salts needed to replace those lost through vomiting. To the enema water add a pinch of sea salt plus a pinch of potassium chloride (KCl, a salt substitute especially for people on low-sodium diets that is sold in supermarkets). This same salt-replacement fluid therapy will help a dog or cat with prolonged diarrhea. Again, administer every four hours or until fluid is no longer retained.

Bathing and cleaning: In some cases an animal is so fouled by vomiting, diarrhea or skin discharges that a cleansing bath is definitely in order. You should, however, take on this task only at the end of an illness, when the animal is well on the way to recovery and its temperature is normal. Otherwise, rely upon the cleaning methods described below. Even then, be sure the animal does not become chilled. Dry him quickly by giving him a good toweling, followed by a warm sunbath or a blow-dry with the dryer set on low. The only exception to the rule of waiting is when the dog or cat, particularly a young one, is so heavily parasitized with fleas and lice that its strength is being sapped. Then a soapy bath that removes and drowns these parasites is in order.

Care of the body openings: Very often, a disease will cause discharges from various body orifices, especially the nose, eyes, ears and anus. Sick animals, particularly cats, are made miserable by accumulations they cannot remove and that can irritate underlying tissues. Here are a few simple cleansing techniques that offer great relief.

The nose: If plugs and secretions have formed, carefully clean the nose with a cloth or gauze saturated with warm water. Sometimes patience is needed in trying to soften the material so you can gradually remove it. Two or three short sessions may be better than a single long one.

Once the nose is clean and dry, smear the area with almond oil, almond oil mixed with vitamin E oil from a capsule, or calendulated oil (which can be purchased from homeopathic pharmacies). Apply two or three times a day.

The eyes: To clean crusts and secretions from the eyes and eyelids, make up a soothing, nonirritating salt solution by mixing ¼ teaspoon of sea salt into a cup of distilled or filtered water. Stir well and use this mixture to clean the eyes the same way described for the nose (above). After the eyes are clean, put one drop of one of the following soothing treatments in each eye: almond oil (for mild irritation), castor oil (for more irritated and inflamed eyes) or cod-liver oil (for eyes that are dry or ulcerated).

Or, instead of the above treatment, bathe the eyes frequently with one of the following two herbal infusions.

An infusion of eyebright (*Euphrasia officinalis*) is useful where there are injuries or irritation of the eyes. To make it, bring 1 cup of pure water to a boil; pour over 1 teaspoon of the herb. Let it steep, covered, for 15 minutes. Then pour off the liquid through a sieve or through cheesecloth, leaving the solid herb pieces behind. For every cup of the infusion, add ¼ teaspoon of sea salt. This makes the solution mild and soothing (like natural tears).

Goldenseal root is helpful when the eyes are infected or discharging thick, yellow material. To make a treatment solution, pour 1 cup of boiling water over ¼ teaspoon of goldenseal powder. Let it steep for 15 minutes; then filter off the liquid part. To this liquid, add ¼ teaspoon sea salt.

When the solution you are preparing has cooled down, gently clean and treat the eyes 3 times a day, or as needed. You can keep these solutions (covered) at room temperature on your countertop for 2 days. To avoid contamination of the whole preparation, always pour off a little into a dish or cup to use for treatment, and then put the cover back on the main batch. Discard this treatment fluid rather than return it to the stock you made.

The ears: If the ears contain much oily or waxy secretion, trickle about ½ teaspoon of almond oil into the ear hole, preferably using a dropper or squeeze bottle. To start, prewarm the oil in a cup or glass that is partly immersed in a sink or bowl of hot water. Firmly lift the ear flap or tip. You may need someone to help you hold the animal's head in place, because if you let go or the animal pulls away before you finish the job, he will shake oil all over you. Let the almond oil run down into the ear for a few seconds.

Then, while still holding the ear flap, reach down with your other hand and massage the ear canal from the outside at the

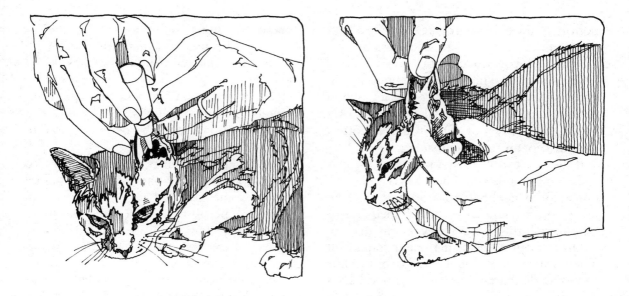

To remove waxy or oily buildup in the ears, trickle a small amount of prewarmed almond oil into the ear. Then massage the ear canal until you hear a squishing sound. Use a tissue to remove the material that has worked its way out.

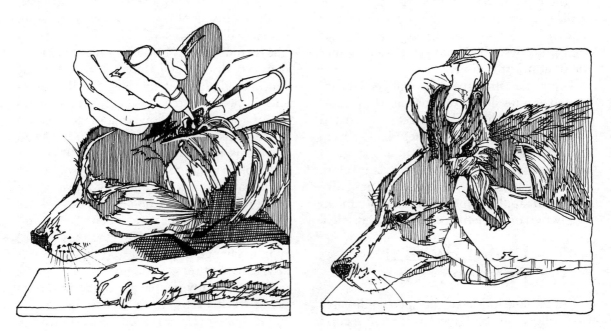

bottom of the ear opening. It feels like a firm plastic tube that you can compress as you massage. If you do it right, you'll hear a squishy sound. This treatment loosens up and dissolves the lodged wax. Use a tissue to remove any excess oil and materials that work their way out. Don't use a cotton swab except around the opening.

If the ear is very red and inflamed, use calendula oil or aloe vera juice. This can be obtained from health food stores or as fresh juice from a plant. It's usually adequate to treat the ear this way once every day or two.

On the other hand, if the ear is painful when touched at the massage point but shows no discharge, some foreign body, such as plant material or a tick, may be inside the ear canal. It is best to have your veterinarian examine the ear and determine the cause of pain. If there is no obvious cause for the ear pain, a good treatment to use is Arnica oil (available at a homeopathic pharmacy or a health food store). Gently treat the ear (as described above) once a day until the discomfort is gone.

The anus: Often the anus will get very inflamed as a result of excessive diarrhea, causing the surrounding tissue to get irritated and sometimes infected with bacteria. To keep this area clean during the diarrhea stage of an illness, sponge it gently with a damp cloth (rubbing can further irritate it). Pat it dry and then apply some calendula ointment. Apply two or three times a day or as needed.

USING HERBAL PREPARATIONS

In the description of the specific diseases that follows in the Quick Reference section on page 227, I have noted many places where you may use various herbs and/or homeopathic preparations. For those who are not familiar with these remedies, I will describe some of the basic methods for making them or obtaining them from pharmacists. Let's start with herbs.

Three basic forms of herbs can be used in preparing treatments.

Fresh herbs: When possible, use an herb that has been freshly harvested right before use. In some areas of the country, useful medicinal herbs can be located easily in vacant lots, along roadsides (avoid heavily traveled areas because of car exhaust contamination), in country fields or woods or perhaps in your own herb garden. Those able to identify herbs in the field can collect them as needed (see "Recommended Reading and Tapes" on page 357 for useful books to help you identify herbs).

For optimal effectiveness, pick an herb when its essential oils are at their peak. In general, that means you should collect any aboveground parts in the morning, after the dew has dried but before the hot sun has evaporated some of the oils. Ideally, leaves should be harvested just before the plant is about to begin its flowering stage. Gather flowers just before they reach full bloom (they have much less value after that).

If you're going for the *whole* aboveground part (leaves, stems and all), pick it just before the flowering stage. Roots and rhizomes are best collected in the fall, when the sap returns to the ground, the leaves are just beginning to change their color and the berries or seeds are mature.

Because many people are unfamiliar with using fresh herbs, the instructions in this book usually refer to dried herbs. But if the fresh plant is available, use about three times the volume indicated for dried herbs in the listings.

Dried herbs: In most cases you will probably just buy the herb dried, either loosely cut or powdered and perhaps packaged in gelatin capsules. Dried herbs can be administered either in these capsules or mixed with water in an infusion, decoction or slurry. You can save some money on capsuled herbs by buying empty capsules from a pharmacy and packing your own. One "00" capsule holds about ½ teaspoon of powdered herb. If you need to powder the herb, use a mortar and pestle to grind it to a fine dust.

If you gather or grow your own herbs, you can dry them for later use. Collect them after the morning dew on the leaves has dried. Tie the herbs in bunches and hang them upside down in a well-ventilated, dry, shaded area. Enclosed attics can be good for this. If you gather roots and barks, scrub them well, then chop them up and dry them on screening in direct sunlight. Once they are thoroughly dried, store them in opaque or brown, capped jars in a cool, dark place. Properly cured and stored, herbs retain most of their medicinal quality for some time. Since these properties are destroyed by heat, sunlight and exposure to air, however, it is best to keep the herbs no longer than a year.

Herbal tinctures: Another way to obtain and use herbs is in the tincture form. The easiest way to get tinctures is to buy them from herbal supply houses or homeopathic pharmacies. But if you have access to the fresh plant, the best form of tincture is one made from freshly collected, organically grown material.

To make your own tincture, macerate and grind the fresh herb (or use a blender). Add 1 rounded tablespoon of herb to ½ cup vodka or brandy (at least 80 proof). Store the mixture in a clean, tightly capped jar and shake it once or twice a day over 2 weeks. Then strain off the solids through a fine cloth or paper, collecting the liquid, which is your tincture. Store it in tightly capped glass bottles in a cool, dark area. (If you used dried herbs instead of fresh, figure 1 rounded teaspoon of the cut or powdered herb for each ½ cup of alcohol.)

Herbal tinctures are a very potent form of medicine and must be used carefully at low dosages, as the specific instructions in the Quick Reference section on page 227 will indicate. Tightly capped, they will keep for three years.

Preparing Herbal Medicines

The fresh or dried forms of herbs can both be used to make infusions, in which boiling water is added to the herb and steeped (like making tea). To make a less strong tasting, more palatable version of an infusion, double the amount of herb used and just soak it in cold water overnight. This is called a cold extract. If the herb comes as a root or a bark, simmer it in boiling water for 15 to 20 minutes (called a decoction). Infusions or cold extracts should be prepared in a covered, nonmetallic container such as pottery or glass (to retain the volatile substances). Decoctions should be simmered in an open, nonmetallic pan (to concentrate the product). Be sure to always use purified water (distilled or filtered) for these preparations. Specific amounts to use in preparation are given in the Quick Reference section on page 227.

Tinctures should always be diluted, three drops per teaspoon of water, just before administering.

How to Give Liquid Medication

There are two techniques I recommend for getting any form of liquid medication (conventional medicine or a diluted tincture, decoction, infusion or cold extract) down an animal's throat.

Pry the mouth open. Lightly grasp the animal's upper jaw with one hand and insert your thumb and fingers in the gaps just behind the fangs. (For a cat or tiny dog, just one finger is needed in addition to the thumb.) Most animals will then relax their mouths slightly so that you can pour the liquid with a spoon or dropper between the front teeth. Tilt the head back when you do this so that the liquid will run down to the throat.

Make a pouch. Use one hand to pull out the corner of the animal's lower lip to make a little pouch, and, keeping the head tilted back, pour the liquid into it with the other hand.

In either instance, if the liquid doesn't go in, it's because the teeth are clenched too tightly. If so, pry them open slightly with your fingers. If your animal backs away, put its rear end in a corner so it can't move away from you during the process, or get someone to help hold your pet. Another way to do this is to sit on the floor or a bed with your pet between your legs. With her rear end toward you and the head facing away, you can keep her positioned more easily for the administration.

For a cat, you may need someone to help by gently but firmly holding its front feet, or you can do the job alone by wrapping the cat quickly and snugly in a towel. Be gentle and positive so your animal doesn't have reason to feel afraid and put up a struggle.

After the medicine is in, induce swallowing by gently holding the mouth almost closed and massaging the throat. Swallowing is signaled by the tongue's emerging briefly from between the front teeth. Alternatively, you can briefly put your thumb over the nostrils to achieve the same purpose.

How to Give Pills and Capsules

To give most solid medications like herbal capsules or vitamin pills, open the animal's mouth by grasping around the upper jaw, as just described for liquids. Hold the capsule or pill between your thumb and the first finger or else between the first and second fingers. Use the remaining fingers to press down the lower front teeth and thus pry the jaw open.

Insert the medication into the throat, pushing it as far back as you can. Then induce swallowing as described above. At first this will seem difficult and awkward. After a few tries, however, you will become more experienced and find it much easier.

Using Homeopathic Medications

To give a homeopathic or tissue salt tablet, use one of two methods.

Give the tablets or pellets whole. Administer them from the cap of the vial or from a clean spoon (it's best not to touch them).

Crush pellets to a powder (use three pellets). To do the crushing, make a crisp fold in a heavy paper. (A small file card is very good for this, or you can take a clean sheet of paper and fold it in half a couple of times.) Pour the tablets from the bottle into the open fold. Fold the paper flat against a hard countertop and tap the pellets with a

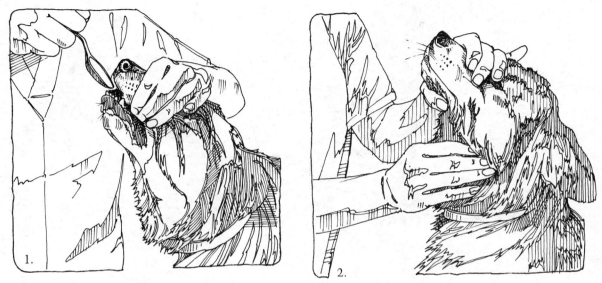

Giving Liquid Medication: Hold the mouth open with your fingers while you pour the medicine between the front teeth (1). Tilt the head back and stroke the throat to make the animal swallow (2).

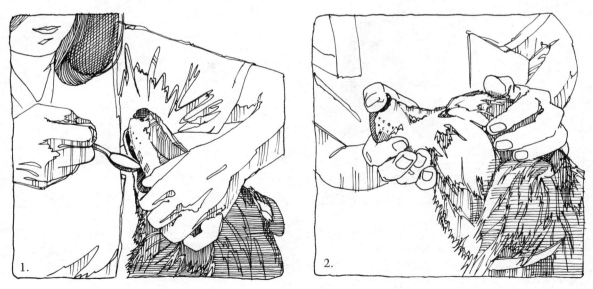

If Your Pet Resists: Pull out the lower lip, forming a pocket to hold the medicine (1). Make the animal swallow by gently and briefly putting your thumb over the nostrils (2).

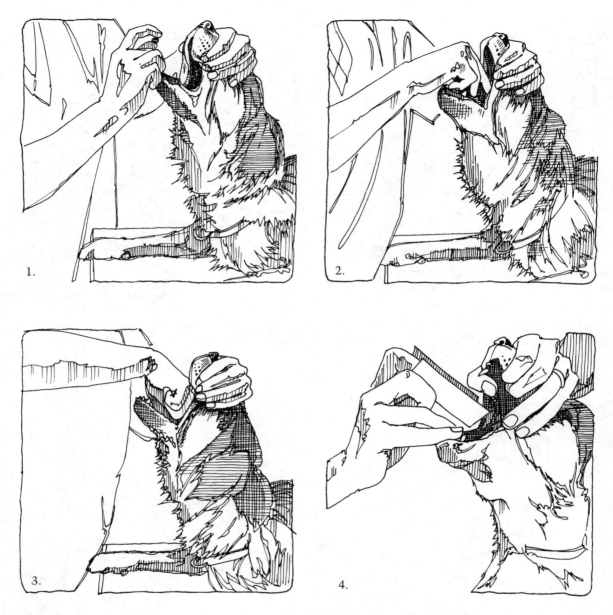

Giving Pills and Powders: Pry the mouth open (1), place the pill on the back of the tongue (2) and quickly push it as far back into the throat as you can (3). Then, hold the muzzle shut and massage the throat to induce swallowing. For powders and crushed pills, slide the contents from a folded paper directly onto the tongue (4).

heavy glass to gradually crush them to a powder. The pellets from some pharmacies can be very hard, so don't try to do this on your antique wooden table.

With a word of encouragement, invite your animal to lick the powder off the paper (it tastes sweet). If he is not interested, use the same holding and prying technique described for other pills and pour or flick the powder from the paper onto the animal's tongue. This method both eliminates the possibility of your pet spitting the medicine out and also keeps it from being contaminated.

There are distinct advantages to using homeopathic drops or tablets. Because only a small number are given, they are easy to administer. Also, in many instances only one or just a few doses are needed during the treatment.

The homeopathic remedies mentioned in the Quick Reference section can either be ordered by mail (see "Suppliers of Homeopathic Remedies" on page 354) or, in some cases, purchased in health food stores. The latter applies mostly to the tissue salts (discussed in chapter 14), a special subgroup of homeopathic remedies made from the basic mineral salts found in the body.

HOW TO PREPARE
THE 38 FLOWER PREPARATIONS
OF DR. BACH

These preparations are available in 38 individual "stock" bottles that are combined and diluted into a formula. Here is how it is done: If you wanted to make a formula of Chicory, Heather and Clematis (three of the flowers out of the available 38), for example, you would first put two drops from the stock bottle for each of these flowers into a clean one-ounce dropper bottle. Then you would fill the bottle with spring water to make the dilution. This is your "treatment" bottle and from this a standard dosage is to give two drops four times a day. The drops can be put on the tongue, inside the lips or added to food or water. Usually, this treatment is done for several days or weeks depending on need.

A HOME REMEDY KIT

Don't wait until your animal needs treatment to track down basic supplies. Like a Boy Scout, be prepared. Some preparations will have to be ordered by mail from the suppliers listed under "Suppliers of Homeopathic Remedies" on page 354. Others can be obtained at your local health food store, herb shop or even grocery store. And, of course, you can grow or collect many herbs yourself. But in all cases, it's best to have a group of commonly used substances on hand. Most are really quite inexpensive.

You can also gather together a kit of basic homeopathic remedies most often mentioned in the Quick Reference section or obtain it ready-made. That way, when the need is immediate, you will already have what you need.

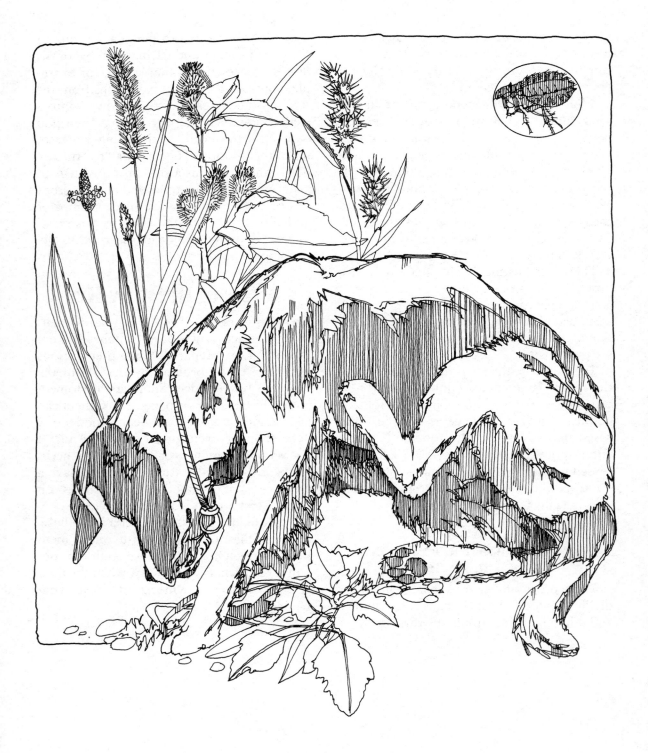

PART TWO
QUICK REFERENCE

How to Use the Quick Reference Section

The very best medicine is prevention. Good diet, exercise and a healthy environment are all essential for excellent health. But sometimes, regardless of what we do or don't do for them, animals get sick. If that happens, what can you do to help care for your pet and optimize its chances for full recovery?

In this section I describe many health problems common to dogs and cats and suggest specific treatments. Some of these treatments can be used in conjunction with conventional veterinary treatment, if necessary. Others, particularly homeopathic medicines, should not be used with drugs. If possible, work with a cooperative, holistically oriented veterinarian or at least one who is sympathetic to your viewpoint.

You may recall from the first part of the book that I believe total health requires a total approach. At the start it's important to consider and address any causative or contributing factors in the lifestyle, environment or diet so that there are no external obstacles to your animal's recovery. Then, as much as possible, select from the treatment choices the one that best fits your pet's particular situation and most accurately corresponds to the animal's symptom complex you observe. This will require careful observation on your part.

For treatment you can use herbs or remedies (like tissue salts) that you can easily obtain at local herb suppliers or health food stores. In other instances, however, I will mention homeopathic remedies that you will probably need to order by mail from one of the pharmacies listed in "Suppliers of Homeopathic Remedies" on page 354. I believe in keeping a ready-to-use kit of common remedies at hand as an aid to timely treatment.

If you also want to learn more about the holistic approach, check the valuable information in the books listed in "Recommended Reading and Tapes" beginning on page 357. Naturally, the more you understand about these treatment methods, the more successfully you can use them.

How to Look Up a Particular Disease

To find an elusive topic, check under a larger grouping. For example, canine distemper, chorea (a common aftereffect of distemper) and feline panleukopenia (often called feline distemper) are *all* listed under "Distemper." Many conditions are grouped according to the body part or organ they affect—"Stomach Problems," "Skin Problems" or "Ear Problems," for example. The cross references should help to lead you to the right category with a minimum of difficulty.

What You Can Expect

Except in some acute conditions that may clear up rapidly, healing generally takes time. It took a while for the body to get out of balance, and it takes time to restore it. Of course, if we give a painkiller or a suppressive drug such as cortisone, we may see some rapid relief, but this is not a true cure. Take away the drug and the symptoms are likely to return eventually, often worse than before.

Since our aim is to address the underlying weakness and restore health permanently, it's important to recognize the progressive stages and understand the gradually changing picture of symptoms in healing. That way we can tell if our treatment is really helping or whether another approach should be tried.

When a treatment is working, an acute illness (sudden, self-limited) generally responds quickly (within a few minutes, a few hours or, at the longest, a day or two). Chronic illness, on the other hand, changes slowly. It often takes several weeks to see a change for the better, and months, or even a year or two, for complete recovery.

The chance of complete recovery depends on several significant factors, including the age, level of vitality and extent of illness in your pet. Though a disease that has progressed far enough to do extensive damage to the body cannot be completely reversed, it can be alleviated, sometimes very significantly. Of course, it isn't reasonable to expect organs or tissues to return to their previous undamaged state. But we may be able to stop the progression of the chronic disease permanently and enhance healing to the limit of the body's abilities.

For example, an old cat with kidney failure can be brought from a state of debilitating illness to one of relative normality. However, the treatment may have to continue for the rest of his life, with occasional use of homeopathic medicines, a restricted protein diet and fluid therapy as needed. Internally, our treatment may only have improved the kidneys' functioning from a level of 25 percent to 30 percent effective use. However, that 5 percent can make all the difference.

On the other hand, if your animal is younger and has been ill only a relatively short time (not years) with little physical damage in the organs or tissues, there is a real chance of restoring the animal to its original healthy state.

Another consideration is the extent of previous drug treatment or surgery. The long-term action of drugs such as cortisone, for example, can damage the glands and organs of an animal so that a healing response cannot be aroused.

Surgery is the most irreversible of all treatments. Obviously, if an organ is removed (a common example is the removal of thyroid glands in cats with hyperthyroidism), it can't be healed. If a client brings such an animal to me, I know at the outset that a cure is not possible. This is because we have to restore the thyroid glands to normal functioning to return this animal to true health. But if there are no thyroid glands. . . .

I can say that in general, however, improved nutrition and use of healing methods like homeopathy, herbal medicine and nutrition will surely improve the quality of your animal's life.

SIGNS OF PROGRESS

Many natural therapies include the notion of the "healing crisis," a brief increase of symptoms that occurs just before the patient really starts to recover. You need to understand the significance of this favorable sign. Otherwise, you might jump to the conclusion that things are getting worse and load the animal down with a host of heavy-duty drugs that could actually interfere with the cure.

How can you tell whether your pet is going through a "healing crisis" or is actually getting worse? Here is a good general rule: If your animal has an increase of (usually) one symptom (diarrhea, for example) but, at the same time, seems to feel better overall, then the change is favorable. Equally important, a healing crisis is almost always over quickly. Typically, in my work with homeopathy, any temporary increase in symptoms in response to effective treatment will be gone in 12 to 24 hours.

In other words, though with a healing therapy some of the symptoms may become worse temporarily, *this is brief and followed by definite improvement*. If your pet goes through something like this and it lasts for days and she still seems sick, it is probably *not* a healing crisis and the situation should be re-evaluated.

Many physicians and healers have noticed certain patterns that the body expresses in its attempt to cope with health imbalances. Homeopaths have formalized these patterns as "Hering's Law of Cure," named after a famous American homeopathic physician, Constantine Hering. Here is the way I understand the process.

There is an underlying intelligence in the body (in homeopathy it's called the vital force) that is in charge of maintenance and repair. To do this, the body utilizes a few basic strategies to limit the problem and protect its most vital and important functions. Specifically, it attempts to:

◆ Prevent disturbances from spreading (by localizing the problem with inflammation and the thickening of tissue, for example).

◆ Keep the disease on the surface of the body rather than let it get to the vital organs.

◆ Focus disease around the limbs, rather than on the trunk.

◆ Confine disease to the lower end of the body, away from the head, and therefore away from the brain and sensory organs.

◆ Maintain the problem at the physical level rather than the emotional or mental level, which would interfere more seriously with the overall functioning of the individual.

Therefore, a patient's health is taking a wrong turn if symptoms start to spread or begin to involve deep-seated organs. Common sense tells us that the more the condition disturbs the functioning of parts of the body that are most crucial to its survival and governing capacities, the worse it is.

Hering's Law can also help you to recognize a turn in the right direction, toward greater health, which can initially require a careful reading of more subtle indications. It is a favorable sign, for instance, if an animal with a chronic degenerative disease affecting vital organs begins to develop a skin rash or discharge. Overall improvement will take place during this process, and, gradually, the surface problem will lessen as the internal disorder is healed. The vital force of the body focuses on this surface lesion as a way to rid itself of the disturbance.

Some cases can be more difficult to interpret, especially those in which the animal begins to re-experience old symptoms that were previously treated in a way that did not really cure them, but simply suppressed them for a time. In such situations it is best to work with a skilled holistic veterinarian.

If you study the principles outlined above, however, you will have an excellent guide for determining whether, as a whole individual, your animal is actually getting better or worse.

Let's look at some examples. Suppose your dog tends to get fungus infections around the feet and lower legs. After months of strenuous drug treatment, the feet have cleared up. Recently, however, little bald patches and irritation have begun to appear on the skin of the abdomen, chest and near the head. Though this new problem may be diagnosed differently, it is really just another expression of the original problem that was suppressed but not really cured. It is the same disease, but it has changed form and location. And it has progressed from a less important, peripheral location (the feet) closer to a more important area (the head).

Here's a more subtle example of a condition getting worse. After repeated treatments and even surgery, your dog's chronically inflamed ears have finally cleared up. But now, several weeks later, you notice that he isn't as friendly as he used to be. He prefers to go off by himself and may even growl or bite. The seat of the disturbance has moved inward, from the physical to the emotional level. Though various drugs may be tried in an effort to control the personality changes, the overall problem will only get worse. Tranquilizers may make him easier to live with, more subdued and passive. But over time, he may weaken at the mental level, perhaps acting sluggish and disoriented. He may have spells of confusion. At this point the disturbance will interfere with the basic mental processes that help him process information and orient himself.

Though this may sound like a farfetched example, I assure you it is not. Cases like this happen all too often. If this same dog were treated in a curative way at the point when his problem became emotional, you would see a return of the earlier physical symptoms after his moods improved. Most likely, it would be a re-emergence of the ear inflammation. Then the ear or any other surface problem could be treated with the methods we discuss in this book. Once you have stimulated the body to move in a curative direction, it is also possible that the ear condition will go away on its own, without further treatment.

As another example, let's say you have a cat with an abscess. She also has been showing emotional signs of trouble—depression and lethargy. After treatment, however, she has begun to run around and act frisky. Even though there may still be a discharge from the abscess, the psychological improvement is a very favorable sign, and it will be followed by physical healing. It is indeed the first sign that healing is under way.

In general, these signs during therapy also indicate good progress.

- An increase in energy and overall playfulness
- Return of a calm, good-natured manner
- Self-grooming (especially true of cats)
- A return of normal appetite
- Re-establishment of normal bowel movements and urination
- Ability to have sound and restful sleep

HEALING DISCHARGES

Let's also look carefully at some of the *methods* the body uses to heal itself. Generally, when a disease is being eliminated you will see signs of discharge. It signals that buildups of toxic materials are leaving the body. The most common ways this elimination occurs are through:

- Formation of a pus-pocket and drainage out of the body
- Development of skin eruptions (a very common route)
- The urine, which may become dark or strong-smelling
- The colon, in the form of dark, smelly feces or diarrhea
- Vomiting (especially during acute conditions)

When using the holistic methods discussed in this book, you may see one or more of these forms of discharge, to a mild degree. This will particularly happen if the problem has gotten well-established in the body.

Sometimes the discharge can be fairly dramatic. For example, I'm reminded of a dog whose owner used herbs and fasting to successfully help her pet recover from a severe attack of distemper. Soon afterwards, however, the animal was covered with red, itchy skin that oozed sticky fluid—clearly a discharge phenomenon. A few more days of supportive treatments were followed by full recovery. Once such a recovery is complete, an animal will be much stronger and better able to withstand future diseases.

Let's summarize the ways to evaluate progress. Supportive, nonsuppressive therapies exhibit two processes: (1) movement of symptoms in a favorable direction (away from the head toward the feet; away from vital organs to surface tissue; from mental and emotional to physical) and (2) some form of discharge. If you see these signs, chances are very strong that the animal is getting better, regardless of which form of therapy you are using.

I should add as a cautionary note, however, that treatment with some drugs, particularly with cortisone, can create a *false* sense of well-being that disappears when the drug is discontinued. So keep in mind that you are looking for a response that comes *from* the animal, *assisted by the treatment.* Such a response will lead to recovery and permanent healing, not a dependence on a drug.

In this Quick Reference section there are several references to small, medium and large dogs—related to diet and kinds of treatments. Here are the criteria for sizes of dogs.

- Small dogs—less than 20 pounds
- Medium-size dogs—20 to 40 pounds
- Large dogs—40 pounds and over

COMMON PET AILMENTS AND THEIR TREATMENTS

ABSCESSES

Abscesses are a common complication of puncture wounds from fights. They plague cats much more than dogs, because cats' needlelike teeth and sharp, penetrating claws inflict narrow but deep wounds. Feline skin seals over very quickly, trapping bacteria, hair or other contaminated material inside. Sometimes, even a broken-off claw or tooth is retained under the skin.

Cat abscesses usually occur around the head and front legs or at the base of the tail. Wounds around the head indicate that your cat was either the aggressor or bravely facing the enemy. Wounds at the tail area or on the rear legs mean that your cat was trying to get away.

In dogs abscesses are usually caused by foxtails or plant awns that get trapped in the hair and work their way through the skin (especially between the toes, around or in the ears and between the hind legs). An abscess that keeps draining and does not heal (called a fistula) usually indicates the presence of a foreign object somewhere in the tissue, sometimes several inches from the place of drainage.

TREATMENT

CATS

I have had several very healthy, well-fed cats that seldom, if ever, developed abscesses after injuries. My experience is that excellent nutrition is the best preventive.

Neutering also greatly reduces the problem. When several intact male cats live in close proximity, there will be frequent warfare as each tries to establish a territory and compete for females. In such circumstances abscesses are a continuous problem.

Often, you can prevent an infection or abscess by giving the homeopathic remedy *Ledum* 30C within a few hours of the fight. Use "Homeopathic Schedule 2," page 348.

If you can't treat it quickly or an infection (or abscess) is already established, however, further symptoms will usually occur, such as swelling, pain and fever (locally or of the whole body). In this case, the cat should fast for 24 hours, taking only liquids—meat and vegetable broth and spring water. Give 250 milligrams of vitamin C three times a day for at least three days to promote the activity of your cat's immune system.

In addition, use *one* remedy from the following list, whichever best fits the situation.

Homeopathic—*Lachesis muta 30C:* Use "Homeopathic Schedule 2," page 348. Useful immediately after the bite to a few hours after. If given early enough, can prevent the abscess from forming.

Homeopathic—*Hepar Sulph Calcareum 30C:* Use "Homeopathic Schedule 2," page 348. Useful for the infection or abscess that is *extremely* painful when touched. The cat will often become angry and try to bite or scratch if the wound is touched.

Tissue Salt—*Silicea 6X:* Use "Homeopathic Schedule 1," page 348. Best for a developed abscess that is ready to burst or is already draining.

Herbal—*Purple cone flower (Echinacea angustifolia):* Use "Herbal Schedule 1," page 346. This remedy is indicated for the animal that is in poor condition, thin, very weak and develops recurrent abscesses. It functions primarily to purify the system, especially the blood, and also restores health to the skin.

If an abscess has actually opened and drained, prevent the drainage hole from closing prematurely by cleaning away any discharge or scab once or twice a day either with hydrogen peroxide or with the herb *Echinacea* used according to "Herbal Schedule 4 or 6" on page 347.

Later, as the abscess is healing and there is no longer any drainage, use the herb Calendula for external treatment, according to the same method as described for Echinacea (above).

If the abscess has been present for a long time and has been draining pus for several weeks, administer the homeopathic remedy *Silicea* 30C, using "Homeopathic Schedule 3," page 348.

DOGS

If the abscess is the result of an animal bite, treat it the same way you would for a cat (above). Just adjust the amount of vitamin C to the size of the dog. Three times a day give about 250 milligrams (small dog), 500 milligrams (medium dog) or 1,000 milligrams (large dog).

However, if the abscess has been caused by plant material, porcupine quills, splinters or other embedded foreign matter, the discharge will not stop until the object is eliminated. Since the tissues cannot "digest" the object, it must either be expelled or removed surgically.

The natural expelling process can be aided by using the tissue salt *Silicea* 6X according to "Homeopathic Schedule 1," page 348. Also, apply hot compresses of a solution made up of Oat Straw (*Avena sativa*). Use "Herbal Schedule 4" on page 347. If the affected area is a paw, soak the whole foot in a jar of the hot solution. Use "Herbal Schedule 6" on page 347.

In natural healing the tendency is for pus or fluid to drain out at a point *lower* than the site of the foreign body. That way gravity helps out. Therefore, apply the poultice not only at the opening but also several inches higher so you cover the probable location of the foreign body. The hot solution will promote the flow of blood into the affected area and keep the process moving. When enough pus has formed around the foreign body to loosen it, it may flow out, right along with the pus. At that point, drainage will stop.

Note: Because of their structure, foxtails and plant awns tend to migrate deeply into the tissues. If you don't get results within a short time, you may have to resort to surgery. (See "Foxtails" for more information.)

ACCIDENTS

See "Handling Emergencies and Giving First Aid" on page 337.

AGGRESSION

See "Behavior Problems."

ALLERGIES

An allergy is an abnormally intense reaction to something that is usually harmless to the body—wheat, house dust or plant pollen, for example. A reaction against some part of the body itself—like the skin, pancreas or thyroid—is called an auto-immune disease.

My impression is that the incidence of allergies and immune disorders has greatly increased since I first entered practice 30 years ago. Now these are among the most common conditions we are asked to treat.

Allergies show themselves differently in dogs than they do in cats. Dogs typically have itchy skin and eruptions, especially on the lower back near the base of the tail. However, these eruptions can occur anywhere and everywhere on the body. Other commonly associated symptoms are inflamed ears, excessive licking of the front feet, digestive upsets (gurgling, gas and a tendency toward diarrhea), inflammation of the toes and an irritated rear end (anus, genitals) with licking and dragging of the rear on the floor. Though other symptoms can also occur, this is a typical picture.

Like dogs, cats can also have skin eruptions, often called miliary dermatitis. Cats are more prone, however, to cystitis (bladder inflammation) and digestive problems. Oftentimes, there is no visible eruption on the skin, but cats will be greatly annoyed by stinging or biting sensations of the skin so that they are always jumping around, frantically licking themselves and pulling hair out in clumps. They act as though fleas were causing it.

Two similar immune disorders that occur—hyperthyroidism and inflammatory bowel disease—are chronic and serious conditions that require careful treatment. In my opinion, the major causes of these immune disorders are the frequent use of combination vaccinations, feeding pets commercial food diets and overuse of cortisone drugs to suppress symptoms—all of which together have greatly weakened the immune system of animals over several generations.

Whatever the causes, once established, the problem is very difficult to eliminate. Successful treatment can be accomplished with the approach outlined in this book, but it takes a long time, usually a year or more.

In mild cases, actions you can take yourself may be sufficient. For instance, some research suggests that about a third of all allergies are caused by substances in foods. You can easily identify the immediate trigger by using a simplified diet for a while. If the symptoms subside but return when you go back to the original diet, you can assume that your pet is allergic to one or more of the ingredients in the daily diet.

Try the following diets as a test. They omit the most common food allergens: beef, wheat, milk, cheese, eggs, nuts, fruits, tomatoes, carrots, yeast and various spices and additives. When given in high doses, vitamin C acts like a natural antihistamine to control allergies. The B complex found in the pet supplements is also very useful to that end.

CAT ALLERGY DIET #1

2 cups brown rice

2 pounds (4 cups) raw lamb or mutton

4 teaspoons bonemeal (or 2,400 milligrams calcium or 1⅓ teaspoon powdered eggshell)

2 tablespoons vegetable oil

   10 days' dose of a complete vitamin-mineral supplement formulated for cats, made without yeast

   Vitamin C in the form of sodium ascorbate powder (200–400 milligrams daily)

Bring 4 cups of filtered or spring water to a boil. Add the rice, cover and simmer for 40 minutes. Meanwhile, trim any excess fat off the lamb or mutton; chop or grind the meat. When the rice is done, thoroughly mix all ingredients except the vitamin C. Give the C fresh each day. (I recommend sodium ascorbate powder because it isn't very tart.)

Substitutes: Instead of rice you may use 2 cups of millet (cooked for 20 to 30 minutes with 6 cups of water until soft) or 4 cups of dry oats (cooked for 10 minutes with 8 cups of water until thick and soft).

Yield: Feeds an average adult cat for 8 to 10 days. Freeze about ⅔ of it to prevent spoilage.

CAT ALLERGY DIET #2

1½ cups millet

2   pounds (4 cups) raw turkey

2   tablespoons bonemeal (or 5,600 milligrams calcium or 1 tablespoon powdered eggshell)

2⅔ tablespoons vegetable oil

    8 days' dose of a complete vitamin-mineral supplement formulated for cats, made without yeast

    Vitamin C in the form of sodium ascorbate powder (give 200–400 milligrams daily)

Bring 6 cups of filtered or spring water to a boil. Add the millet, cover and simmer for 20 to 30 minutes or until soft. When done, thoroughly mix all ingredients except the vitamin C (see Cat Allergy Diet #1).

Substitutes: Instead of millet you may use 1½ cups of brown rice (cooked for 40 minutes with 3 cups water) or 2½ cups of dry oats (cooked for 10 minutes with 5 cups water).

Yield: Feeds an average adult cat for about 8 days. Freeze about ⅔ of the finished product to prevent spoilage.

DOG ALLERGY DIET #1

4 cups brown rice

2 pounds (4 cups) raw lamb or mutton

4 teaspoons bonemeal (or 2,200 milligrams calcium or 1¼ teaspoons powdered eggshell)

2 tablespoons vegetable oil

   Complete daily vitamin-mineral supplement formulated for dogs, made without yeast

   Vitamin C in the form of sodium ascorbate powder (give 200–1,000 milligrams daily, depending on dog's size)

Bring 8 cups of filtered or spring water to a boil. Add the rice, cover and simmer for 40 minutes. Meanwhile, trim any excess fat off the lamb or mutton; chop or grind the meat. When the rice is done (indicated by tender, firm grains), thoroughly mix all ingredients except the daily supplement and the vitamin C. Add these at the time of feeding. See supplement label for amount.

Substitutes: Instead of rice you may use 4 cups

of millet (cooked for 20 to 30 minutes with 12 cups water) or 8 cups of dry oats (cooked for 10 minutes with 14 to 16 cups water). Cooked grains should be soft and mushy. For a higher-protein feed, you may reduce the amount of grain to 3 cups dry rice or millet (or 6 cups oats).

Yield: Enough to feed a small dog for 6 to 8 days, a medium dog for 3 to 4 days or a large dog for a couple of days. Freeze any of this food that can't be eaten in 3 days.

DOG ALLERGY DIET #2

6 cups millet

2 pounds (4 cups) raw turkey

2⅔ tablespoons bonemeal (or 5,200 milligrams calcium or 1 scant tablespoon powdered eggshell)

¼ cup vegetable oil

   Complete daily vitamin-mineral supplement formulated for dogs, made without yeast

   Vitamin C (give 200–1,000 milligrams daily, depending on dog's size)

Bring 9 cups of filtered or spring water to a boil. Add the millet, cover and simmer for 20 to 30 minutes or until soft and fluffy. Thoroughly mix millet with all ingredients except the vitamin C and daily supplement. Feed these supplements fresh each day, as in Dog Allergy Diet #1.

Substitutes: Instead of millet you may use 5 cups of brown rice (cooked with 10 cups of water for 40 minutes or until grains are tender, firm and separate) or 10 cups of dry oats (cooked with 18 to 20 cups of water for 10 minutes or until grains are soft and mushy).

Yield: Makes about 4,600 calories, enough to feed a small dog for 6 to 8 days, a medium dog for 3 to 4 days or a large dog for a couple of days. Freeze any of the batch that can't be eaten in 3 days.

◆

Be sure to use filtered, spring or other nonchlorinated water. To give this diet an adequate chance, keep your animal on it for at least two months. If the problem clears up or improves, slowly reintroduce the omitted foods one at a time to find out which one or ones are causing the problem. By determining which ingredients are causing a reaction, you may be able to switch to a quality kibble that excludes the problem food. This is especially helpful with a large dog, where cooking in such quantities can be challenging. Your best bet would be one of the lamb-rice kibbles formulated for dogs with skin problems. Read the label carefully.

If your pet's condition has not improved after a couple of months on a restricted diet, the cause of its problem may not be a food allergy. Bear in mind that allergies can be triggered by a variety of environmental factors, such as chlorine and other contaminants in water, household cleaning chemicals, outgassing of formaldehyde and other chemicals from furniture and buildings, synthetic carpets and upholstery, plastic food bowls, certain plants or grasses, regularly administered drugs like heartworm preventive medicine or flea chemicals and, of course, flea bites. Also, while many people have heard that they can be allergic to their pets, few realize that their pets can be allergic to them!

Determining exactly what substances are causing an allergic reaction can be difficult. Certain diagnostic procedures can be used, but I haven't found them very helpful. They do not always correlate with the clinical situation. Also, if you do find some offending substances, it may not be possible to eliminate them completely anyway.

The approach that works best for me is to put the animal on a natural diet (which by itself clears up a lot of problems) and to use homeopathic treatment to remove the underlying allergic tendency. In many cases that I handle, allergic tendencies can be greatly mitigated or eliminated completely.

The things you can do that will be most helpful are to use a strictly home-prepared, raw-meat diet (raw meat does not cause the same allergic reaction that cooked meat does) and to stop vaccinating (or greatly reduce frequency). Animals with allergies do not respond well to vaccination, and I find that it accelerates the intensity and frequency of allergy symptoms (see "Vaccinations" for further advice on this). See "Skin Problems" for specific advice on dealing with that aspect of allergy disease.

ANAL GLAND PROBLEMS

Difficulties with the anal glands are primarily canine problems. Dogs have a pair of small scent glands on either side of the anus, under the tail. Similar in structure to the scent gland of the skunk, they contain a strong-smelling material which is apparently used to mark territory or to express extreme fear.

Problems manifest either as abscesses that form within the glands themselves or as what is called impaction, in which the glands become inactive and overfilled with secretion. In the latter case the dog will often "scoot" along the floor or ground in an attempt to empty these glands, which have exceeded their normal capacity. Some of the factors that may play a role in the development of these problems are:

◆ Frustration in trying to establish a territory, perhaps from being crowded with other animals or from having inadequate space for exercise and exploration.
◆ Constipation or infrequent bowel movement, especially as a result of not being allowed outside frequently. Many an indoor animal will hold its urine or feces to the very limit rather than soil the house and displease its people.
◆ Toxicity because of poor food and inadequate exercise. In such a case a disorder of the skin or ears frequently occurs as well (also see "Allergies").

PREVENTION

Make sure your animal has adequate exercise, the opportunity to go outside and have frequent bowel movements, and psychological "space." Good nutrition is important also, as it is in most conditions. Especially useful are those nutrients that help promote healthy skin: zinc, the B complex, vitamin A, lecithin and unsaturated vegetable oil.

Olive oil is a good source of unsaturated fatty acids and, by promoting muscular contraction of the bowels, has the advantage of being a slight laxative.

TREATMENT

ANAL GLAND ABSCESS

Homeopathic—First use the remedy *Belladonna* 6C, using "Homeopathic Schedule 2," page 348. Follow it the next day with *Silicea* 6X (tissue salt) using "Homeopathic Schedule 1" on page 348. The Belladonna helps with the initial inflammation and *Silicea* 6X promotes the discharge of pus and encourages healing. Also apply warm or hot calendula solution (see "Abscesses") twice a day for at least five minutes each time. Continue the calendula treatment about three days, though a longer period is fine, if necessary.

IMPACTED ANAL GLANDS

Since this condition is associated with sluggishness of the tissues and often with toxicity and obesity as well (see "Weight Problems"), regular vigorous exercise is an important part of the treatment. If you add vegetables and a little bran mixed with olive oil to the food, it will help to regulate the intestines and encourage bulky bowel movements. Copious evacuation will stimulate the natural emptying of the glands.

In addition, a hot fomentation of either Marigold flower (*Calendula officinalis*) solution or Red clover (*Trifolium pratense*) blossoms will stimulate the glands and soften their contents. Immediately after the application, use gentle pressure with a "milking" action to help to empty the glands manually. Consider the manual emptying as a temporary measure, not something to do continually. It's much better (I'm sure you would agree!) if the glands empty naturally.

A useful adjunct to the above measures is to give the tissue salt *Silicea* 6X according to "Homeopathic Schedule 6(a)" on page 349 for at least ten days.

ANEMIA

Anemia is often caused by blood loss from wounds or parasites such as fleas and worms. The problem is characterized by white (or pale) gums, weakness and a fast pulse. Occasionally, it indicates more serious diseases like feline leukemia or a toxicity resulting from drug exposure. Here, however, we'll consider only the more common and simple anemia caused by losing blood, with a view toward promoting the growth of new red blood cells.

TREATMENT

A diet rich in iron, protein and vitamin B_{12} is important. That's why the following foods are particularly helpful.

- Beef liver (for protein, B complex, B_{12} and iron)
- Nutritional yeast supplemented with B_{12} (same benefits as liver)
- Green vegetables (for iron and other minerals)
- Kelp powder (for iodine and other trace minerals)
- Vitamin C, 500 to 2,000 milligrams a day, depending on the animal's size (promotes the absorption of iron from the intestinal tract)

In addition to the nutritional supports, give *one* of these remedies (whichever seems best indicated) for ten days.

Homeopathic—*China officinalis* 6C, using "Homeopathic Schedule 6(a)" on page 349. This is most indicated after blood loss that has resulted in marked weakness and loss of strength.

Homeopathic—*Nux vomica* 6C, using "Homeopathic Schedule 6(a)" on page 349. Try this remedy when your pet has become withdrawn and irritable after the blood loss.

If the anemia is caused by parasites, these must be controlled (see "Skin Parasites" or "Worms"). In such a case use the nutritional advice given for anemia, but instead of using the anemia remedies suggested, follow the treatment guidelines under the appropriate section. (For an anemic animal, however, do *not* use the fasting program.)

Flea infestations are most safely controlled by frequent bathing with a nontoxic soap (such as products containing d-limonene from citrus), controlling fleas in the environment and using the lemon skin tonic, as described in chapter 7. When the animal is stronger, you can use more strenuous flea-control methods if required, but I do discourage the use of poisonous chemicals, because they are not really effective in a long-term way and are very toxic to both humans and animals.

Sometimes very young kittens or puppies are so besieged by fleas that they are almost drained of their blood. In such cases it is essential not to use flea powders or sprays, even though the temptation is great. The young animals are much too small and weak to handle such an assault. Instead, bathe them often and use the lemon tonic rinse. To prevent them from getting chilled, dry them thoroughly afterward. Towel them off and then use a hair dryer set on low or place them in a warm sunny spot. Keep them warm and quiet in general and, if the weather allows, give them some fresh air and sunlight. Also use a flea comb to remove fleas not killed by the baths. Feed only natural foods—no commercial fare—and follow the treatment program suggested for anemia. You will be amazed at how quickly these little creatures can respond.

APPETITE PROBLEMS

Changes in normal appetite often show up as an aspect of an illness. This is a problem more common in cats than in dogs, probably because cats have such stringent nutritional requirements. The thing to understand about this is how gradually an inadequate appetite can creep up with a cat. Usually the first indication is what most people would call a finicky cat, one who rejects many different foods and prefers just one or two brands. Most people just give in to this demand and don't think much about it. However, especially if it is coupled with regular water drinking, you have the beginnings of a more serious condition.

The next stage is a fluctuation in preferences. Maybe your cat no longer relishes what it once did. Or perhaps you find it necessary to open a different brand of food at each meal. Even this variation is not always totally acceptable, and your cat may pester you frequently for more food, only to reject what you offer. It is no wonder that some people end up feeding their cat tuna or liver exclusively.

If this deterioration continues, the next stage is inadequate eating with a gradual loss of weight. You may see a skeleton cat that eats just barely enough (with coaxing and indulgence) to maintain life. Cats like this do not eat enthusiastically. They just lick at their food or eat around the edges, leaving the less desirable parts in the bowl. Over time, these cats will waste away until they are finally diagnosed with some disease that is the end product of this long decline.

How will you know if your cat has started into this pattern? Ask yourself some questions: Is your cat addicted to a particular brand of food? Will she eat only dry food? Must you open a new can at every feeding (can't use any leftovers)? Do you find yourself adding irresistible foods like tuna or liver to get your cat to eat? Are you required to sit there with your cat while he eats (perhaps petting him the whole time) lest he will go away from his food?

If the answer to any of these questions is yes, you probably have a problem. Another test is to hold back on the food your cat always wants. Instead, offer a home-prepared diet or another good brand of canned food. If your cat does not accept the new food within five days, then you definitely have a problem.

Resolving this situation usually requires a specific homeopathic treatment (called constitutional therapy) or an equivalent method of alternative treatment best undertaken by a well-trained professional. Sometimes, however, appetite problems are just one symptom of a specific disease for which you will find treatment suggestions in this section.

ARTHRITIS

Arthritis and bone disease are much more common in dogs than in cats and usually take one of several forms.

Hip dysplasia: a malformation of the hip sockets that allows excessive movement in the joint, causing chronic inflammation, calcium deposits and further breakdown. This was first seen in the larger breeds of dogs, but now is seen in any breed. Larger dogs, however, have more trouble with it because they weigh more (see "Hip Dysplasia").

Dislocation of the kneecap: a malformation of the leg bones that causes the kneecap to repeatedly pull out of position, slip back and forth and set up a continuous low-grade inflammation. Mostly seen in small breeds, it is fostered by poor breeding practices and low-quality food.

Degeneration of the shoulder joint: the breakdown of cartilage in the shoulder, leading to inflammation and pain on movement. Mostly found in medium to large breeds, it is always an aspect of an overall chronic disease condition that affects other parts of the body as well.

Arthritis of the elbow: a condition that is caused by improper bone formation and is considered to be hereditary. It is generally seen in German shepherds. Like shoulder joint problems, it is part of a larger chronic disease condition.

Swelling and pain in the leg bones: seen in young dogs (a few months of age) of the large breeds. It is apparently partly caused by inadequate production of vitamin C and is the result of poor nutrition and heredity.

PREVENTION

Most of these conditions could be prevented if the female were properly fed throughout her pregnancy. The time of growth in the uterus is critical in terms of the formation of structure and essential tissues. Inadequate nutrition is most detrimental at this time (see "Pregnancy, Birth and Care of Newborns"). Avoiding commercial foods and feeding a natural, wholesome diet is an important part of a preventive program. Homeopathic treatment during pregnancy is also an excellent means of minimizing the likelihood of this problem in the next generation. Of course, the mother should not be vaccinated while she is pregnant.

In addition, the regular use of vitamin C minimizes or prevents some of these problems. Depending on the size of the animal and its age, give 250 to 2,000 milligrams a day. For instance, a small puppy (like a

Pekingese) would get 250 milligrams, a large puppy (like a German shepherd) 500 milligrams. After the dog matures give 500 to 1,000 milligrams daily for most sizes and perhaps up to 2,000 milligrams for a giant breed like the Great Dane or Saint Bernard.

Prevention is very important in arthritic conditions, because once the joints are distorted, the damage has been done.

TREATMENT

Even in the face of an already-established condition, there are several things you can do to minimize your animal's arthritic discomfort. But the first step is to feed the natural diet, as described in chapters 4 and 5.

Add vitamin C to the diet, using 500 to 2,000 milligrams a day, depending on the animal's size. It's best to divide the daily amount and give it twice a day. Other vitamins and supplements that are especially important are vitamin E and a vitamin A and D combination. Increase the amounts in the recipes by an additional 50 to 100 IU of vitamin E. Double the vitamin A and E supplement (or cod-liver oil).

Be sure to include raw grated vegetables in the diet, particularly carrots, beets and celery.

In addition to these nutritional guidelines, one of the following remedies may help. Choose the one which best fits your situation.

Herbal—*Alfalfa (Medicago sativa):* Indicated for the thin, nervous animal with a tendency toward digestive problems as well as arthritis. Depending on its size, add 1 teaspoon to 3 tablespoons of ground or dry blended alfalfa to the daily ration. Or you can administer alfalfa as a infusion using "Herbal Schedule 3," page 347. A third choice is to give your pet 2 to 6 alfalfa tablets a day.

Herbal—*Garlic (Allium sativum):* Garlic is suited for the overweight animal with hip pain, especially a pet that has been on a high-meat diet. Include fresh grated garlic with each meal, using ½ to 3 cloves, depending on the body size.

Homeopathic—*Rhus toxicodendron 6X (poison ivy):* Do not use the herbal form, of course, but the safe homeopathic preparation, which you can order by mail in tablet or pellet form (see "Pet Supplies" beginning on page 352). Rhus tox. is indicated for a dog or cat with chronic arthritis, pain or stiffness which is most apparent when the animal gets up after a long rest (for example, overnight). When it first starts to move, the animal shows discomfort or stiffness, but after a few minutes it seems to loosen up and feel better. If the pet also has a tendency toward red, swollen, itchy skin, Rhus tox. will work on both problems (see "Skin Problems"). Use "Homeopathic Schedule 6(a)," page 349.

Tissue Salt— *Silicea 6X:* This medicine fits many dogs that have inherited joint and bone disease problems. Typically, the symptoms become more severe as the dog gets older, with stiffness, pain and even distortion of the joints and legs in severe cases. I use this medicine for hip dysplasia, elbow dysplasia, joint arthritis and arthritis of the spine (spondylitis). Use "Homeopathic Schedule 6(a)," page 349.

A disease that affects young dogs, hypertrophic osteodystrophy causes pain and inflammation of the bones of the legs. It is best treated by one of two remedies.

Homeopathic—*Pulsatilla 30C:* This medicine is suited to the dog that, once ill, wants lots of comfort and affection and likes to be held. Typically this type of dog will drink less water than usual. Use "Homeopathic Schedule 3," page 348.

Homeopathic—*Silicea 30C:* Try this remedy if Pulsatilla (above) was not sufficient to resolve the problem or if your dog does not fit the picture described for Pulsatilla. Use "Homeopathic Schedule 3," page 348.

BEHAVIOR PROBLEMS

Behavioral abnormalities can be complex and difficult to change, but often you can help considerably. Poor breeding practices, especially in purebred dogs, have fostered the development of many such disturbances, including viciousness, epilepsy, repetitive habits and other signs of nervous system imbalances. It is also my impression that many behavior problems have their roots in one or more of the following: poor nutrition and associated toxicity, chronic encephalitis (brain inflammation) following vaccination, inadequate exercise, insufficient psychological stimulation and attention, and the influence of the owner's personality patterns, expectations or conditioning. For instance, family conflict, excessive attachment to a pet as an attempt to escape loneliness or the desire to have an aggressive animal to feel safer from other people can all have a strong adverse influence on an animal's personality.

TREATMENT

In this brief discussion we'll focus on general measures that can be very helpful and, in some cases, may be sufficient to treat the disturbance, provided that the contributing environmental factors are understood and eliminated. Start with nutrition.

Take your pet off commercial food, if you have not already done so. Any food that contains artificial preservatives, coloring agents or other additives contains chemicals that can irritate the brain tissue and cause abnormal responses. Feed our fresh foods diet.

Provide a complete vitamin supplement that is especially rich in the B complex. I would use a multi-vitamin tablet with the major B vitamins at the 5- to 20-milligram level for a trial period of at least two months.

Use supplements to help eliminate and counteract the effect of substances that may be irritating the brain cells. If you suspect a buildup of toxic material, give your pet the following: zinc (2 to 20 milligrams a day, depending on the animal's size); vitamin C (250 to 2,000 milligrams a day); lecithin (½ teaspoon to one tablespoon of granules in the food daily); and bonemeal (an extra ⅛ teaspoon to one tablespoon daily).

Algin (sodium alginate) is also useful. It's a natural substance which works to remove heavy metals such as lead from the body. Depending on the animal's size, use from ¼ teaspoon to 1 teaspoon a day, mixed with the food.

The zinc and the vitamin C work as a team to eliminate toxic heavy metals, while lecithin protects the nerve cells against irritation. With the addition of bonemeal, this group as a whole helps to detoxify the body and to protect the nerves.

Minimize exposure to toxic substances. Make sure your animal is protected from accidental poisoning by various household chemicals. Just as important, minimize its exposure to such pollutants as cigarette smoke, car exhaust and antiflea chemicals (which affect the nervous system).

In addition to these measures, one or more of the following treatments may be useful.

Tissue Salt—*Kali phosphoricum 6X (Kali phos.):* Indicated for a hyperactive, overly sensitive animal whose problem seems to stem from psychological or hereditary factors rather than toxic exposures. Use "Homeopathic Schedule 6(a)," page 349.

Herbal—*Common oat (Avena sativa):* Oats are well suited as a general nerve tonic and are particularly useful where nerve weakness or irritability may have appeared after other stressful diseases. This remedy is good for animals that have received a lot of drugs, are old or have a tendency to epilepsy. It is also helpful for the animal with weak legs, muscle twitching or a trembling associated with weakness. All of this, of course, will be in addition to any particular behavior problems exhibited (this applies to all of the herbs to be described).

Though feeding rolled oats as a cooked grain in the diet is helpful, a more potent preparation is the tincture. Use "Herbal Schedule 1," page 346.

Herbal—*Blue vervain (Verbena hastata):* Vervain is suited for animals that are depressed and have weak nervous systems. It's also for those with irritated nerves and muscle spasms and is especially appropriate for those whose abnormal behavior is associated with epilepsy; in such cases it will strengthen the brain function. Use "Herbal Schedule 1," page 346.

Herbal—*Skullcap (Scutellaria lateriflora):* This herb is useful for behavior disturbances that center around nervous fear. The animal may also show one or more of the following signs: intestinal gas, colic, diarrhea, muscle twitching and restless sleep. Use "Herbal Schedule 1," page 346.

Herbal—*Valerian (Valeriana officinalis):* Valerian suits the animal that tends to get hysterical, associated with a hypersensitivity. The animal shows a changeable mental disposition and an irritable temperament. Like skullcap, valerian may be most successfully used for animals that have digestive disturbances like gas and diarrhea, because of nervous derangement, and those that may also have a history of leg pains or joint inflammation.

Since valerian is one of those herbs that can cause a toxic reaction if given in large doses over a long period of time, I advise that you try "Herbal Schedule 1" on page 346 for no more than a week. If you don't see beneficial results by then, discontinue use and try one of the other suggested remedies, such as the oat tincture.

Herbal—*German chamomile (Matricaria chamomilla):* Animals that will benefit from this herb are noisy, whining, moaning and complaining. They will let you know about their pains or discomforts. They are sensitive, irritable and thirsty and may snap or try to bite. Such animals don't like to be hot and are often mollified or quiet only when being carried or constantly petted. Use "Herbal Schedule 1," page 346.

Use the suggested schedule for the herb you have chosen for two to three weeks (except for valerian, which should not be used for more than a week). If you see an improvement in that time, even a slight one, continue the treatment as long as the improvement goes on, up to a maximum of six weeks. Then discontinue the regular use of the herb, but give a few more doses of it whenever symptoms return or worsen.

Also, the herb can be used preventively. Give it to your pet before an event you know will trigger the problem behavior, for example, before leaving him alone for long periods. In this way it can be used occasionally, as needed, over several weeks or months.

What if you don't see a good response over the trial period? Then discontinue the selected herb and either try it again after a few weeks on a better diet or use one of the alternative herbs suggested.

I would like to suggest one additional alternative for those who are willing to go a little further. In my own work I find that the best "herbal" system for behavior problems with psychological roots is the use of the 38 flower preparations discovered by Dr. Edward Bach. These were originally developed for human use by Dr. Bach in England in the 1930s. I have found them just as effective for animals. They are dilute extracts of selected flowers given orally over a long period (weeks to months), often with remarkable improvements (see chapter 14 for more information).

It is beyond the scope of this book to cover this extraordinary system in depth, but interested readers will find a relevant supplier and books in "Supplier of Bach Flower Remedies" on page 355 and "Recommended Reading and Tapes" beginning on page 357. For those who want to explore the system or who are already acquainted with it, I want to call special attention to the following flower essences (but not to the exclusion of the others).

- ◆ Chicory: for the overly attached, possessive animal
- ◆ Holly: for the vicious, aggressive, suspicious or jealous animal

- ◆ Impatiens: for the uptight, impatient or irritable pet
- ◆ Mimulus: for the animal afraid of specific things, like the dog afraid of men or of thunder
- ◆ Rock rose: for use where attacks of terror or panic are part of the disturbance
- ◆ Star of Bethlehem: for use where physical or emotional shock seems to have initiated the imbalance
- ◆ Walnut: for the animal that is overly influenced by a strong personality (human or animal) or apparently under the influence of bad heredity

Select up to four (no more) of the best-suited essences. Add two drops from the stock bottle of each of these essences to a clean one-ounce dropper bottle. Then fill the bottle with spring water. Store it at room temperature. If the solution clouds up in a few days, make a fresh batch.

Regardless of the size of your animal, give two drops of this diluted medicine orally four times a day until the desired results are obtained. If you can, drop it directly in the mouth. If not, mix it with a little food or milk. There is no unfavorable side effect or possible toxicity with this system.

BIRTH

See "Pregnancy, Birth and Care of Newborns."

BLADDER PROBLEMS

Inflammation of your pet's bladder lining and urethra or the formation of urinary mineral deposits and stones is not unusual, particularly for a cat (see "Allergies"). Symptoms show up as increased frequency of urination, the appearance of blood in the urine and, in severe cases, extreme discomfort with straining and partial or complete blockage of the bladder.

Though conventional veterinary treatment usually includes antibiotics, research shows that bladder problems are not caused by bacteria. In my own practice I have not found it necessary to use antibiotics for over 17 years.

Another common but erroneous idea is that the ash in food is responsible for urinary tract trouble. The latest findings show that ash doesn't cause the problem; rather, it occurs because the urine becomes too alkaline. Some commercial foods now add extra acid to make the urine more acid. There are side effects from use of these acid formulations, however, and all they do is cover up the tendency to this problem without curing it.

It is clear to me that much of this problem originates in feeding pets poor-quality food with a resulting toxicity and excessive elimination load on the linings of the urinary system. Almost invariably, the first attack follows a history of feeding dry commercial foods over a long period. Sometimes I say (as a way to make a point) that if you want to increase the chance of a bladder problem, feed dry food and leave it out all the time.

I've found that, once through the crisis, the condition is very responsive to diet changes and natural therapies, resulting in a stable cure rather than a temporary relief.

TREATMENT

First, change your pet's diet. If it mostly centers on commercial foods, the condition is almost sure to recur. During the acute phase of the condition (below), put the animal on a liquid fast, offering a broth. For cats use a broth made from meat or fish. For dogs use vegetables and meat. You may add a small amount of natural tamari soy sauce to season it and to supply easily digested amino acids. In addition, provide your pet with pure water (without chlorine or fluorine) at all times.

After improvement or recovery, adopt the natural diet as advised in chapters 3 and 4. Feed your cat only twice a day—morning and evening. Don't leave the food out for more than 30 minutes. If she does not want to eat at these times, let a natural hunger develop until the next feeding time. This is very important. Frequent feeding alkalizes the urine, leading to formation of "sand" and "stones." Cats, as carnivores, are meant to eat infrequently and fast in between.

For one month, also use these measures.

Give vitamin C, 250 milligrams twice daily. This will help maintain an acidic urine, which makes mineral salts more soluble and counters the formation of crystals.

Increase the amount of vitamin E to minimize or prevent scarring of tissues that are healing. Add an extra 25 to 50 IU daily to your cat's food.

Give vitamin A. Add four drops of cod-liver oil (to the food) once a day or 10,000 IU of vitamin A once a week.

Besides diet, here are some specific treatments. Let's start with cats, who are more prone to bladder trouble. There are three different phases of the problem.

CATS

ACUTE CASES

If the urethra has become thoroughly plugged up, the cat cannot pass urine, and the bladder will become enlarged and hard from urine accumulation. It feels like a large stone in the back part of the abdomen.

This is a problem for male cats, because they tend to have narrow urethras. (A female cat may have bladder problems, but she isn't likely to get a plugged urethra.) The condition is quite serious, since urine and poisonous waste products are backing up into the bloodstream. Make an emergency run to your veterinarian to have a catheter put in, a plastic tube that relieves the obstruction and allows urine to come out. If you are too far from a veterinarian or can't reach one right away, however, try one of these treatments while you are waiting for help (assuming you have the remedies on hand).

Homeopathic—*Nux vomica 30C:* Give 1 pellet every 15 minutes for a total of 3 treatments. This remedy is best for the cat that is irritable, doesn't want to be touched and withdraws from company, preferring to be by himself.

Homeopathic—*Pulsatilla 30C:* Give 1 pellet every 15 minutes for a total of 3 treatments. This remedy is best for the cat that becomes quiet and unusually affectionate, wanting to be held.

Homeopathic—*Coccus cacti 30C:* Give 1 pellet every 15 minutes for a total of 3 treatments. This remedy is most useful where there is a lot of straining and likely obstruction of the bladder from stones (known as calculi) or mucous.

Homeopathic—*Cantharis 30C:* Give 1 pellet every 15 minutes for a total of 3 treatments. The cat that needs this medicine will be very upset, angry and growling with almost constant and intense attempts to urinate. Often there is also frequent licking of the penis after (or between) urination attempts.

Homeopathic—*Sarsaparilla 30C:* Give 1 pellet every 15 minutes for a total of 3 treatments. Use this remedy if your cat has to stand up to pass urine. Some cats will start out squatting but then rise up and only pass a little urine on standing up.

With any of these treatments, improvement will mean a sudden passing of a large quantity of urine with considerable relief for your cat. If this happens, you may be through the crisis and catheterization will be unnecessary. Watch closely for the next several days to make sure that urination continues unimpeded. Follow the crisis with the nutritional changes already discussed above.

If your cat needs to be catheterized, an additional treatment that will assist recovery from this procedure is:

Homeopathic—*Staphysagria 6C (stavesacre):* Use "Homeopathic Schedule 2," page 348.

SUBACUTE CASES

Here the problem is not obstruction but inflammation. The cat feels a frequent urge to urinate, but the flow is scanty or blood-tinged. This misery can go on for days, perhaps with temporary improvement (especially with antibiotics). However, the problem continues or recurs every few weeks. The remedies that follow are often useful for this stage of the problem. From the three remedies below choose the *one* that best suits the condition. Don't mix them.

Homeopathic—*Pulsatilla 30C:* This remedy is useful for the cat that does not like heat in any form. Here is how you can tell. Put out a hot water bottle or heating pad wrapped with a towel. If your cat is not interested in huddling next to it and prefers to lie on something cool like cement, tile, linoleum or even the bathtub or sink, then you will know it prefers coolness to heat. Usually the urine is passed in small amounts and contains blood. Use "Homeopathic Schedule 2," page 348.

Homeopathic—*Rhus toxicodendron 30C (poison ivy):* This remedy (which will not cause poison ivy problems in this dilute form) is indicated for the cat who likes to sit around on cold cement, stones or steps when it is well. But then it may get chilled and have an attack of cystitis (bladder inflammation). So the problem often crops up after cold, wet, rainy weather. When sick, this cat will prefer to be warm, will like a hot water bottle and wants to be touched or rubbed. However, a cat with this problem does not rest quietly, but constantly changes position or stretches its limbs. Its urine will be dark and scanty and may contain blood. Urination is difficult and painful. Use "Homeopathic Schedule 2," page 348.

Homeopathic—*Sepia 30C:* This medicine is indicated for the cat that has recurrent attacks associated with an attitude of "touch me not." These cats are often unfriendly fellows, with a tendency to be aggressive to other cats and to be difficult to handle or medicate. Getting pills down them is almost impossible. There are also appetite problems—rejecting many foods and being very "finicky." Many of the cats needing this remedy will continue to produce a lot of "crystals" that are found in the urine. Use "Homeopathic Schedule 2," page 348.

Homeopathic—*Mercurius vivus (or solubilis) 30C:* The cat needing this remedy will act very annoyed with his rear end, doing a lot of licking after urinating, thrashing the tail around and straining to produce small quantities of urine. Sometimes the straining is associated with passing stool. If the cat also has become unusually thirsty before the attack, this is probably the remedy to use. Use "Homeopathic Schedule 2," page 348.

Note: If you do not see any improvement after 24 hours of using one of these homeopathic preparations, discontinue the treatment and reassess the situation. If antibiotics and other drugs were used at any time, they may have altered the symptom picture. Think back to the symptoms that were present before treatment was started. Use these as your guidelines in choosing a remedy.

CHRONIC CASES

Try the following herbal treatment for a cat who never has a severe bladder problem, just a weakness in that area, such as a tendency toward urinary frequency or urinating outside the litter box. Or use any *one* of the medications as recommended for subacute cases in cats, if the symptoms displayed match those described for the particular medication.

Herbal—Use shave grass, also known as horsetail grass or scouring rush (*Equisetum arvense*). To use the medication, use "Herbal Schedule 2," page 347, for 2 to 3 weeks.

DOGS

Though bladder problems are more common in cats, dogs do get them too. Their most common disturbances are either cystitis (as in cats) or stone formation.

If your dog has a case of cystitis resembling the symptoms described above for cats (increased frequency of urination, discomfort, blood in the urine), use the feline treatment program, adjusting nutritional supplements to your dog's body size. Use the same remedies for the same indications.

What if it's a stone problem? They occur in two forms—small, pellet-size stones that form in the bladder but move down and block the urethra, and very large stones that fill the bladder.

Small stones are most troublesome to the male dog. They pass down into the urethra and get caught at the point where it passes through the bone in the penis. When this happens, the unfortunate fellow will attempt to urinate frequently, without success, or will give off little spurts of urine instead of a full flow. In such cases immediately use:

Herbal—*Shepherd's purse (Thlaspi bursa pastoris):* Use "Herbal Schedule 1," page 346. Sometimes the stone will pass through when this herb is used. More than likely, the herb will give some temporary relief until surgery or other correction can be done.

Homeopathic—*Coccus cacti 30C:* Give 1 pellet every 15 minutes for a total of 3 treatments. This remedy is (like shepherd's purse) a treatment for obstruction of the urethra with a stone. The remedy will not make the stone dissolve, of course. But it may reduce the spasms and inflammation from the presence of the stone. If it is small enough, the stone may then pass through. Remember, however, that it may simply be too large to get through and will need to be surgically removed.

Large stones are another matter. Numerous large stones can grow to fill the bladder and eventually irritate the lining, causing bleeding and recurrent bacterial infection. This form of large stone formation is more common in dogs than in cats. The stones can be surgically removed. They usually will recur at shorter and shorter intervals, however, which necessitates repeated surgery.

The causes for this condition are not really understood. There are various ideas about the role of calcium and other minerals, and the relation with vitamin D and other nutrients, but nothing is (in my opinion) really clear about the etiology.

The animals I have worked with have done well on a natural diet program with appropriate homeopathic treatment. Considering the many kinds of stones that can form and the many clinical problems that they can be associated with, however, I can give only general advice that will be helpful regardless of the type of stone involved. More specific, individualized treatment will be needed for persistent and recurrent problems.

First improve the diet. This will help the animal by strengthening the urinary tract, normalizing liver function and adjusting the animal's metabolism. A home-prepared diet with the following supplements will be of great help.

Cod-liver oil: The lining of the bladder and urinary tract is kept in top condition by adequate vitamin A in the diet. In addition, vitamin D, which is produced by the animal's body in the presence of sunlight, can be deficient in many animals that live indoors much of the time. Use cod-liver oil or another source of both vitamin A and vitamin D. Give 2,500 IU per day of vitamin A to small dogs, 5,000 to medium dogs and 10,000 to large dogs (see page 226).

Vitamin C: Give this vitamin to aid detoxification and to acidify the urine, which helps control bacterial infection and reduces the likelihood that stones will form. Twice daily give 250 milligrams to small dogs and 500 milligrams to medium dogs. Large dogs get 500 milligrams, three times daily (see page 226).

B complex: The most important B vitamins for this condition are B_2 (riboflavin) and B_6 (pyridoxine). However, don't give them alone. Always use a complete natural formula so no imbalances of the B complex occur. Give small dogs a daily tablet with the major B vitamins (including B_2 and B_6) at the 10-milligram level, for medium and large dogs make it the 20-milligram level.

Do not restrict calcium in the diet. Sometimes people are advised to follow a low-calcium diet with the idea that restricting calcium will reduce the formation of stones. However, there is no evidence that this is effective; in fact, insufficient calcium actually makes the problem worse by increasing the amount of oxalate (a common component of bladder and kidney stones) in the urine.

Magnesium: This mineral helps prevent reformation of stones. Magnesium chloride or other magnesium chelates are good supplements to use, given at levels of 50, 100 or 300 milligrams a day, depending on the animal's size (see page 226).

Avoid exposure to cadmium, which is known to increase the formation of stones. The most common source of cadmium exposure for pets is cigarette smoke (even more reason to quit).

In addition to these dietary measures, I would use *one* of the following treatment programs for the tendency to form stones, either small or large in size.

Homeopathic—The treatment most likely to be effective, in my experience, is this sequential homeopathic treatment: First give the remedy *Thuya occidentalis* 30C (arborvitae) using "Homeopathic Schedule 5," page 349.

Wait for one month and then do the same treatment (Schedule 5) with *Calcarea carbonica* 30C. This treatment program will not be effective in every case, but will with many and is worth trying.

Herbal—*Barberry (Berberis vulgaris):* This herb is good for an animal with arthritic or rheumatic (muscle and joint soreness) tendencies in addition to bladder or kidney stones. Use "Herbal Schedule 1," page 346, for a month to give it an adequate try.

Herbal—*Sarsaparilla (Smilax officinalis):* Useful in cases where "gravel" and small stones are in the urine, accompanied by bladder inflammation and pain. Urination may be painful and blood may be passed. Often the animal suited to this herb will also have dry, itchy skin that flares up most in the springtime. Use "Herbal Schedule 1," page 346, for a month to give it an adequate try.

If your dog needs surgery to remove bladder stones, here's a treatment to relieve pain and assist recovery. Start it the day after surgery, if possible.

Homeopathic—*Staphysagria* 6C *(stavesacre):* Use "Homeopathic Schedule 3," page 348.

BREAST TUMORS

Breast tumors are more likely in older females that have not been spayed. Spaying your pet while it's young not only helps to ease the pet population problem, it also helps to prevent breast tumors. Like any problem with growths or tumors, it is best to avoid vaccinations and to emphasize the purest foods. A pure diet is especially important because the hormones that stimulate cancer growth are more likely to be higher in meat by-products. By using organic meats (or even just human-grade meats from a market), you significantly reduce exposure.

TREATMENT

In many cases breast tumors are malignant and radical surgery involving removal of associated lymph nodes is recommended. My experience, however, is that this is not always the best thing to do. Surgery will result in a weakened immune system and can result in a decline in health. I find that the animals that have had surgery or chemotherapy cannot usually be helped by the alternative methods I use. You can try a more natural approach first, however, and, if there is no progress, consult a veterinarian about the possibility of surgery or other treatment.

It is difficult to give you general advice because this is a serious problem that requires professional evaluation. If your dog develops such tumors, I suggest that you have her examined by your veterinarian. If the tumors are not thought to be malignant, you certainly could try one of the following treatments. If they *are* thought to be malignant, however, you should work with your veterinarian rather than go it on your own.

One of these treatments may be suitable.

Homeopathic—Use this sequential homeopathic treatment: First give the remedy *Thuya occidentalis* 30C (arborvitae) using "Homeopathic Schedule 5," page 349. Wait for 1 month and then give *Silicea* 30C, also using Schedule 5.

Homeopathic—*Lachesis muta 30C (venom of bushmaster snake):* This is suitable for a tumor that is in the *left* breast, and the skin over the tumor is dark or blackish. Use "Homeopathic Schedule 4," page 348.

Herbal—Poke root (*Phytolacca*) is a very important herb for treating inflammation, infection and drainage from the breast. It is indicated for tumors or hardening of this tissue with discharge of pus or bad smelling fluid. Use "Homeopathic Schedule 1," page 348, for as long as is necessary.

Herbal—Goldenseal (*Hydrastis canadensis*) is generally useful in treating any kind of cancer, especially if it is associated with a loss of weight. Use "Homeopathic Schedule 1," page 348, for as long as it seems helpful. When using this herb for long periods, supplement the diet with extra vitamin B complex, as goldenseal tends to deplete the body of these vitamins.

Note: Remember that nutrition is all-important. Besides the natural diet, offer large amounts of vitamin C (500 milligrams to 5 grams daily, depending on the size of your animal) as well as vitamin E (50 to 200 IU) and vitamin A (2,000 to 5,000 IU) each day. All three vitamins are useful for detoxification.

BRONCHITIS

See "Upper Respiratory Infections."

CANCER

The dreaded disease cancer is becoming increasingly common in our time. Research suggests that environmental pollutants and chemicals in food are major factors in the development and support of this group of diseases. The way I see it, there are many factors that seem to "cause" cancer, but they don't take effect unless the individual is in a weakened, susceptible condition.

The condition of the thymus gland and its associated lymphatic tissues and immunological functions is extremely important. If an animal can be kept in excellent health with good food, adequate exercise, access to fresh air and sunshine, and a stable emotional environment, this immune system will be strong. Whereas a weaker animal might succumb to the effects of carcinogens, the strong one will more likely resist and detoxify them. Prevention is really the most we can do, and it is very important. No drug or vaccine can ever take the place of good health.

PREVENTION

Certain influences in animals' lives increase their exposure to carcinogens, and you should help your pet avoid them as much as possible. They include chronic exposure to cigarette smoke, riding in the back of a pickup truck (and inhaling car fumes), resting on or close to a color TV set, drinking water from street puddles (which can contain hydrocarbons and asbestos dust from brakes), frequent diagnostic work with x-rays (all radiation effects are cumulative in the body), use of strong toxic chemicals over long periods (as with flea and tick control) and consuming pet foods high in organ meats and meat meal (concentrators of pesticides, and growth hormones used to fatten cattle, which can promote cancer growth) as well as in preservatives and artificial colors known to cause cancer in lab animals.

Unfortunately, for a pet that already has cancer, the time for prevention has passed. By avoiding these toxins, however, we will at least not be adding stress to an already burdened body.

In addition to these precautions, a fresh natural diet is imperative. (Cancer is difficult enough to deal with. Don't compromise when dealing with a disease of this seriousness.) Supplement the diet with vitamins C, A and E as well as yeast and fresh raw vegetables (particularly sprouts and grasses, notable for their B vitamin and trace mineral contents).

TREATMENT

What can we expect in treating cancer? Helpful treatments have three possibilities: maintaining good-quality life during the time remaining, extending life beyond what is usually expected or curing the condition with diminution or disappearance of the tumors.

The majority of my cases fall into the first two groups because most of the animals I work with are older and not particularly healthy to start with. But even then the animal's quality of life usually remains good, much better than expected, during nutritional and homeopathic treatment. However, the animal may not live much longer than was expected when diagnosed. This outcome is true of about a third of my cancer cases.

Another third of my patients live longer than expected, sometimes considerably longer, especially if they are younger and have not had prior surgery. Eventually, they do succumb to the disease. This is more likely to happen with some types of cancers than others, of course.

The remaining third do better than this, with the tumors no longer growing—perhaps even regressing and disappearing. As you would expect, this improvement is more likely to occur in a younger animal with more vitality. It seems to be very important that there be no prior use of corticosteroids or surgery if I am to obtain results like this. The use of nutrition and homeopathy depends on a vigorous immuno-defense system, so this system must be kept in tip-top condition.

Though chemotherapy, radiation and surgery can have dramatic and rapid results, the quality of life for the animals afterwards does not impress me. Life is more than just physical duration. To me it is not enough for the patient to be alive—there must also be some pleasure in that life. From the beginning of my career in veterinary medicine, I have been averse to the harsh treatments used for cancer. It just doesn't feel right to me.

Further, I don't think that conventional treatment is effective in prolonging life. Recent evaluations of research into cancer treatment methods show that, contrary to popular belief, the overall death rate from cancer has stayed the same over the last 35 years. (Because of earlier diagnosis, the survival rate only appears to be longer than it used to be.) Considering the discomfort entailed in conventional treatment, I don't think it is worth it.

So, let's say you have thought about this and still opt for the conventional program. Then, I suggest the following measures to help support the body during conventional cancer therapy.

- Avoid commercial foods completely. Feed only fresh, unprocessed foods, including as much raw fare as the animal is willing to accept (see the discussion about food under "Breast Tumors"). Use only organic meat, if you can get it.
- Give high levels of vitamin C (one gram daily for every 15 pounds of body weight). Give half of this in the morning and half in the evening.
- Give oat tincture as described under "Behavior Problems."

- Use only spring, distilled or other pure water, not tap water.
- If your animal becomes ill from the drugs used during treatment, feed cooked oatmeal (with milk and honey) if possible and give the homeopathic remedy *Nux vomica* 6C using "Homeopathic Schedule 2," page 348.
- Avoid all vaccinations. Giving a vaccine to an animal with cancer is like pouring gasoline on a fire.

On the other hand, if you decide to forgo conventional treatment, follow the instructions above and do the following treatments as well. Start with the goldenseal and the treatment with thuya.

Herbal—Goldenseal (*Hydrastis canadensis*) is generally useful for treating any kind of cancer, especially if it is associated with a loss of weight. Use "Herbal Schedule 1," page 346, for as long as it seems helpful. When you use this herb for long periods, you will need to supplement the diet with extra vitamin B complex.

Homeopathic—*Thuya occidentalis 30C:* Use "Homeopathic Schedule 4," page 348. This treatment should be done at the outset of any cancer case, as it removes the influence of prior vaccinations which may stimulate the growth of tumors.

If there is not enough improvement after three or four weeks, then try one of these treatments using "Homeopathic Schedule 6(b)," page 349.

Homeopathic—*Natrum muriaticum 6C (salt, sodium chloride):* This is most helpful to cats that have solid tumors or lymphosarcoma, especially if associated with appetite problems.

Homeopathic—*Silicea 6C (silicon diox-*

ide, quartz): This is most helpful to dogs that have solid tumors or lymphosarcoma, especially if associated with a ravenous appetite and weight loss.

Homeopathic—*Conium maculatum 6C (poison hemlock):* This is indicated for the animal that has very hard tumors.

Homeopathic—*Phosphorus 6C:* Useful where the tumors tend to hemorrhage or bleed persistently.

CATARACTS

See "Eye Problems."

CHOREA

See "Distemper, Chorea and Feline Panleukopenia."

CONSTIPATION

Constipation sometimes occurs when animals don't get enough bulk in their diet or don't get enough exercise. If a dog or cat is not allowed to evacuate when the urge is there, the animal may develop the habit of holding its stool. A dog that is not let out often enough or a housebound cat with a dirty litter box is most likely to develop this habit. In relatively simple cases like this, the following treatments generally will suffice.

TREATMENT

Feed a natural diet that includes fresh vegetables for adequate bulk. Raw meat seems to be a natural laxative for dogs and cats. Milk sometimes is the same for cats.

If the animal's stools seem dry, add ½ teaspoon to 1 tablespoon of bran to each meal (depending on the animal's weight). It will help the stools hold additional moisture. A similar treatment is to use ¼ teaspoon to 2 teaspoons of powdered psyllium seed, which is available in health food stores.

Use mineral oil temporarily where there is a large buildup of hard stools. Depending on the animal's size, add ½ teaspoon to 2 teaspoons to the food twice a day, for no more than a week. Continued use is inadvisable because the oil will draw reserves of vitamin A from the animal's body and may also create a dependency on its use for normal evacuation.

Give the animal plenty of opportunity to relieve itself. Make sure your cat has a clean, accessible litter box and let your dog out several times a day.

Make sure the animal gets plenty of exercise. This is very important for massaging the internal organs and increasing blood flow throughout the body, often stimulating a sluggish metabolism. Long walks or runs or a game of fetch are excellent. For a cat try games involving pouncing, such as "thing-on-a-string."

DOGS

CHRONIC CASES

If your dog has chronic constipation, try one of these remedies in addition to the advice just given. Pick the one that most closely matches your pet's situation.

Homeopathic—*Nux vomica 6C (poison nut):* This is an effective treatment for constipation caused by poor-quality food in the diet, eating too many bones, or emotional upset (frustration, grief, scolding). It is best suited to a dog that has repeated but ineffectual straining and may show irritability, pain and a tendency to hide or be alone. Use "Homeopathic Schedule 3," page 348.

Tissue Salt—*Silicea 6C (silicon dioxide, quartz):* Silicea is best for the constipated animal that seems to have a weak rectum. With this weakness the stool, though partly expelled, slips back in again. It's also good for a dog that has trouble getting the whole bowel movement out and for the poorly nourished animal. Use "Homeopathic Schedule 3," page 348.

Where the rectum is weak, you should also consider the possibility of aluminum poisoning. Signs include chronic constipation with straining, and stools that are sticky and messy rather than hard. Even though the stool is soft, weak rectal muscles make passage difficult. Consider the possibility of aluminum poisoning in all recurrent cases, even though the symptoms may be different from those given.

If you suspect this problem, stop using aluminum cooking pots or dishes for your animal's food. Avoid pet food sold in aluminum cans. Also, do not feed processed cheeses (which may contain sodium aluminum phosphate as an emulsifier), table salt (which often contains sodium silicoaluminate or aluminum calcium silicate to prevent caking), white flour (which may be bleached with an aluminum compound, potassium alum) and tap water (aluminum sulfate may be used as a precipitant to remove water impurities).

To help remove the aluminum from the body, use high levels of vitamin C (500 milligrams to 3 grams daily) along with a zinc supplement (5 milligrams for cats and small dogs, 10 milligrams for medium dogs and 20 milligrams for large dogs—see page 226). A chelated form of zinc is best.

Please understand that not all animals are adversely affected by aluminum; however, there are some individuals that are very sensitive to it.

CATS

CHRONIC CASES

For the cat with chronic constipation, use the basic treatment described above. In addition choose the *one* remedy below that best suits your cat's condition.

Homeopathic—*Nux vomica 6C (poison nut):* Use for the cat that strains ineffectually or passes only small amounts without relief. It may act irritable, withdraw to be alone in another room or avoid your touch. Constipation may follow emotional upset, stress or too much rich food. There may be a history of nausea and vomiting. Use "Homeopathic Schedule 3," page 348.

Homeopathic—*Sepia 30C:* This is indicated for the most severe and persistent forms of constipation in cats. When the case is this severe, it is often called obstipation. Some cats never empty their bowels adequately, going two or three days between inadequate bowel movements. Use "Homeopathic Schedule 4," page 348.

Herbal—*Common garlic (Allium sativum):* For the cat with a big appetite that likes a lot of meat and tends to constipation, add ½ to 1 clove of freshly grated raw garlic to the daily food. Many animals like the taste.

Herbal—*Olive oil (Olea europaea):* This oil serves as a tonic for the intestinal tract and stimulates the flow of liver bile and the contraction of intestinal muscles. Any excess oil will also lubricate the fecal mass and soothe the mucous membrane linings of the intestine and rectum. Give ½ to 1 teaspoon twice daily, mixed with food, until the movements are regular. (You also can give it once a week as a tonic or to prevent hair balls.)

Note: Also consider the possibility of aluminum sensitivity, as described for dogs.

CORNEAL ULCERS

See "Eye Problems."

CYSTITIS

See "Bladder Problems."

DEMODECTIC MANGE

See "Skin Parasites."

DENTAL PROBLEMS

The mouth and its associated structures are very important to animals, not only for eating but also for grooming and manipulating things. This part of the body contains many nerves and is served by a plentiful blood supply, making dental problems more serious than you might expect. Mouth pain can keep an animal from eating enough or grooming properly.

Four problems are most common: accidents that damage the teeth or gums, congenital or developmental disorders, periodontitis (calculus on the teeth and associated gum disease) and tooth decay. Let's look at each in turn.

Accidents

If a pet is hit by a car, it's not unusual that teeth are broken off or knocked out. In most cases, after the initial inflammation has subsided, the animal feels no real discomfort. Generally, a broken tooth can be left in place, at least until a convenient occasion for removal occurs, such as another need for surgical anesthesia. Sometimes, however, the root will become abscessed and require removal.

As for injured gums, an excellent immediate treatment to stop bleeding and promote rapid healing is:

Herbal—*Calendula tincture (Calendula officinalis):* Apply it directly to the bleeding gum with a saturated cotton swab or dilute the tincture with 10 parts water and use it as a flushing mouthwash, applied with a syringe or turkey baster.

An excellent treatment for mouth pain from injuries is:

Homeopathic—*Arnica* 30C (Leopard's Bane) using "Homeopathic Schedule 2," page 348. The next day give *Hypericum* 30C (St.-John's-wort) also using Schedule 2.

Congenital or Developmental Disorders

Problems of this sort are so common in some breeds of dogs that they seem to be standard equipment. Cats, however, have very few congenital mouth problems, probably because they've been less modified by intentional breeding.

Some dogs, especially toy breeds, have teeth that are simply too crowded, often overlapping in position. Sometimes the jaw is too long or too short. Worst of all is the fate of breeds like the bulldog and Boston bull terrier, who have very short jaws with teeth that are crammed together, turned sideways and completely out of position. They really have a mouthful of problems.

What can you do about it? I recommend extracting some of the permanent teeth as they develop, preferably while the dog is still young. Left untreated, the crowding and poor fit may lead to gum disease and loose teeth.

Some dogs have relatively straight, uncrowded teeth, but one jaw is longer or shorter than the other. As a result the teeth don't meet properly, causing discomfort and premature breakdown of both teeth and gums. If the difference between the jaws is ¼ inch or less, removal of some of the deciduous (baby) teeth before the arrival of the permanent set may restore proper alignment. But if the difference is greater, little can be done preventively.

Other structural problems include supernumerary (extra) teeth, which should be removed to prevent accumulation of food and debris, and retained baby teeth, which force the permanent teeth to grow beside or in front of them (trapping debris and perhaps distorting the jaw formation). They, too, should be removed by a veterinarian.

Periodontal Disease

This is the most common tooth and gum problem. It results from a change in the normal saliva, which creates a buildup of calcium salts, food, hair and bacteria on the animal's teeth. These deposits put pressure on the gums, causing inflammation, swelling, pulling away and receding gums. A pocket opens up between the gums and teeth, which collects still more debris and further worsens the problem. Eventually, the process can loosen the teeth and cause them to fall out.

Of course, periodontal disease doesn't destroy teeth overnight. It may take months or years. A serious complication is the development of an abscess which destroys the root of the tooth.

If your pet has periodontal disease, it will show these symptoms: bleeding gums, foul breath, excessive salivation, painful chewing (dropping food while eating or turning its head to the side to chew only on one side) and possible loss of appetite or weight. You can see heavy brown deposits (calculus) on the teeth, particularly on the back ones. And the teeth may be loose.

The usual causes for the buildup of calculus are misaligned teeth, overfeeding, poor-quality food, lack of hard, chewable things to exercise the teeth and gums and frequent nibbling. Once the deposits have formed, they are rock-hard and can only be removed adequately by your veterinarian (under anesthesia) with careful hand-scraping or an ultrasonic cleaner. Often the infected and loose teeth must also be extracted and hemorrhage controlled.

After any dental work at the hospital, you can do a lot with follow-up care both to promote rapid healing and to prevent recurrence. The gums will be very sore and inflamed. Certain herbs will be very helpful. Pick *one* of the following that seems best suited (or, if indicated, you may use both the goldenseal and the myrrh, ½ teaspoon of each).

Herbal—*Purple cone flower (Echinacea angustifolia):* This is useful where teeth were found to be infected, and the animal is thin and run down. Boil 1 teaspoon of fresh-smelling rootstock in 1 cup of water for 10 minutes. Cover, remove from heat and let steep for an hour. Strain and apply this decoction directly to the gums with a swab (or use it as a mouthwash). It promotes saliva flow, so don't worry if your pet begins to drool.

Herbal—_Goldenseal (Hydrastis canadensis):_ This herb is antiseptic and helpful for new gum tissue growth. Steep 1 teaspoon of powdered rootstock in a pint of boiling-hot water until cool. Pour off the clear liquid and use it to flush out the mouth and gums.

Herbal—_Myrrh (Commiphora myrrha):_ Myrrh is indicated for loose teeth. Steep 1 teaspoon of the resin in a pint of boiling water for a few minutes. Strain it and paint the infusion on the gums or flush them using a syringe or turkey baster.

Herbal—_Plantain (Plantago major):_ This herb helps when the condition is not serious enough to require major cleaning but when you see minor deposits on the teeth and the gums are inflamed. Bring 1 cup of water to a boil. Turn off heat and add 1 tablespoon of the leaves. Steep for 5 minutes. Strain and use as a mouthwash.

General directions for herbs: Whichever herb you pick, use it twice a day for 10 to 14 days. Alternatively, use the herb in the morning and apply vitamin E (fresh out of the capsule) to the gums with your fingers at night. (This treatment is very soothing.)

Diet is also extremely important in the period after teeth cleaning. Without proper nutrition the gums can't repair themselves or maintain necessary resilience. Emphasize those vegetables rich in niacin, folate and minerals—leafy greens, broccoli, asparagus, lima beans, potatoes and lettuce. Also, serve fresh liver twice weekly for its folate, vitamin A, protein and other richly supplied nutrients. Other good folate sources are eggs or plain peanuts (which can be given as unsalted peanut butter).

Also add ⅛ to ½ teaspoon of bonemeal powder (for extra calcium and phosphorus), 100 to 1,000 milligrams of vitamin C twice daily and a B-complex tablet or capsule with the major vitamins at the 5- to 10-milligram level (amounts depend on the animal's size). Use these extra supplements for the next three weeks.

Also give your pet its own natural "toothbrush"—either bones or a hard raw vegetable like a carrot. For dogs I advise that one day a week you feed nothing but one large _raw_ bone. There is no better natural cleaner for teeth. But avoid cooked bones (which splinter) and small or easily splintered bones from chickens and turkeys. These can be dangerous.

Some dogs that have trouble digesting bone fragments get irritation and either diarrhea or constipation; this is usually a result of weak stomach acid from improper feeding. Good diet and a B-complex supplement will likely clear up the problem. For the first few weeks limit bone chewing to 30 minutes a day and watch to make sure that large pieces are not swallowed.

Cats can be given small raw bones as well but do not really pick up on this practice unless they are started quite young. Somewhat more accepted is to feed part of a raw game hen once a week instead of the regular meals. Unfortunately, having lost their natural instincts, many mature cats will not adapt to this. It is worth trying, however, because it will keep their mouths quite clean and healthy.

Tooth Decay

This is primarily a problem in cats that develop decay of the sides of the teeth (near the gums) or in the roots. This is an increasingly common problem and, in my opinion, is a direct outcome of generations of eating commercial foods. There is little that can be done to reverse this once it happens. Often, the affected teeth need to be removed, though some veterinarians have learned to fill these cavities much as your dentist does. Prevention is essential and the advice given in this book about nutrition is most important.

One more thing: If you're about to get a new pet, look for one with properly formed teeth and jaws (and parents with the same). See chapter 9 for information on hereditary defects.

DERMATITIS

See "Skin Problems."

DIABETES

Seen in both dogs and cats, the type of diabetes animals get is similar in most ways to the diabetes seen in humans. It has now been determined that human diabetes is an immune disorder in which the body attacks the pancreatic cells that make insulin. It is likely this same process that destroys the insulin-producing ability of our pets.

This failure of the pancreas to secrete insulin does not allow proper use of blood sugar. Instead of reaching the body tissues, the increasing levels of blood sugar spill over into the urine and are lost from the body. Thus, despite adequate caloric intake, the tissues are in a condition of semi-starvation all the time.

Thus, the animal eats a lot, but still gets thinner and thinner. The continuous presence of sugar in the urine also causes fluid loss. That's because the sugar must be dissolved in water to be eliminated, so it carries the water out with it. As a result, the animal is abnormally thirsty and passes large volumes of urine.

There is apparently more to this condition than just lack of insulin, however, because even if insulin needs are carefully met with injections of this hormone, there are still progressive changes and weaknesses that may persist. These sometimes include recurrent pancreatic inflammation, formation of eye cataracts and an increased susceptibility to infection (particularly of the urinary tract).

TREATMENT

The usual treatment consists of strictly regulating sugar intake and using daily injections of insulin (derived from the glands of other animals). Feeding is usually restricted to canned food fed once a day, about 12 hours after the insulin is given (when its activity is highest).

The diabetic dogs I have treated have generally done well on the basic fresh and raw natural food diet given as two or three meals during the day rather than one large one. Their insulin needs seem to stabilize, rather than going through erratic ups and downs from day to day. You may need to experiment with your animal to find the best frequency of feeding, also taking into account the advice of your veterinarian.

Above all, avoid the soft-moist dog foods that come in cellophane bags and don't need refrigeration. These products are very high in carbohydrates like sugar that are used as preservatives, as well as artificial colors and other preservatives.

A supplement that is quite helpful is glucose tolerance factor, a natural chromium-containing substance found in yeast. It can assist the body in using blood glucose more effectively. I always recommend supplementing the natural food diet with this element. Give one teaspoon to one tablespoon of brewer's yeast with each meal.

Vitamin E is also important because it reduces the need for insulin. Give 25 IU to 200 IU of this vitamin each day.

In addition to the nutritional advice given here, see that your animal gets lots of exercise, which has the effect of decreasing insulin needs. Erratic exercise could destabilize the insulin needs, though, so a regular, sustained program of exercise is best. It is also important for your pet to maintain a normal weight. Obese animals have a much harder time with this disease.

SEVERE DIABETES

The more severe cases need to have stringent dietary regulation. If your animal is not responding to the above program or is already quite ill with difficulty stabilizing its condition, then the following will be helpful.

Dietary guidelines: The main goal of a special diet to control diabetes is to reduce the stress placed on the pancreas. That means strict avoidance of foods that contain sugar as well as a low fat intake (because the pancreas produces a number of enzymes particularly involved in the breakdown of fat). Therefore, use the natural diets given in this book, but avoid fatty meats and give only half of the fat or oil called for in the recipe.

Certain foods are particularly beneficial for diabetes, so emphasize them in your selections—especially millet, rice, oats, cornmeal and rye bread. Excellent vegetables are green beans (the pods of which contain certain hormonal substances closely related to insulin), winter squash, dandelion greens, alfalfa sprouts, corn, parsley, onion, Jerusalem artichoke and garlic (which reduces blood sugar in diabetes). Garlic also stimulates the abdominal viscera and increases digestive organ function. Use it regularly in some form (fresh or in capsules).

Milk and milk products are helpful because they are alkalizing (as are vegetables and most fruits), which helps to counter overacidity. They are best fed raw, as are meat, eggs, fruits and some vegetables, because uncooked foods are much more stimulating to the pancreas. Fruits in season are fine, if acceptable to your animal; the natural fruit sugar (fructose) can be used by the diabetic animal. Feed them separately from other foods.

Specific treatments for diabetes include:

Homeopathic—*Natrum muriaticum* 6X (salt, sodium chloride) is sometimes helpful to cats. Those it is suitable for usually have appetite problems and a marked weight loss. Sugar will be detectable in the urine, and there will be a tendency to anxiety and fearfulness. Use "Homeopathic Schedule 6(a)," page 349.

Homeopathic—*Phosphorus* 6X is useful for some dogs with this condition. They tend to have ravenous appetites with a tendency towards being overweight. There may be a history of pancreatitis (inflammation of the pancreas). Use "Homeopathic Schedule 6(a)," page 349.

DIARRHEA AND DYSENTERY

Diarrhea, though common, is not a very specific condition. That is, many things can *cause* diarrhea, and yet the clinical appearance (frequent, soft or fluid movements) is about the same. It helps to understand the general purpose of diarrhea, which is that the gastrointestinal tract has one major defense against irritants of many sorts—moving its contents along more quickly than usual. The cause of the irritation may include worms, bacteria, viruses, spoiled or toxic food, food sensitivities (see "Allergies"), bone fragments or indigestible material like hair, cloth or plastic.

The body's primary response to these irritants is to increase bowel contraction (called peristalsis) in order to flush them out of the system. Because the intestinal contents move along so quickly, the colon does not absorb the amount of water it usually does. Thus, the bowel movement is abnormally fluid.

Depending on what part of the tract is irritated, you may see certain additional symptoms. If there is inflammation and bleeding in the upper part of the small intestine, near the stomach, then the bowel movement will be very dark or black from digested blood. You also may notice a buildup of excess gas that causes belching, a bloated stomach or flatulence. The animal in this pattern usually shows no particular straining when passing a stool.

A different picture appears when the inflammation is lower down in the colon. Generally, there is no problem with gas buildup. The diarrhea tends to "shoot" out of the rectum with force and obvious straining. If there has been bleeding in the colon, the blood will appear as a fresh red color mixed with the stool. The bowel movements tend to be more frequent than when the disturbance centers in the small intestine. Often you may notice excessive mucus that looks like clear jelly.

Because diarrhea can be associated with so many causes and other disorders, we must be alert to the possibility of other conditions lurking behind this symptom. Most of the time, however, diarrhea is caused by eating the wrong kind of food or spoiled food, overeating, parasites (in young animals especially) or virus infections.

The following guidelines are useful for treating simple or mild conditions that fall in the above categories. If they don't clear it up or if conditions are severe or otherwise seem to warrant it, seek professional help—sooner rather than later.

TREATMENT

Most importantly, do not feed any solid food for the first 24 to 48 hours. A liquid fast will give the intestinal tract a chance to rest and do its job of flushing things out. Make sure that plenty of pure water is available at all times and encourage drinking. A danger of excessive diarrhea is that the body can get dehydrated from the loss of water, sodium and potassium. So provide these in the form of a broth made from vegetables, rice and some meat or a bone. You may also add a small amount of naturally brewed soy sauce to enhance flavor and provide easily assimilated amino acids and sodium. Use just the liquid part of the soup, serving it at room temperature several times a day during the fast period.

If the condition is mild or is a sudden attack following consumption of spoiled food, this treatment alone may suffice. In more severe cases, however, it will be wise to use *one* of the following as well.

Kaopectate solution: Made from finely powdered earth and pectin from plants, this over-the-counter pharmaceutical absorbs irritating substances and soothes inflamed tissue without slowing down the intestinal activity. Depending on body size, give 1 teaspoon to 3 tablespoons every 4 hours for a couple of days.

Activated charcoal: Sold in drugstores as a powder or in tablets, this type of charcoal prepared from plant matter has the ability to absorb toxins, drugs, poisons and other irritating material. It's especially useful for treating diarrhea that was caused by eating spoiled food or toxic substances. Mix it with water and give it by mouth every 3 or 4 hours for a 24-hour period (except during sleep). Because overuse of charcoal could interfere with digestive enzymes, a short course is best. Depending on the animal's size, use ½ to 1 teaspoon powder or 1 to 3 tablets.

Roasted carob powder: Available in health food stores, this plant substance is commonly used as a chocolate substitute. However, it is also a popular and soothing aid to diarrhea. Give ½ to 2 teaspoons 3 times a day for 3 days. Mix it with water and perhaps a little honey, giving it by mouth.

Slippery elm powder: Available in most health food stores, this material from the inner bark of the slippery elm tree is an excellent treatment for diarrhea of any cause, and I use it frequently with the animals I treat. To make it, thoroughly mix 1 slightly rounded teaspoon of slippery elm powder

to 1 cup of cold water. Bring to a boil while stirring constantly. Then turn down the heat to simmer and continue to stir for another 2 to 3 minutes while the mixture thickens slightly. Take it off the heat, add 1 tablespoon of honey (for dogs only) and stir in well. Cool to room temperature and give ½ to 1 teaspoon to cats and small dogs, 2 teaspoons to 2 tablespoons for medium dogs and 3 to 4 tablespoons for large dogs (see page 226). Give this dose 4 times a day or about every 4 hours. Cover the mixture and keep at room temperature. It will keep for a couple of days.

Homeopathic—*Podophyllum 6C (mayapple):* This remedy is often useful for the typical diarrhea with a forceful, gushing type of stool, especially if it smells unusually bad. Use "Homeopathic Schedule 2," page 348.

Homeopathic—*Mercurius corrosivus 6C (corrosive sublimate):* The typical dysentery (frequent, bloody stools with much straining) is suited to this medicine. This type of diarrhea can come on after eating toxic substances or from a viral infection. Use "Homeopathic Schedule 2," page 348.

Homeopathic—*Arsenicum album 6C (arsenic trioxide):* Use this remedy for diarrhea from eating spoiled meat. Usually there are frequent bowel movements, rather small in quantity. Also there is weakness, thirst and chilliness. Use "Homeopathic Schedule 2," page 348.

Tissue Salt—*Natrum muriaticum 6X (salt, sodium chloride):* This is appropriate for longer-lasting diarrhea of cats. It is usually dark and offensive smelling and associated with the cat acting uncomfortable after eating—sitting hunched up on all fours. Use

"Homeopathic Schedule 2," page 348.

Homeopathic—*Pulsatilla 6C (windflower)*: This is a good remedy for dogs or cats that have overeaten or had food that is too rich or fatty. They will get diarrhea from an upset stomach, generally becoming subdued and timid. Typically, they do not have any thirst with the diarrhea (which is unusual). Use "Homeopathic Schedule 2," page 348.

General advice: During the treatment it is important to be watchful for the possibility that some causative factor remains, such as an irritating chemical (for example, a new flea collar), the use of milk (which bothers some animals), polluted water or access to spoiled food in somebody's garbage can or a compost pile. An animal's lack of response to treatment can sometimes be traced to the persistence of such a cause. Also, consider worms and infectious diseases and treat them at home or with your veterinarian's help, as is appropriate.

Once recovery seems to be on its way, feed small amounts of plain yogurt to help replenish the intestinal tract with friendly bacteria. Always provide yogurt when antibiotics are being used, as the antibiotics kill off normal bowel inhabitants and leave a space for the growth of nasty things like yeast and fungus. Yogurt or acidophilus milk will provide protection.

When you are breaking your pet out of the fast (after a couple of days), start with the broth, mixed with the solid vegetables used to make it. After 24 hours you can introduce the yogurt and begin to reestablish a regular diet, using white rice (just for a few days, then brown rice) as the grain, because it is generally good for slowing down diarrhea.

DISTEMPER, CHOREA AND FELINE PANLEUKOPENIA

We will consider all three of these diseases together, since they are related. Chorea (uncontrollable twitching or jerking) is a possible result of distemper. Panleukopenia is commonly known as cat distemper. Let's discuss each in turn.

Canine Distemper

Distemper is so common that few dogs escape exposure to the virus, which is spread through the air (from exhaling or sneezing) or by contact with contaminated bowls, toys, bones and such. Most, however, do escape the disease.

Distemper progresses in stages. After a six- to nine-day incubation (usually not noticeable), the dog contracts a brief initial fever and malaise. Afterward, the dog is apparently normal for a few days or a week, and then it will suddenly show the typical distemper symptoms: fever, loss of appetite and energy and perhaps a clear discharge from the nose. Within a short time the condition advances and the dog develops one or more of the additional symptoms: severe conjunctivitis (eye inflammation) with a thick discharge that sticks the lids together, heavy mucus or yellow discharge from the nose, very bad-smelling diarrhea and skin eruption on the belly or between the hind legs.

Though I have treated many distemper cases with the orthodox approach of antibiotics, fluids and other drugs, I have not seen it do much good. Indeed, sometimes it seems to increase the likelihood of encephalitis, a severe inflammation of the brain (or smaller areas in the spinal cord) that often arises after apparent improvement or recovery. At this point dogs are usually put to sleep because medical treatment is almost always ineffective. I am convinced that the use of drugs increases the likelihood of encephalitis, while natural methods make it less probable. I have witnessed many successful recoveries in distemper cases treated with homeopathy and nutritional therapy. The suggestions that follow are gleaned from this experience.

TREATMENT

In order to prevent complications like encephalitis, it is crucial to withhold solid food while the dog is in the acute phase of distemper with a fever. (The normal rectal temperature is 100.5 to 101.5°F. It might be a little higher at a veterinarian's office because of excitement.) Fast the dog on vegetable broth and pure water as described in chapter 15, until at least a day after the temperature becomes normal. If the fever returns, fast again. Because fevers tend to rise in the evening, record temperatures both morning and night to get a better overview.

In case you are wondering how long dogs can go without solid food before starving, the normal healthy animal can get along all right for several weeks. A dog that is sick with distemper can profitably fast for seven days, provided it is an adult of normal weight and general condition. However, few will need to fast this long. Make sure you have fresh, pure water available at all times.

Vitamin C is an important aid. Many distemper cases can recover without ill effects by using vitamin C along with fasting. (However, I always use homeopathic treatment as well in my practice.) Dose as follows: 250 milligrams every two hours for puppies and small dogs, 500 milligrams every two hours for medium dogs, 1,000 milligrams every three hours for large or giant dogs. Don't continue the dosing through the night, because rest is also important. Once the acute phase and fever have passed, double the interval between doses. Continue until recovery is complete.

Special eye care may be necessary because the lids can get severely inflamed. Bathe the eyes in a saline solution (see chapter 15). Then put a drop of sweet almond oil, cod-liver oil or olive oil in each eye to help heal and provide protection.

During the early stages of distemper, use of *one* of the following remedies should help considerably.

Homeopathic—*Distemperinum 30C:* Specially prepared from the distemper virus, this is the most effective remedy for the early stages. I've seen it produce recoveries in just a day or 2. Give 1 pellet morning and evening until improvement is evident. Then give only if symptoms flare up again.

Tissue Salts—*Ferrum phosphoricum 6X (iron phosphate)* or *Natrum muriaticum 6X (sodium chloride):* You may want to use cell salts instead since they are easier to obtain than Distemperinum. Use Ferrum phosphoricum for the early state that shows fever. Natrum muriaticum is for the early stage with a lot of sneezing.

Homeopathic—*Pulsatilla 6C (windflower):* This remedy is suitable for the stage of conjunctivitis with thick, yellow or greenish eye discharge. Use "Homeopathic Schedule 1," page 348.

Homeopathic—*Arsenicum album 6C:* This remedy is indicated for the dog that is very ill with rapid weight loss, loss of appetite, weakness, restlessness, frequent thirst and a slight clear discharge from the eyes that causes irritation of the eyelids and surrounding areas. Use "Homeopathic Schedule 1," page 348.

If none of these work, there are many other remedies worth trying if you are able to consult with a homeopathic veterinarian.

During the later stages of distemper, select one of the following treatments (in case you did not treat earlier or it has gotten worse despite treatment).

Homeopathic—*Hydrastis canadensis 6C (goldenseal):* Indicated for advanced distemper with a thick, yellow discharge of mucus from the nose or down the back of the throat. Often there will be loss of appetite and emaciation. Use "Homeopathic Schedule 6(a)," page 349.

Homeopathic—*Psorinum 30C:* This is most useful for the dog that has survived distemper but cannot completely recover. Often there is a poor appetite, skin eruptions or irritated skin and a bad smell to the body. Use "Homeopathic Schedule 5," page 349.

RECOVERY

With proper treatment distemper is not too severe, and you can generally expect recovery in a few days to a week. The initial state of health of the animal and the degree of immunity acquired from the mother (in the case of puppies) seem to be important factors in the severity of individual cases.

If recovery is not easy or complete or leaves the animal in a weakened condition, the following measures should help. Feed a convalescence diet (see "Feeding Dogs with Extra Needs" on page 64) emphasizing oats (which strengthen the nervous system) and B vitamins (give a natural B-complex tablet

in the 10- to 50- milligrams range for a few weeks).

For the dog weakened with distemper, give a tincture of the common oat (*Avena sativa*), which is a good nerve tonic available from herb stores, natural food stores or homeopathic pharmacies. Twice daily give 2 to 4 drops for small dogs or puppies, 4 to 8 drops for medium dogs or 8 to 12 drops for large ones.

If the animal is left with a weakened digestive system, residual diarrhea or chest complications, give fresh grated garlic *(Allium sativum)* three times daily. Use ½ small clove for small dogs or puppies, ½ large clove for medium dogs and 1 whole clove for large ones. Add the grated garlic to the food or mix it with honey and flour to make pills.

Chorea

Usually an aftereffect of the distemper virus infection, chorea is a condition in which some muscle in the body (usually a leg, hip or shoulder) twitches every few seconds, sometimes even during sleep. It results from damage to part of the spinal cord or brain. Most pets with chorea are put to sleep because it is not considered curable; however, once in a rare while a spontaneous recovery occurs. I think it is worth giving alternative therapy a try, as it will improve the odds. See relevant information about diet and herbs under "Behavior Problems." In addition, try this more specific treatment.

Homeopathic—*Nux vomica 30C:* Use "Homeopathic Schedule 3," page 348. After doing this treatment, wait and observe for 2 weeks. If there is no change for the better, then use the next treatment.

Homeopathic—*Hyscyamus 30C:* Use "Homeopathic Schedule 3," page 348. Again watch and wait for a 2-week period. If this does not resolve the problem, there are other medicines that can be used, but you will need guidance from a homeopathic veterinarian.

Feline Panleukopenia (Feline Distemper; Infectious Enteritis)

This disease of cats comes on suddenly and severely, without apparent warning, commonly killing young kittens within 24 to 48 hours. The associated virus is thought to be spread through urine, feces, saliva or the vomit of an infected cat. Epidemics are prevalent.

After an incubation period of two to nine days (usually six), the first signs are a high fever (up to 105°F), *severe* depression and severe dehydration. Vomiting often follows soon afterward. Initially, it is a clear fluid; later, it's tinged yellow with bile. Typically, the cat will lie with its head hanging over the edge of its water dish, not moving except to lap water or vomit.

Apparently, it's not the panleukopenia virus itself that produces these severe symptoms, but a secondary infection that results from the destruction of various tissues including the white cells (which protect the body against infections). In many cases they are almost eliminated, which opens the door to the growth of other bacteria or viruses. In many ways this disease is very similar to the parvovirus infection of dogs.

TREATMENT

The most crucial factor in successful treatment is to catch the disorder in its earliest stages. Since young animals can die very quickly, there often isn't enough time to get a home treatment under way. Clinical methods like whole-blood transfusion, fluid therapy and antibiotics can be successful if started early, so get professional care if possible.

If you aren't able to get such care right away and you are prepared with supplies, here is a regimen I suggest: As long as there is fever or vomiting, fast the animal on liquids (chapter 15). Administer high doses of vitamin C, about 100 milligrams per hour to very small kittens and 250 milligrams per hour to young and adult cats. It's easier to give it as sodium ascorbate powder. Use a pinch to make a 100-milligram solution or $\frac{1}{16}$ teaspoon for a 250-milligram solution. Mix the sodium ascorbate with water and give orally.

If vomiting causes both the loss of essential fluids and the vitamin C you have administered (characterized by a rough hair coat, dry-looking eyes and skin that is stiff when pulled up), focus on using the following homeopathic treatment alone until symptoms are improved. Then go back to giving vitamin C along with the homeopathic treatment.

Homeopathic—*Veratrum album 6C (white hellebore):* Use this if the cat is weak, depressed and cold, with vomiting (aggravated by drinking water) and diarrhea. Use "Homeopathic Schedule 1," page 348. If there is improvement, gradually decrease how often you give it over the next couple of days. Eventually, give 1 tablet at a time when there is any recurring nausea or lethargy.

Homeopathic—*Phosphorus 6C:* Use "Homeopathic Schedule 1," page 348. This is the best choice for a cat that is limp, with extreme lethargy and apathy. It will also be thirsty for cold water, yet vomit about 10 to 20 minutes after drinking. The cat that should be treated with phosphorus has less coldness but more listlessness than the cat treated with *Veratrum Album*. If you find that despite either treatment the vomiting is very severe and life-threatening, then follow the advice under "Vomiting."

Herbal—If you have them in stock, consider this alternative herbal treatment: Mix 1 teaspoon of the tincture or decoction of purple cone flower (*Echinacea angustifolia*) with 1 teaspoon of the tincture or decoction of boneset (*Eupatorium perfoliatum*). Give 1 drop of the mixture every hour until you see improvement, then reduce to every 2 hours until recovery.

If the cat is already very ill and close to death, you'll need a different approach. Such a cat will lie in a comatose state, hardly moving. Its ears and feet will feel very cold to the touch. Its nose may have a bluish look. As an emergency measure, administer camphor. Use an ointment containing camphor, such as Tiger Balm. Hold a small dab in front of the cat's nose so that a few breaths will carry in the odor. Repeat every 15 minutes until there is a response.

Once you see improvement you can go to one of the other treatments outlined. Be sure to discontinue the camphor and remove it from the vicinity when homeopathic or herbal remedies are used, or it will counter their effects.

RECOVERY

Once the cat is obviously getting well and the fever is gone (a temperature less than 101.5°F rectally), give solid food once again. Follow the diet and supplement instructions for canine distemper. Offer raw beef liver for a few days, which is a good "tonic" for cats. Take care to minimize stress and avoid chilling for several days after the initial recovery, as a relapse is possible. Continue the vitamin C at reduced levels (250 to 500 milligrams twice daily) for two weeks to prevent complications or residual effects.

DYSENTERY

See "Diarrhea and Dysentery."

EAR MITES

See "Ear Problems."

EAR PROBLEMS

Inflammation, irritation, pain and swelling of the ears are common problems of both dogs and cats, often reflecting allergy or skin problems that also manifest in other parts of the body. Such allergies express themselves periodically as a sudden redness or flushing of the skin, perhaps after a meal during certain times of the year, such as pollen season. A dog with ear problems is likely an allergy victim if it also chews its front feet excessively and scoots its rear end along the floor or ground.

Cats can develop a similar problem, with an accumulation of dark wax or oily material in the ears, itching and head shaking. Ear mites are another possible cause of cat ear trouble, but more often it's allergies.

"Allergy Ears"

It's important to understand that the larger issue of allergies usually underlies an ear problem. Otherwise, you might just focus on the ears and ignore the rest of the problem or even make the situation worse if the ear treatment is suppressive. For more information on the underlying problem, see "Allergies." Here we will look at helpful ways to care for the ears, whether or not they are part of that larger problem.

Keeping the ears clean of discharges and secretions is very helpful in reducing irritation. Chose one of these three alternatives.

Herbal—*Calendula:* If the discharge is watery, smelly and thin, flush and massage the ear canal once or twice a day with a solution of 1 cup of pure water (distilled, spring or filtered), 1 teaspoon of a tincture or glycerin extract of Marigold flower buds (*Calendula officinalis*) and ½ teaspoon sea salt (see chapter 15 for more information on treatment of the ears).

Herbal—*Aloe vera:* For ears that are very painful or sensitive but have little discharge, treat in the same way as above but use fresh juice. Use a liquid preparation of gel made from the leaves of the aloe vera plant.

Herbal—*Sweet almond oil:* To soften and dissolve dark, waxy, oily ear discharge, flush and massage the ear canal with sweet almond oil (*Prunus amydalus*), which is also soothing and healing to the skin. If the ear is painful as well, alternate with the aloe treatment.

Along with one of these cleaning methods, it's helpful to use:

Homeopathic—*Pulsatilla 6C (windflower):* Indicated for the dog or cat that becomes submissive and "pitiful" with the ear problem. The animal will want to be held or comforted. Use "Homeopathic Schedule 6(c)" on page 349. Continue only if it is helping.

Homeopathic—*Silicea 30C:* This remedy is very helpful for dogs with recurrent ear inflammation and excessive wax production or fluid that accumulates in the ear canals. The irritation is severe with head shaking, pawing at the ears and a raw redness of the ear tissues. Usually the veterinarian will diagnose the problem as a bacterial or yeast infection. Use "Homeopathic Schedule 5" on page 349.

Homeopathic—*Sepia 30C:* Helpful for cats with waxy, dirty and itchy ears. They will shake their heads and react violently having their ears cleaned—struggling to get away or scratching uncontrollably with their feet. Use "Homeopathic Schedule 5" on page 349. Often these cats will be thought to have ear mites, though none will be found on microscopic examination.

There are several other factors that can complicate and aggravate allergy-related ear problems or that may be problems in their own right. For many breeds of dogs, the major factor has to do with the shape of their ears. Other minor and associated causes are water in the ear canal, which predisposes the ear to infections, trapped foxtails or other plant awns, and ear mites (a parasite, more often found in cats). Let's examine each of these.

Anatomical Problems

In nature canine ears evolved to stand upright from the head—the best design both for hearing and for ear health. An upright ear like that of a wolf or coyote works well to funnel sounds directly into the ear canal. It also allows a proper exchange of air and moisture between the ear canal and the outside. If water should get in the ear, head-shaking and free flow of air will soon reduce the humidity to the proper level. Throughout thousands of years of raising domestic dogs, however, people selected many with heavier, hairier ears that tended to fold over or hang down a bit. Maybe they seemed cute, or perhaps they just happened to accompany some other feature the people desired.

In any case, floppy ears have caused a great deal of unnecessary suffering for dogs and expense for people. A hanging ear creates an effective trap. It closes off the ear canal from the free exchange of air and moisture and makes it easier for stickers and debris to get stuck inside. Some breeds, like poodles, even have hair growing inside the ear canal, making the problem worse. With this in mind, now let's look at three complicating factors in ear problems. While they may afflict any dog, all three are inevitably worse in dogs with floppy ears.

Water in the Ear Canal

Many dogs enjoy a good swim. Invariably, they get water (sometimes not so clean) down their ears. In excess such moisture can lead to a condition much like swimmer's ear in people, a low-grade irritation which can occasionally develop into more serious infections.

If your dog has this tendency, flush out the ears after a swim with a slightly acidic solution of warm water and lemon juice (figure about half a small fresh-squeezed lemon to a cup of water; alternatively, use about a tablespoon of white vinegar to a cup of water). This will diminish the chance of bacterial or fungal infection and is also healing to the ear tissue. If either preparation seems to "burn,"

dilute the mixture further with warm water. With the help of a dropper or small cup, fill and then massage the ear canal from the outside (see ear care instructions, above). Afterward, allow the animal to shake its head well (it's hard to *keep* them from it!). Blot off all the excess moisture from the inside ear with a tissue and gently swab out just inside the ear opening with a cotton swab. Remember, you are just taking up moisture; do not rub against the skin.

As an additional precaution you can clothespin or tie the ears up behind the head to allow them to dry out further. Do not pin or tie the ear itself, only the hair at the end. Also, if hair grows inside your dog's ears, ask your vet or groomer to show you how to pull it out every so often.

Trapped Foxtails

Floppy ears are much likelier to trap foxtails and other plant stickers. The flap is like a hinged trapdoor that directs the stickers right into the ear canal. Though you can do little to prevent stickers (other than cutting down your weeds and controlling where your animal runs), here is how to deal with them if they get trapped in your dog's ears.

After the dog has an excursion in a field, immediately check the ears (and between the toes as well). If you see foxtails, pull them out. If you can't see any but think there is one deep down in the ear, *don't* try to remove it yourself. The ear can easily be damaged or the foxtail pushed right through the eardrum. Try pressing gently on the ear canal, which feels like a small plastic tube under the ear. If the dog cries out in pain, there is a good chance a foxtail is trapped inside.

If you can't get immediate veterinary care, put some warm oil (almond or olive) into the ear to soften the sticker and make it less irritating. There's also a slight chance that your dog can shake the foxtail out after this procedure, but don't count on it. As soon as possible, take your dog to a veterinarian, who will remove the culprit with the proper instruments (sometimes under anesthesia). Otherwise, very severe damage can occur.

Ear Mites

These parasites are very common in cats, and when dogs get them it is usually from cats. If you have a cat with ear mites and your dog shows symptoms, there's a good chance he has them too.

Though the mites are not possible to see with the naked eye, the discharge that forms in the ear is. It looks much like deposits of dried coffee grounds down in the ear canals. A cat will scratch like mad whenever you rub its ears.

A dog will shake its head and scratch its ears frequently. Usually, there is no bad smell or any discharge like that seen in cats, but the ear canal looks quite red and inflamed (different than in cats who have less irritation) when your veterinarian peers in with an otoscope.

Generally, low vitality invites infestation, so an improved diet will indirectly aid in both prevention and recovery (see chapters 3 and 4). Garlic and brewer's yeast are especially helpful.

A mixture of ½ ounce of almond or olive oil and 400 IU vitamin E (from a capsule) makes a mild healing treatment for either cats or dogs. Blend them in a dropper bottle and warm the mixture to body temperature by immersing it in hot water. Holding the ear flap up, put about ½ dropperful in the ear. Massage the ear canal well so that you hear a fluid sound. After a minute of this, let the animal shake its head. Then gently clean out the opening (not deep into the ear) with cotton swabs to remove debris and excess oil. The oil mixture will smother many of the mites and start a healing process that will make the ear less hospitable for them. Apply the oil every other day for six days (three treatments in total). Between treatments cap the mixture tightly and store at room temperature. After the last oil treatment let the ear rest for three more days. Meanwhile, prepare the next medicine, an herbal extract which is used to directly inhibit or kill the mites.

Herbal—Once the ears are cleaned out, one of the simplest ways to kill mites is with the herb Yellow Dock (*Rumex crispus*). Prepare it as described in "Herbal Schedule 1," page 346, and apply it in the same way as the oil, above. Treat the ears once every three days for three to four weeks. Usually, this is enough to clear up the problem. If you observe irritation or inflammation during the treatment process, then also use the treatment for allergy ears, above.

In a very stubborn case you may need to thoroughly shampoo the head and ears as well. The mites can hang out around the outside of the ears and crawl back in later. Also shampoo the tip of the tail, which may harbor a few mites from when it is curled near the head. Use a tea infusion of yellow dock as a final rinse. Remember also that toning up the skin with a nutritious diet is absolutely necessary for the pet with a stubborn mite problem.

If there is no improvement, the problem

may not be mites at all. It's just as likely to be an expression of an allergy. Here's how to tell the difference: Ears with mites have a dry, crumbly "coffee ground" discharge seen only (with a light) down in the ear canal; allergy ears exude an oily, waxy, dark brown fluidlike discharge that comes up out of the ear canal and is also seen around the outside of the ear.

ECLAMPSIA

See "Pregnancy, Birth and Care of Newborns."

ECZEMA

See "Skin Problems."

EMERGENCIES

See "Handling Emergencies and Giving First Aid" on page 337.

ENCEPHALITIS

See "Distemper, Chorea and Feline Panleukopenia."

EPILEPSY

Epilepsy has become fairly common in dogs, though it is rather unusual in cats. Often it's difficult to find the cause. In some cases it seems to be an inherited tendency, probably tied to intensive inbreeding. I think the biggest factor, however, stems from yearly vaccinations. I have seen many dogs that first developed epilepsy within a few weeks after their annual shots. Apparently, it is triggered by allergic encephalitis, an ongoing, low-grade inflammation of the brain caused by a reaction to proteins and organisms in the vaccine. This condition was discovered many years ago and has been well documented in laboratory animals. Some have even pointed to it as a significant cause of human behavior and learning problems. Fortunately, now that we know that annual vaccinations are not necessary, it will be easier to avoid this possible cause (see "Vaccinations").

In general, the health of the nervous system and brain is influenced by heredity, nutrition during the mother's pregnancy, lifelong nutrition and any toxic or irritating substances that reach the brain. Also, certain brain diseases (for example, distemper) or a severe head injury can result in epilepsy.

For most animals, however, it's hard to point to an obvious cause. The convulsions may start without warning and continue with increasing frequency. An epileptic animal may be either young or old at the time of the first attack. The diagnosis of epilepsy is usually made only after other possibilities—like worms, hypoglycemia (low blood sugar), tumors and poisons—have been eliminated. Thus, it is a sort of diagnosis by default, and the epilepsy may actually be caused by a mixed bag of things.

TREATMENT

My own approach is to use a natural diet to promote nutrition for the brain tissues, to detoxify or eliminate possible toxins in the environment and to use homeopathic remedies to control the seizures.

Nutrition should be geared toward preventing the intake of substances that may irritate the brain tissue. Work with hyperactive children indicated that food additives, for instance, may affect the brain this way. Thus I recommend that you put your animal on a strict regimen that excludes all commercial foods, snacks or foods containing additives or coloring agents. Use the basic diet described in chapters 3 and 4, with certain modifications.

- ◆ Limit organ meats (especially liver and kidney) to once a week or less. They are more likely to be contaminated by pesticides, antibiotics, heavy metals and hormonal substances.
- ◆ Consider a vegetarian diet for a dog (or using low-meat recipes for cats, as in chapter 5). Many human epileptics are significantly helped by avoiding meat, and it may help pets as well. Give it a trial of at least three months to see if it helps.
- ◆ Use special supplements. Since the B vitamins are very important to nerve tissue, use a natural, *complete* B complex in the 10- to 50-milligram level, depending on your pet's size. Niacin or niacinamide should be a minimum of 5 to 25 milligrams. Also supplement with ¼ to 2 teaspoons of lecithin and 10 to 30 milligrams of zinc (the chelated form is best). Give about 250 to 1,000 milligrams of vitamin C daily to assist detoxification. Again, use the level best suited to your pet's size.

Protect your animal's environment. Avoid exposing your epileptic pet to cigarette smoke, car exhaust (rides in the back of pickup trucks are particularly harmful), chemicals (especially flea sprays, dips and collars, which affect the nervous system) and excessive stress or exertion (but moderate regular exercise is beneficial). Don't let your animal lie right near an operating color TV or close to an operating microwave oven.

Use treatments that strengthen the nervous system. See the herbs suggested under "Behavior Problems," giving special attention to common oat, blue vervain and skullcap.

As an alternative to herbal treatment, there are certain homeopathic remedies that are often quite useful in this condition.

Homeopathic—*Thuya occidentalis 30C (arborvitae):* Use "Homeopathic Schedule 4," page 348. Start with this treatment, observe for a month and if the problem is no better, go to the next remedy (if the animal is better, do not give further remedy but continue with the nutrition and other supportive methods discussed above).

Homeopathic—*Silicea 30C (silicon dioxide):* Use "Homeopathic Schedule 4," page 348. Wait another month to observe. If there is improvement, further treatment will not be needed. If there is no improvement, you will need to consult with a veterinarian who practices alternative medicine.

Homeopathic—*Arnica montana 30C (mountain daisy):* Use "Homeopathic Schedule 5," page 349. This remedy is indicated for the animal that has developed seizures after a head injury. It is an alternative to the two remedies just discussed and is appropriate only if you know that the cause of the problem is an injury (also see Tissue Salt, Natrum sulphuricum, below).

If the above remedies have no effect, then try one of the following, whichever seems best suited.

Tissue Salt—*Kali phosphoricum 6X (potassium phosphate):* Consider it where there are other nervous disturbances, like insomnia, irritability or excessive nervousness. Very strengthening to the nervous system. Use "Homeopathic Schedule 6(a)," page 349.

Tissue Salt—*Ferrum phosphoricum 6X (iron phosphate):* Best for the type of seizures accompanied by head congestion (that is, the head feels hot and the whites of the eyes look bloodshot). Use "Homeopathic Schedule 6(a)," page 349.

Tissue Salt—*Natrum sulphuricum 6X (sodium sulphate):* Use if the epilepsy began after an injury to the head (also see use of Arnica, above). Use "Homeopathic Schedule 6(a)," page 349.

Tissue Salt—*Silicea 6X (silicon dioxide):* Indicated for an attack that occurs during sleep or at night. Use "Homeopathic Schedule 6(a)," page 349.

EYE PROBLEMS

Five major problems can affect animals' eyes: cataracts, corneal ulcers, injuries, inflammation (infection) and ingrowing eyelids (called entropion). We will consider each of these in turn.

Cataracts

This condition is just like what happens with people. The round, clear lens in the interior of the eye (behind the pupil) which transmits and focuses light becomes cloudy or white (milky). Sometimes this happens as a result of injury to the eye. This condition, however, is also a frequent accompaniment of chronic disease and immune disorders in dogs. Many of the dogs with chronic skin allergies, hip dysplasia and ear problems will develop this as they get older. Cataracts are also more common in animals that have diabetes mellitus, even with insulin treatment.

Veterinarians sometimes remove the lens surgically, and this may help. Unless the underlying condition is satisfactorily addressed, however, the eye is never really healthy. Prevention, by treatment of the chronic illness, is really the only effective method.

TREATMENT

See "Allergies" and "Skin Problems" for treatment suggestions, even though these do not deal directly with the eyes. You must take the approach of healing from the inside out. If the cataract is the result of an injury of the eyes, however, use this treatment.

Homeopathic—*Conium maculatum 6X (poison hemlock):* Use "Homeopathic Schedule 6(a)," page 349.

There are other remedies that can be used for eye problems that are the result of injury. If this one is not effective, contact a homeopathic veterinarian.

Corneal Ulcers

Ulcers of the cornea are usually the result of an injury such as a cat scratch. When the surface of the eye is broken, it hurts and tears will form. The injury itself can be so small you can't even see it unless a light is cast upon it from the side or a special dye is used. Bacteria may infect the scratch, but in the healthy animal a rapid, uncomplicated recovery is common.

TREATMENT

If the injury is deep or there is debris or a splinter stuck there, it will need careful professional treatment under anesthesia. Superficial injuries do not bleed. If you see blood, suspect penetration into and damage of delicate internal structures. This kind of injury can be very serious. The following recommendations are for treating slight irritations, shallow ulcers or noninfected scratches only.

Nutritional—*Cod-liver oil:* Add ¼ to 1 teaspoon, depending on size, of cod-liver oil to the diet. Also add vitamin E to the diet, 100 to 400 IU daily depending on size.

Every 4 hours apply a drop of cod-liver oil directly onto the eye or into the lower lid. The oil has protective functions, and the vitamin A in it will stimulate healing. Or, instead of dropping the oil into the eye, you can use an infusion of the herb eyebright.

Herbal—*Eyebright (Euphrasia officinalis):* Use the extract (which is available as either tincture or glycerin), 5 drops to 1 cup pure water. To this mixture also add ¼ teaspoon of sea salt. Mix well and store at room temperature. Put 2 to 3 drops in the affected eye 3 times a day to stimulate healing.

An immediately useful homeopathic treatment for the pain and inflammation is:

Homeopathic—*Aconitum napellus 30C (monkshood):* Use "Homeopathic Schedule 4," page 348.

Injuries

Other eye injuries include scratches, abrasions and bruising of the eyeball. If this is the problem, use one of these homeopathic treatments.

Homeopathic—*Euphrasia officinalis 30C (eyebright):* Use "Homeopathic Schedule 2," page 348. This is especially useful for scratches and abrasions of areas other than the cornea (see "Corneal Ulcers," above).

Homeopathic—*Symphytum 30C (comfrey):* Use "Homeopathic Schedule 2," page 348. This remedy is indicated for blows or contusions of the eyeball (for example, from being hit by a rock, a car or a club).

Inflammation

This is often part of a viral or bacterial infection. Use the eye cleansing treatment methods discussed in chapter 15 (with saline washes).

Ingrowing Eyelids (Entropion)

In this condition the lids turn in and press the eyelashes against the corneal surface. The constant rubbing of the hairs causes a large (sometimes white), long-lasting ulcer to appear. This problem is not as easy to see as you might suppose. Gently pull the lids away from the eye and let them fall back. Repeat several times. If the animal has ingrowing eyelids, you should be able to see the cuffing in of the lids as they are released. Some dogs are born with this condition, so you can see it when they are quite young. Others develop it after a long period of low-grade conjunctivitis (inner eyelid inflammation). The repeated inflammation and contraction cause the lids to turn in. Ingrowing eyelids are more common in dogs than cats.

TREATMENT

The usual correction is surgery, which is quite easy to perform and usually successful. I have also had very good results in young animals with this condition using:

Homeopathic—*Calcarea carbonica 30C (calcium carbonate):* Use "Homeopathic

Schedule 5," page 349. If after a couple of weeks there is no change, then surgery is indicated. It will help, temporarily, to put a drop of almond oil in the affected eye 3 times a day.

Of course, if the underlying cause is chronic inflammation, then you must deal with that. A helpful treatment is:

Herbal—*Goldenseal (Hydrastis canadensis):* Use the extract (tincture or glycerin) and add 5 drops to 1 cup of pure water. To this mixture also add ¼ teaspoon of sea salt. Mix well and store at room temperature. Put 2 to 3 drops in the affected eye 3 times a day to stimulate healing.

If the lids have become hardened through scarring, use:

Tissue Salt—*Silicea 6X (silicon dioxide):* Use "Homeopathic Schedule 6(a)," page 349.

FELINE IMMUNODEFICIENCY VIRUS (FIV)

This recently recognized disease of cats is also called Feline AIDS because it causes a depression of the immune system just like AIDS (acquired immunodeficiency syndrome) in human beings. The virus is in the same family as human HIV (retroviruses), but fortunately it's different enough that it doesn't affect people. Since its discovery in a California cattery in 1986, the virus has been found in every part of the United States and in other countries as well.

The incidence of infection is surprisingly high—14 percent of sick cats brought to veterinarians in the United States are positive for the virus; 44 percent is the rate among sick cats in Japan. As far as is known, FIV is spread only through bite wounds—from fighting—not from close physical or sexual contact. So it is not surprising that the disease is more common in unneutered males and in cats that roam outdoors. Reports indicate a wide range of ages affected—from two months to 18 years.

If the virus is not resisted, the disease is very serious, usually causing lifelong chronic illness with a wide range of symptoms. Typically, four to six weeks after becoming infected from a bite, the cat develops fever and swollen lymph glands (for example, those under the jaw) along with suppressive effects on the immune system. Often this will clear up, and the cat can seem normal for months or years, until there is too much stress or some other factor which depresses the immune system. Then the disease is reactivated and the chronic phase begins—a process that ends in death six months to three years later (without alternative treatment).

It is difficult to fully describe all the different ways in which symptoms can manifest. This is because a major effect of the virus is to depress the immune response, and, as is the case with human AIDS, many other infections get established and persist—infections that ordinarily would be brief and insignificant. For example, colds can lead to permanent upper respiratory symptoms with runny eyes and a plugged up nose (or discharge).

A common symptom is an inflamed mouth with periodontal disease and loose teeth. However, examples of other problems include: blood disorders, anemia, bacterial infections, skin eruptions and infection, persistent mange (skin parasites), chronic diarrhea (and wasting away), inflammation of the interior of the eye, fevers, lymph gland enlargements, chronic abscesses, recurrent urinary tract infections (cystitis) and loss of appetite and weight. In addition, there can be other persistent infections, like fungal diseases or toxoplasmosis (see "Toxoplasmosis"). One of the most alarming expressions of the disease affects the brain. Cats will act demented, have convulsions or attack people or other animals.

Prevention

Prevention is the most important way to approach this disease because, once established, it is very difficult to eliminate. If you can keep your cat healthy by using a raw, fresh diet—along with the rest of the general program in this book—its chance of resisting the disease is very high. Of course, preventing your cat from roaming and fighting significantly reduces the chance of infection.

Another important point is that any cat suspected of having FIV (or feline leukemia or other chronic viruses) should never be vaccinated. That's because the vaccine viruses stress the body (possibly triggering the latent state) and depress the immune system in many cats (again allowing the virus to get started). The principle is to avoid anything that will disturb or weaken the immune system. I know this advice runs counter to that of many veterinarians who encourage vaccination as a way to protect a weakened cat. My clinical experience and background in immunology, however, convince me that this is the worst thing to do.

Treatment

It is possible to greatly help cats with this problem. Success depends on how much damage has already occurred and the age of the cat. Some will need treatment the rest of their lives and never regain their health. Others, younger and less advanced in the disease, may recover—at least in the sense that the disease goes into remission.

Because of the tremendous variability of symptoms, I will not give specific treatments here. You can apply the different treatments described in other parts of this Quick Reference section as appropriate to the symptoms your cat has. It will be best, however, if you can work with an alternative veterinarian.

Feline Infectious Peritonitis (FIP)

This serious infection can be fatal for almost all cats that develop symptoms. It seems to come on after something depresses the immune system. For example, I have seen many cases occur within a few weeks of the cat receiving a vaccine against feline leukemia—probably from a temporary immunosuppressive action of the vaccine (an effect known to occur with several vaccines). It is not that the vaccine causes the disease directly, but rather that the cat was already carrying the FIP virus and the vaccine gave it an opportunity.

FIP is caused by a coronavirus, a group of viruses that also cause disease in pigs, dogs and humans. As far as is known, however, the FIP virus does not spread to humans or other animals.

It is thought that cats become infected through the mouth and throat, the upper respiratory tract or, perhaps, the intestinal tract. People often don't realize when their cats begin to get FIP because they may show no particular symptoms or may run just a mild fever and seem like they're not feeling well for a few days. During this period (one to ten days after initial infection) the virus can be shed from the throat, lungs, stomach and intestines and spread to other cats. After this the virus incubates anywhere from a few weeks to several years before symptoms appear.

Once symptoms appear and the disease progresses, the cat gradually loses its appetite (and weight), develops a persistent fever and becomes depressed (inactive, subdued). Meanwhile, the virus spreads throughout the body tissues, especially affecting blood vessels. It is interesting to note that by this time (when symptoms are so evident) the cat is no longer shedding the virus and is not contagious.

This points up one of the real problems in control. When the cat is the most contagious, you don't realize anything is wrong; but once there are symptoms it does no good to isolate the cat. It does help to know, however, that the virus can persist in the environment (soiled floors, food or water bowls) for a long time—up to three weeks in home conditions. So sanitation can be very helpful in limiting the spread of disease from one cat to another. It is no surprise that this disease primarily impacts multiple-cat households or catteries.

The most common symptoms are fever, loss of appetite, weight loss, rough hair coat and, possibly, accumulation of fluid in the chest or abdomen. Early symptoms can also resemble a common cold, with sneezing and watery discharges from the eyes and nose. (Some of the very chronic upper respiratory problems in multiple-cat households can be caused by this virus.) In other cats the first symptoms may involve the gastrointestinal tract (vomiting, diarrhea); this is a serious form that can rapidly become fatal.

FIP can also affect the eyes, causing one pupil to be larger than the other or causing fluid or blood to accumulate in the eyeball. Like the other serious cat virus diseases in this section, FIP can sometimes affect the brain or interfere with reproduction.

PREVENTION

See the prevention advice for Feline Immunodeficiency Virus (FIV), above.

Unfortunately, the diagnostic test to see if a cat is carrying the virus is extremely inaccurate. There are too many other related viruses that are mild and insignificant that will give false positives on the test, indicating a problem where there is none. Many veterinarians no longer even test for this virus.

TREATMENT

Since FIP takes many forms, I can give only some general guidelines for its most common manifestations. The more severe forms require very careful and persistent treatment under the guidance of a veterinarian. I strongly suggest not using antibiotics or corticosteroids, however, as these drugs do not help at all and only further weaken the cat.

As severe as the disease can be, I have had very satisfying results in the majority of cases I have treated with homeopathy and nutrition. Inevitably, I will be asked if the cat is completely cured and free of the virus. Clinically, and by their appearance, many cats can become normal. As there is no way to be sure that the body is free of the virus (by testing or other means), however, this aspect of the question cannot be answered. But most people are satisfied when their cat begins to act normally and look well.

Here are some guidelines for treatment.

◆ In the early stages of FIP (which are characterized by fever and loss of appetite), try the treatments for feline leukemia (below).

◆ If the symptoms are primarily of a cold, that is, if there are primarily upper respiratory symptoms, then refer to the section "Upper Respiratory Infections."

◆ In the intestinal form with vomiting and diarrhea, use the treatments under the corresponding sections.

◆ If your cat has the very unfortunate form of FIP with accumulation of fluid in the chest and abdomen (hydrothorax or pleural effusion in the chest, ascites in the abdomen), the following treatments may help. However, this form is usually eventually fatal.

Homeopathic—*Arsenicum album* 6C: Indicated for the anxious, chilly, thirsty and restless cat. Use "Homeopathic Schedule 6(a)," page 349.

Homeopathic—*Mercurius sulphuricus* 6C: Tremendous difficulty with breathing. The cat has to sit up all the time because of the fluid in the chest. Use "Homeopathic Schedule 6(a)," page 349.

Both of these remedies have their place in treatment. Try one and if it doesn't help after a few days, try the other.

FELINE LEUKEMIA (FeLV)

This serious disease of cats is caused by a retrovirus similar to the ones that cause Feline Immunodeficiency Disease (see above) or human AIDS. About 21 percent of sick cats that are brought to veterinarians are ill from feline leukemia, which is the greatest killer of cats after accidents. FeLV occurs mostly in cats aged one to five years. It affects males and females equally, but occurs more often in neutered animals (no one knows why).

The virus is spread from one cat to another through body fluids (saliva, urine, blood, feces). For the same reason, mother cats can give it to their young during pregnancy or nursing. Fortunately, it takes close or prolonged contact between cats for the virus to spread. Most contagion occurs from bites, grooming or sharing water and food bowls. It is not transmitted through the air or via human handlers.

Actually, about 70 percent of all cats are exposed to FeLV, and nearly all of them recover spontaneously—most showing little or no illness. Those that are weak, however, are affected more severely. The incidence of serious illness is also much higher in multi-cat households.

There are several types of feline leukemia virus, and they cause slightly different symptoms. The most common signs of illness, especially early on, however, are weight loss, fever and dehydration (lack of water in the tissues). Other possible symptoms include anemia, immune suppression (like FIV, see above), bleeding disorders, kidney inflammation (and deterioration), arthritis, ulcers forming at body openings (mouth, anus, vagina, eyes), immune diseases like inflammatory bowel disease or eosinophilic granuloma complex and persistent bladder inflammation (cystitis).

Other peculiar, less common symptoms

are skin growths (like "horns"), deposits of cartilage, skin disease (with oily coats) and nerve damage (paralysis, urinary incontinence). With some cats an odd symptom is that one pupil is smaller or larger than the other.

Many affected cats cannot reproduce properly, having spontaneous abortions, stillbirths or what is known as fading kittens, kittens that waste away in spite of the best care.

As if this were not enough, many affected cats develop tumors or cancer. It is estimated that 30 percent of all cat tumors are a result of this virus.

Infection with FeLV goes through six recognized stages.

- Stage 1—Infection of the mouth tissues. (The disease stops here in healthy cats.)
- Stage 2—The virus is spread from the mouth by certain blood cells.
- Stage 3—The virus infects lymph glands (such as the tonsils and glands under the throat or in other parts of the body—like when we get colds). Even if it reaches this point, most cats can still block the infection from going further.
- Stage 4—Infection of the bone marrow. Once infection is established here, the cat will be infected the rest of its life (though the disease may still be controllable with proper treatment).
- Stage 5—The infection spreads again into the blood, through circulating cells.
- Stage 6—Various tissues in the body are persistently infected, especially the tear glands, salivary glands and urinary bladder. These cats are now shedding the virus and are infectious to other cats.

PREVENTION

Follow the same preventive guidelines given above for Feline Immunodeficiency Virus (FIV).

TREATMENT

Nutrition: This is a serious illness with many possible forms of expression, which means that complete guidelines for treatment could fill a whole book. Since the symptoms usually include loss of appetite, nutritional treatment is very difficult. You *can* force-feed your cat, however. It's not pleasant, but it can be life-saving in a crisis (see "Appetite Problems" for guidelines). If your cat is still eating, then it is essential that you feed a raw-meat, home-prepared diet. I realize that your cat may not accept such a diet, so you will have to do what is possible. But this is the very best.

Vitamin C can be very helpful to cats with this disease; give 250 milligrams twice a day. Often sodium ascorbate, the salt form of vitamin C (ascorbic acid), is best tolerated. Add the powder to food or, if necessary, dissolve it in water or broth and give it with a syringe. Pureed raw liver is often accepted by these cats and provides some very useful nutrition. Give several tablespoons a day if possible.

Other useful treatments include:

Homeopathic—*Nux vomica 30C (poison nut):* Use "Homeopathic Schedule 3," page 348. This is especially indicated for the cat that becomes irritable and withdraws to a quiet part of the house or apartment.

Homeopathic—*Pulsatilla 6C:* Use "Homeopathic Schedule 6(a)," page 349. Most useful for the cat that becomes "clingy," wanting a lot of attention and to be held. She will act sleepy and sluggish and perhaps vomit easily if the food is too rich. There may be a tendency to lie in the bathtub or other cool places.

Homeopathic—*Phosphorus 30C (phosphorus):* Use "Homeopathic Schedule 3," page 348. This remedy is indicated for the cat that is extremely lethargic, like a wet washrag, or vomits about 10 to 20 minutes after drinking water (but not after eating food).

Homeopathic —*Sepia 6C (cuttlefish ink):* This suits the cat with very red or inflamed gums. Sometimes there will be a red line along the border of the teeth with the rest of the mouth looking fairly good. Use "Homeopathic Schedule 6(a)," page 349.

Homeopathic—*Nitricum acidum 30C (nitric acid, aqua fortis):* Like the remedy above (Sepia), this medicine is a good choice for a cat with a very painful, inflamed mouth. If she is also very irritable or angry when ill, then this medicine may be especially helpful. It is also suitable for lesions on the lips, anus or eyelids. (The lesions look like ulcers or painful, raw areas.) Use "Homeopathic Schedule 4," page 348.

Tissue Salt—*Ferrum phosphoricum 6X (iron phosphate):* Use "Homeopathic Schedule 1," page 348. Most helpful for those cats with fever and not many other symptoms.

There are many other remedies that can be used. Consult an alternative veterinarian. (See "Holistic Veterinary Training and Organizations," beginning on page 355, for references.)

FELINE PANLEUKOPENIA

See "Distemper, Chorea and Feline Panleukopenia."

FELINE UROLOGIC SYNDROME

See "Bladder Problems."

FLEAS

See "Skin Parasites."

FOXTAILS

See also "Ear Problems."

The number-one enemy of dogs and cats could well be the numerous foxtails, plant awns and wild oat seeds that get caught in the hair and crevices of their bodies. Because of the way these stickers are constructed, they will not easily dislodge. Instead, they tend to migrate through the skin or into body openings (eyes, ears, nose, mouth, anus, vagina, sheath) where they cause tremendous problems. If a foxtail works through the skin, the body cannot digest it; even years later it will look fresh on removal.

Thus, although the body makes every effort to eliminate the sticker, it clings tenaciously to the tissue. The result is a constantly inflamed tract that drains pus and never heals completely. The plant material can migrate a foot or more into the body, making it difficult, if not impossible, to find. Toes are a favorite lodging place, as are the ears (see "Ear Problems") and eyes, where they can get behind the "third eyelid" and cause a lot of irritation.

PREVENTION

Always check over your animal after it has run in fields, vacant lots or other weedy places. Check all the body openings, and run a comb or brush through the hair. Be sure to check between the toes, too. If you clip the hair between the toes during foxtail season, your job will be much easier and your animal's life much more comfortable. Also, have the hair coat trimmed to a short length, an inch or less, and trim away any hair growing around the ear hole or inside the ear flap. Stickers are much likelier to get into the ears of dogs with hanging ears. See "Ear Problems" for treating foxtails in the ears. Also, see "Abscesses."

TREATMENT

If your animal already has a foxtail under the skin with chronic discharge from a small opening, and your veterinarian is not able to find and remove it, the following treatment may help as a last resort, only if surgery fails.

Tissue Salt—*Silicea 6C (silicon dioxide):* Use "Homeopathic Schedule 6(a)," page 349. If the sticker does not work its way out, your veterinarian must keep trying to remove it surgically. Remember, in the case of foxtails an ounce of prevention is worth *at least* a pound of cure.

HAIR LOSS

See also "Skin Problems."

Hair loss is often the result of skin allergies and excessive licking and chewing. Sometimes, however, the hair falls out without any sign of skin irritation. This can signal inadequate protein intake, as in cats that eat poorly. It can also indicate an inadequate diet.

There are two remedies that are especially useful for simple hair loss unaccompanied by other symptoms.

Homeopathic—*Selenium 30C (selenium):* Use "Homeopathic Schedule 5," page 349. If this treatment is successful, you will see signs of hair growth within a month.

Homeopathic—*Sepia 30C (ink from the cuttlefish):* Use "Homeopathic Schedule 5," page 349. This remedy suits a female that loses hair after giving birth and nursing the young. This is not necessarily a nutritional problem; it's more likely a hormonal imbalance, which can be corrected by this remedy.

HEART PROBLEMS

Disorders of the heart are relatively common in aging pets, both dogs and cats. They do not have atherosclerosis and the type of heart attacks that afflict humans, however. Rather, the problem is usually a weak heart muscle with enlargement of one or both sides of the heart. Sometimes there is inadequate heart valve action or a rhythm that is too quick or too slow.

Typical signs of a heart problem include one or more of the following: becoming easily tired by exercise, bluish discoloration of the tongue and gums upon exercise, sudden collapse or prostration, difficult breathing or wheezing, a persistent dry cough that produces little expectoration, and an accumulation of fluid in the legs or abdomen (a potbellied look).

TREATMENT

Conventional veterinary treatment includes the use of digitalis, a diuretic and a low-sodium diet. The assumption is that the condition is progressive, and so treatment aims to control symptoms rather than to cure.

I prefer an alternative approach emphasizing nutrition and homeopathic, herbal or mineral remedies. Though complete recovery may not be possible, these measures do more than just counteract symptoms; they can actually strengthen the affected tissues. Of course, the chance of help from any treatment depends upon the degree of tissue damage and the age of the animal.

The best route of all is prevention, in the form of a healthy lifestyle with nutritious food and regular exercise. If symptoms have already developed, however, here is what I suggest.

Nutrition should emphasize the basic natural foods diet (chapters 3 and 4). Feed the meat raw, rather than cooked, for its superior nutrition. Do not add any salt, soy sauce, bacon or other salty foods or flavorings to the food. Use spring water or other water that is nonchlorinated and unfluoridated. If the animal is overweight, slim it down with the diet under "Weight Problems." Weight reduction is important because more heart energy is required to push blood through all that fat.

Supplement with a complete B-complex tablet with all the B vitamins, but especially niacin and pyridoxine. Major components should be at the 10-, 25- or 50-milligram level (depending on size). It's also helpful to give a trace mineral supplement containing chromium and selenium (scale the recommended human dose on the label to your animal's size) and chelated zinc (5, 10 or 20 milligrams daily, depending on size).

Other important measures are regular, daily exercise that is not too strenuous or exciting (a walk is ideal) and the avoidance of cigarette smoke. In the sensitive animal, many of the symptoms of heart disease can be caused by exposure to secondary cigarette smoke—including irregular pulse, pain in the heart region, difficult breathing, cough, dizziness and prostration.

Specific remedies may be helpful. Where the condition is not too severe, try the following:

Tissue Salt—*Calcarea fluorica 6X (calcium fluoride):* Helps to restore strength to the heart muscle, especially when it is dilated and the action is weak. Use "Homeopathic Schedule 6(a)," page 349.

Tissue Salt—*Kali phosphoricum 6X (potassium phosphate):* Suited for the problem that seems more functional (rather than the result of tissue changes or pathology). That is, such things as nervousness and physical or emotional excitement seem to lead to symptoms. Use "Homeopathic Schedule 6(a)," page 349.

For more severe or persistent symptoms that are not controlled by nutrition and other measures (above), pick one of the following treatments, whichever seems best indicated. (Don't skip the other measures and expect good results, however!)

Homeopathic—*Crataegus oxycantha 3X (hawthorn berries):* Indicated for the animal with a dilated heart, weak heart muscle, difficult breathing, fluid retention and (often) a nervous or irritable temperament. Use "Homeopathic Schedule 6(a)," page 349.

Homeopathic—*Strophanthus hispidus 3X (Kombe seed):* For the weak heart with valvular problems. The pulse is weak, frequent and irregular, and breathing is difficult. There may also be fluid retention, loss of appetite and vomiting. Obesity and chronic itching of the skin also point to this medicine. Use "Homeopathic Schedule 6(a)," page 349.

Homeopathic—*Digitalis purpurea 6X (foxglove):* Give one tablet of the 6X potency after an attack in which the animal collapses or even faints after exertion, with the tongue turning blue. Often the pulse or heart rate is abnormally slow. There may be heart dilation and fluid retention. Liver disturbances may be evidenced by a white, pasty stool. If you give a tablet after each attack, the attacks will become less frequent (if treatment is helping).

Homeopathic—*Spongia tosta 6X (roasted sponge):* For the animal whose crises are characterized by a rapid pulse, difficult breathing and fearfulness. It may have difficulty lying down and may breathe easier sitting up. A dry, persistent cough is an indication for this medicine. Use "Homeopathic Schedule 6(a)," page 349.

General directions for the homeopathic remedies are to use the medicine that seems best suited to the situation. If it helps for a while, use it as long as it does. If it stops helping or the symptoms change, then re-evaluate and use another of the medicines listed. Many animals with this problem need ongoing treatment, especially if they are quite old. Some will gradually get better, however, and you will be able to discontinue treatment.

HEARTWORMS

The heartworm parasite actually lives in the heart of a dog, where it can grow as long as 11 inches, and, in a minority of infestations, cause persistent coughing, difficult breathing, weakness, fainting and sometimes even heart failure. Adult heartworms produce young ones (called microfilaria) which circulate through the dog's bloodstream in greatest numbers when hungry mosquitoes are most likely to come a-biting (especially summer evenings). When a mosquito bites the dog, it can ingest these microfilaria and later infect another dog.

When a mosquito carries them to a new dog, the microfilaria go through two more developmental stages under the skin, after which they enter the bloodstream via nearby veins. After reaching the heart they settle into their new home, where they mature and reproduce their own babies, renewing the cycle about six months after the original mosquito bite.

A heartworm diagnosis is made when a veterinarian finds microfilaria in the blood, but not necessarily any symptoms of illness. Just a few worms are insignificant and may not require treatment. Only a small percentage of dogs in an area may be noticeably sick from heartworm, which usually requires infestation with a considerable number of worms.

Once a dog does show clinical symptoms, treatment can be very involved and almost always requires hospitalization. The drugs used in treatment are very toxic and hard on the animal. Thus, the preferred route is prevention, for which veterinarians prescribe drugs like Diethylcarbamazine to inhibit the microfilaria while they are growing just under the skin. Most doctors recommend daily doses, starting several weeks before mosquito season and continuing until two months after its close. In some areas this means all year. The other major preventive drug, Ivermectin, is given once a month, killing all the baby worms that have accumulated during that month.

Though these preventive drugs are widely used, it does not mean that they are without problems. Side effects for diethylcarbamazine include headache, general malaise, weakness, joint pains, loss of appetite, nausea, vomiting and an eruption on the scrotum. Many of these symptoms are subjective, making them hard to detect in animals and easy to overlook.

Ivermectin can lead to even more side effects: vomiting, diarrhea, seizures, paralysis, jaundice and other liver problems, coughing, nose bleeds, high fevers, weakness, dizziness, nerve damage, bleeding disorders, loss of appetite, breathing difficulty, pneumonia, depression, lethargy, sudden aggressive behavior, skin eruptions, tremors and sudden death. Though a minority of dogs experience these reactions, they are seen in many breeds. Veterinarians also report that many dogs get stomach and intestinal upsets, irritability, stiffness and seem to just feel "rotten" for the first one or two weeks after each monthly dose of heartworm protection. An American Veterinary Medical Association report on adverse drug reactions showed that 65 percent of all drug reactions reported and 48 percent of all reported deaths caused by drug reactions were from heartworm preventive medicine.

I am reluctant, however, to tell people to stop the use of heartworm preventives, particularly in highly infested areas, partly because I cannot guarantee that their dogs will not get heartworm. However, I dislike the use of these drugs, and I think they cause much more illness than we realize.

What other choice do we have? Unfortunately, almost all heartworm research is directed toward finding new drugs to kill the microfilaria. Very little attention goes to enhancing the dog's natural resistance to the parasite. However, we do know several things which make that a promising direction to pursue: One is that wild animals are quite resistant to the parasite. That is, they get very light infestations and then become immune. Another factor is that an estimated 25 to 50 percent of dogs in high-heartworm areas become immune to the microfilaria after being infested and cannot pass heartworms to other dogs. Finally, after being infested by a few heartworms, most dogs do not get more of them even though they are continually bitten by mosquitoes carrying the parasite. In other words, they are able to limit the extent of infestation.

All this points to the importance of the *health and resistance mounted by the dog itself*. That takes us back to the central thesis of this book: If we care for our pets so as to maximize their health, their resistance to parasites (and disease) will be much higher. Isn't this a much more attractive way to go than to continually poison them with drugs? Clearly, we need serious research in this direction.

Another overlooked factor arises when we ask why there has been such an extensive spread of heartworm in dogs all over the United States in the last 30 years. I agree with the authorities who say that the incidence of heartworm increases whenever we upset the natural balance in a way that increases the mosquito population. For example, this happens when we expand irrigation acreage in farming areas.

Wild animals like coyotes, however, thrive in the very same conditions, even without preventive drugs. The major difference is lifestyle—fresh raw foods, plenty of exercise, no drugs and no toxic flea products.

So it is likely the combination of environmental upset coupled with a deteriorating level of health through several dozen generations of dogs fed on commercial foods and poisoned with drugs and insecticides that has created this unnatural explosion of parasitism. It is particularly frustrating that recent research shows the incidence of heartworm infestation in dogs in any particular geographic area is the same now as it was in 1982 even after all these years of preventive treatment. It doesn't take too much contemplation to realize that the path of continued drug use is a dead-end road.

Some veterinarians who practice holistic medicine, myself included, have been experimenting with a homeopathic preventive made from microfilaria-infected blood, called a heartworm nosode. Though we have only been able to do small clinical studies, early results are very encouraging. This may eventually provide a true alternative to drug use. Much more research is needed, however, to decide this question.

PREVENTION

For those committed to a natural, non-chemical approach, here are some suggestions to help prevent heartworm. Use a completely natural (preferably organic) raw food diet fortified with raw garlic and liberal amounts of yeast. These foods may help to repel mosquitoes from the skin in some animals. To further minimize exposure to mosquitoes, you can keep your dog indoors in the evenings and night. Use a natural insect repellent when she does go outside: Rub one drop of eucalyptus oil, diluted in one cup of warm water, over the muzzle and the area between the anus and genitals (favorite mosquito-biting areas). Be careful to avoid rubbing the oil on the sensitive tissues of the eyes and mucous membranes.

TREATMENT

Remember that the presence of one or two heartworms is not serious in itself. But the dog who has a large number of worms and has also developed heart problems is in trouble. The treatment of such a condition requires experienced supervision because the dog could undergo heart failure or embolisms (internal blood clots). So follow your veterinarian's treatment program. If you can, find one who uses herbal treatment, acupuncture or homeopathic medicine (see "Holistic Veterinary Training and Organizations" on page 355 for referral sources). In addition, use the diet under "Heart Problems."

I do not like the conventional treatment for this condition because strong poisons such as arsenic compounds are injected intravenously, and sometimes the treatment is worse than the disease. I have treated dogs whose health was permanently ruined by these drugs. Fortunately, these are in the minority and most dogs will do well. Still, the whole way of handling the problem is unappealing. But it is difficult to recommend gentler alternatives without supportive scientific data. While I have treated a few dogs ill from heartworms who are too sick or too old to undertake conventional treatment, I do not yet have a body of experience sufficient to establish a true alternative. We hope for this to come.

HEPATITIS

See "Liver Problems."

HIP DYSPLASIA

This term describes a poorly formed hip joint. The veterinary profession generally regards hip dysplasia as a genetic problem complicated by a variety of environmental influences. The cause, however, is not really understood. Unfortunately, it is common among dogs.

Hip dysplasia is not present at birth. It develops during puppyhood, as the hip joint forms in a loose or "sloppy" way that allows too much movement of the leg bone in the hip socket. Irritation and scarring occur because the weak ligaments and surrounding joint tissues aren't able to stabilize the joint adequately. In addition, there tends to be a rheumatic tendency—inflammation and pain of the muscles in the legs. Untreated, gradual loss of function will result. Some older dogs actually lose use of their rear legs.

PREVENTION AND TREATMENT

Orthodox treatment centers on a number of surgical procedures that involve cutting certain muscles, repositioning the joint, removing the head of the leg bone or completely replacing the hip joint with an artificial device. But there are other avenues of greater promise.

Prevention is the best place to start. Generations of poor feeding practices have contributed greatly to the development of hip dysplasia, the effects magnifying with each generation. If possible, you should avoid selecting an affected dog in the first place (see chapter 9). Apart from that, good prevention means feeding the pregnant female or newly acquired puppy a wholesome, fresh, well-supplemented diet as outlined in this book (see chapter 5). Be sure to include plenty of bonemeal. Don't succumb to the fallacy that too much calcium in the diet causes this problem.

Another foolish idea is that hip dysplasia is caused by dogs growing too fast. Some people actually advocate restricting food or protein to prevent the puppy from developing normally. They think that keeping it small will somehow prevent the problem. It does not.

There is, however, a good preventive: Give lots of vitamin C (ascorbic acid), particularly if either parent had the condition or the pup is of a commonly affected breed, such as a German shepherd or other large purebreds. Indeed, there is some good evidence that hip dysplasia is in part caused by chronic subclinical scurvy (a lack of adequate vitamin C). In this view, the hip forms incorrectly as a result of weak ligaments and muscles around the joints. Vitamin C is essential to these tissues.

Wendell Belfield, D.V.M. reported in *Veterinary Medicine/Small Animal Clinician* that high amounts of vitamin C provided 100 percent prevention of hip dysplasia in eight litters of German shepherd pups coming from parents that either had the condition themselves or had previously produced offspring with it. He used the following program.

- The pregnant female is given two to four grams of sodium ascorbate crystals in the daily ration (½ to 1 teaspoon of the pure powder; ascorbic acid could also be used).
- At birth the puppies are given 50 to 100 milligrams of vitamin C orally each day (using a liquid form).
- At three weeks of age, the dose is in-

creased to 500 milligrams daily of sodium ascorbate (given in the feed) until the puppies are four months old.

♦ At four months the dose is increased to one to two grams a day and maintained there until the puppies are 18 months to two years of age.

For older animals that already have the problem, feed our natural diet (see chapters 3 and 4), including ample amounts of vitamin C, 500 milligrams to two grams a day. In arthritic cases see if there is a suitable

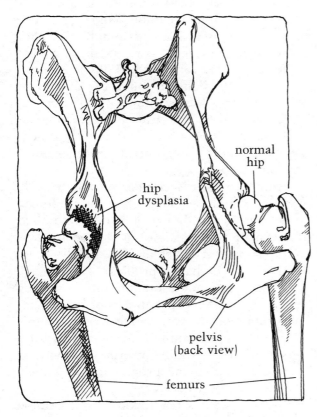

Hip dysplasia is a condition in which the hip's ball-in-socket joint does not form properly. Severe arthritis may result.

normal hip

hip dysplasia

pelvis (back view)

femurs

remedy among those described under "Arthritis." If you have access to acupuncture or chiropractic treatment, you may find your dog will experience marked improvement. See chapter 14 for some interesting case examples.

INFECTIOUS PERITONITIS

See "Feline Infectious Peritonitis."

INJURIES

See "Handling Emergencies and Giving First Aid" on page 337.

INTERVERTEBRAL DISK DISEASE

See "Paralysis."

JAUNDICE

Jaundice, which can be caused by many factors, creates a visible yellowing of the tissues. We usually think of it as a liver disease, but it occurs for other reasons. If there is a rapid breakdown of red blood cells (because of, for instance, blood parasites, certain chemicals or drugs, various infections or poisonous snakebites), the liver can't process all the released hemoglobin quickly enough. The result is a release of yellow pigment (which makes up part of hemoglobin), which backs up and stains the tissues yellow.

Your veterinarian will have to distinguish between jaundice caused by such factors and the type associated with liver disease. If the liver is ailing, the stool often looks pale in color. If the jaundice is from red blood cell breakdown, however, the stool is typically very dark from extra bile flow.

The type of jaundice caused by a sudden loss of intact red blood cells also leads to a form of anemia, even though no blood was lost to the outside. To help the body form new red blood cells, follow the advice under "Anemia." Apart from dealing with any of those underlying causes of red blood cell breakdown, you can treat this type of non-inflammatory jaundice simply by exposing your animal to direct sunlight (or indirect if it's too hot) for several hours daily for a few days. Sunlight stimulates the elimination of the pigments responsible for the jaundice. In addition, it may help to use the remedy *Natrum sulphuricum* as indicated under "Liver Problems" for a few days to stimulate liver function and enhance a return to normal.

KENNEL COUGH

See "Upper Respiratory Infections."

KIDNEY FAILURE

See "Bladder Problems" for a discussion of kidney stones.

Deterioration of the kidneys is a common problem of old age for both dogs and cats. It is the second leading cause of death in cats (after feline leukemia and not counting accidents). Why or how kidney disease starts (often in young or middle age) is not known. It is very difficult even to be aware that it is happening because of the tremendous capac-

ity of the kidneys to compensate for loss of tissue. As long as one-third of the kidney tissue is still all right, there are no obvious signs of sickness. Past this point, however, illness gradually develops—until death comes, when only 15 to 20 percent of the kidney tissue is still functional.

Early signs of kidney problems are increased thirst, frequent urination with large quantities of pale urine, inability to hold urine all night and occasional periods of low energy, lack of appetite and nausea or vomiting that last for a few days at a time.

How much thirst is too much thirst? For dogs, use your common sense and notice any increases not attributable to hot weather or exercise. For cats, drinking water every day (or even less often) is suspicious, even if it's a young cat of two or three years. Because they evolved in dry regions, healthy cats drink little or no water by nature. The only exception to this rule is if your cat is eating only dry food (which I don't recommend). Dry food is so low in water (15 to 20% compared to 80 to 85% of a natural diet) that some cats are forced to drink even though it is not natural to them. If your cat is on a canned food or home-prepared diet and is still drinking, however, you have a problem.

Another indication of future kidney problems is repeated attacks of bladder inflammation (cystitis). Treatment of this condition with antibiotics and the use of a special diet to acidify the urine does nothing to slow down the progression of kidney disease; it only masks the symptoms.

If you are observant, you can detect these signs of kidney failure early. That way you stand a much better chance of prolonging your animal's life with a special diet and other natural treatments than if you wait until an emergency.

TREATMENT

Once a kidney problem appears, the strategy is to avoid further deterioration, if possible, and to assist the function of what is left of the kidneys. We do the former by homeopathic, herbal and nutritional treatment and the latter by reducing or eliminating the toxic load on the kidneys.

Let's consider the question of toxicity first. Anything in the food or in the environment which is not usable by the body must be eliminated. This includes food preservatives, coloring agents, insecticides, pollutants and the like. This elimination is primarily done through the kidneys.

The cleansing function of the kidneys is related to that of the skin, which is another important eliminative organ. Skin irritations and eruptions often precede eventual kidney failure in old age. This process is accelerated if the skin discharge is repeatedly suppressed with corticosteroids.

Early symptoms of kidney disease progress into uremia (blood poisoning) characterized by low energy, frequent vomiting, dehydration, complete loss of appetite, foul breath and, perhaps, an inflammation of the mouth or presence of mouth ulcers. At this point the animal needs an emergency intravenous infusion of large quantities of fluids to save its life. Afterwards, things return to normal, but it's a fragile normality, for in many cases 60 to 70 percent of the kidney tissue has been destroyed and cannot be regained. The kidneys can cope with this for a while by moving everything along faster. The fluids are pushed through much more rapidly (up to 20 times faster), resulting in a loss of essential salts, water and other nutrients. Think of it like this: If a major freeway were blocked and everyone had to drive on surface streets to get around it, one way to keep traffic moving would be for the police to stand at intersections waving everyone on at higher than normal speeds. Imagine them yelling "Let's go! Move it along. We've got to get the job done!" This is what the kidneys do to compensate. Let's see what we can do to help as well.

Nutrition: Our main dietary goal is to reduce the load of metabolic wastes on the kidneys; this waste results from excess protein, phosphorus and sodium. Since most of the waste (urea) results from protein, you must feed a minimal level of protein of maximally usable quality. Also, it is vital to replace water-soluble vitamins that get flushed out of the body easily, especially vitamins B and C, and to supply plenty of vitamin A, which is good for the kidneys.

The following recipes meet these needs. They provide about 24 percent protein for cats and 16 percent protein for dogs; all the protein is of high quality. We use enriched white rice because it is better digested than brown rice and also contains higher levels of iron and major B vitamins, which are hard to supply in a low-meat diet.

Choose a well-assimilated form of calcium, such as calcium lactate, calcium gluconate or chelated calcium. If you can't find one of these, use calcium carbonate or eggshell powder in the recipe (¾ teaspoon for cats, ⅓ teaspoon for dogs). Avoid calcium supplements containing phosphorus.

The pet vitamins insure adequate amounts of essential nutrients which could become low in this diet.

These diets are also low in ash, which

makes them suitable for pets prone to stone formation and urinary obstruction.

Note: It is important to avoid feeding special acid-forming diets to cats with kidney disease. These are the commercial foods formulated to prevent cystitis and are advertised as such. Chemicals have been added to these diets to force the urine to be acid; one side effect is that the body becomes too acid, and kidney function is reduced.

CANINE DIET FOR KIDNEY PROBLEMS

½	cup (¼ pound) regular-fat hamburger
2¾	cups cooked white rice, enriched
1	egg
2	tablespoons cold-pressed safflower, soy or corn oil
	600 milligrams calcium
⅛	teaspoon iodized salt
2	tablespoons parsley, finely grated carrot or other vegetable (optional)
½–1	clove garlic, minced (for flavor)
	Dog vitamins (as recommended on label for medium-size dog)
	20-milligram-level B complex
	5,000 IU vitamin A
	1,000 milligrams vitamin C (¼ teaspoon sodium ascorbate)

Mix all ingredients together and serve raw if the dog will accept it. Otherwise, mix all but the vitamins together, bake about 20 minutes in a moderate oven and then wait until it cools to mix in the vitamins. Occasionally, substitute 1 to 3 teaspoons of liver for part of the meat. Be sure to provide plenty of fresh, pure water (filtered or bottled) at all times.

Yield: Generally, feed as much as your dog will eat, but, as a guideline, this recipe should feed a 10-pound toy for three days or a 40-pound dog for a day. By tripling it you can feed a 60-pound dog for two days. Multiply the recipe as needed for convenience.

Note: If your dog isn't eating well, force-feed vitamins separately, using these daily levels: toys and small dogs—10 milligrams B complex and 250 milligrams vitamin C; medium-size dogs—as indicated in recipe; large and giant dogs—50 milligrams B complex and 2,000 milligrams vitamin C.

FELINE DIET FOR KIDNEY PROBLEMS

1⅓	cups (⅔ pound) ground chicken, turkey or lean heart
4	cups cooked white rice, enriched
4	eggs
2	tablespoons cold-pressed safflower, soy or corn oil
	1,500 milligrams calcium
⅛	teaspoon iodized salt
⅛	teaspoon potassium chloride (optional, for a saltier flavor)
1	teaspoon parsley, finely grated carrot or other vegetable (optional)
	5,000 IU vitamin A
	Taurine and other cat vitamins (about 5 days' worth)
	50-milligram-level B complex (or 10 milligrams per day)
	2,500 milligrams vitamin C (½ teaspoon sodium ascorbate)

Mix everything together in a large bowl. Serve raw if the cat will accept it. Otherwise, mix all but the vitamins together, bake about 20 minutes in a moderate oven and then wait until it cools to mix in the vitamins. Your cat may have a poor appetite, so to some extent you will need to cater to him to keep him alive. Occasionally, substitute 1 to 3 teaspoons of liver for part of the meat. Be sure to provide plenty of fresh, pure water (filtered or bottled) at all times. Also encourage drinking by providing meat or fish broth (warm) once or twice a day.

Yield: Feed as much as your cat will eat. This makes about 5 to 6 days' food for the average cat.

Note: *If your cat isn't eating well, force-feed the vitamins separately. Follow the label directions for the cat vitamins and give 5 to 10 milligrams B complex per day and 250 milligrams vitamin C ($^{1}/_{16}$ teaspoon sodium ascorbate) twice daily.*

Many cats with kidney disease will develop a state of low potassium levels in the body, which further complicates the situation and creates symptoms in its own right. If your cat does not respond adequately to the treatments suggested here (and below), consult your veterinarian about adding a potassium gluconate supplement to this diet.

◆

Other therapeutic measures are to avoid cigarette smoke; chemicalized or chlorinated water (use filtered or bottled); highly processed, overcooked, spoiled or commercial foods; stress; excessive heat and unnecessary exposure to chemical products, car fumes and polluted environments in general.

Vigorously brush the coat and skin regularly and give a weekly bath with a natural, mild, nondrying shampoo. Provide regular, mild outdoor exercise and exposure to fresh air and sun. Always allow easy access to a place for urination and defecation. Make lots of pure water available for drinking at all times and feed the daily rations as two meals instead of one (if that has been your practice).

Herbs and remedies that may strengthen your animal's kidney tissue are listed below. Pick one of them to try.

Herbal—*Alfalfa (Medicago sativa):* Using the tincture, 3 times daily give 1 or 2 drops to cats or small dogs, 2 to 4 drops to medium dogs and 4 to 6 drops to large dogs (see page 226). Continue until you see an improvement, then reduce to once a day or as needed. Alternatively, you may use alfalfa tablets, giving 1 to 4 twice a day (depending on the animal's size). Crush and mix with the food.

Herbal—*Marsh mallow (Althaea officinalis):* Prepare an infusion by adding 2 tablespoons of the flowers or leaves to 1 cup of boiling water. Let steep 5 minutes. Or make a decoction (which is more potent) by simmering 1 teaspoon of the root in a cup of boiling water for 20 to 30 minutes. Twice a day give ½ teaspoon to cats or small dogs, 1 teaspoon to medium dogs and 1 tablespoon to large dogs (see page 226). Try mixing it in the food. Continue for several weeks and then taper off to twice a week.

Homeopathic—*Nux vomica 30C (poison nut):* Use "Homeopathic Schedule 4," page 348. This remedy is useful as an occasional treatment for uremia. Often, it will help with the symptoms of toxicity, especially nausea, vomiting and feeling generally ill.

Tissue Salt—*Natrum muriaticum 6X (sodium chloride):* This treatment will help with the body's use of water. It is indicated for the cat that is very thirsty and prefers cool surfaces to lie on. Use "Homeopathic Schedule 6(a)," page 349.

Homeopathic—*Sepia 6C (cuttlefish ink):*

This is helpful to the cat that has primarily stomach symptoms, such as nausea, vomiting or loss of appetite. Use "Homeopathic Schedule 6(a)," page 349.

Homeopathic—*Pulsatilla 6C (windflower):* Useful for the dog or cat that shows no sign of thirst (in spite of the kidney disease) and prefers cool surfaces to lie on. Use "Homeopathic Schedule 6(a)," page 349.

CRISIS THERAPY

A severe crisis in an animal with weak or failed kidneys is best handled by your veterinarian. Often the technique of intravenous fluid administration is critical to survival because anything given by mouth is immediately vomited. Your veterinarian may show you how to give daily fluid injections, which can help many cats to survive for additional months or years—often much longer than dogs survive with similar treatment.

An additional supportive treatment is that adapted from herbalist Juliette de Bairacli-Levy, who advises that you withhold all solid food until the crisis passes. Instead, give:

Cool parsley tea: Steep a tablespoon of fresh parsley in a cup of hot water for 20 minutes. Give 1 teaspoon to 2 tablespoons 3 times a day.

Barley water: To make this, pour 3 cups of boiling water over a cup of whole barley. Cover and let steep overnight. In the morning strain and squeeze out the liquid through muslin or cloth. Add 2 teaspoons each of honey and pure lemon juice. Feed your animal ¼ to 2 cups of this liquid twice a day. (Make a bigger batch if necessary.)

Parsnip balls: Combine raw, grated parsnips (which help to detoxify the kidneys) with thick honey (an energy source).

Roll into balls and give as desired. This combination is more likely to be accepted by dogs than cats.

Enemas: Make pure water available at all times. If your pet has trouble keeping fluids down, however, give 1 to 3 enemas per day until vomiting stops. For every 20 pounds of weight, make a solution combining ½ teaspoon sea salt, ½ teaspoon potassium chloride (a salt substitute), 1 teaspoon lemon juice and 500 milligrams vitamin C, well-dissolved in a pint of lukewarm water. (See instructions for administration in chapter 15.) When an animal is dehydrated it will retain the enema rather than discharging it, and this will help replenish the blood.

After the crisis stage you can slowly return the animal to food, utilizing the maintenance program already described. Remember, the single most important thing is to give large volumes of fluids to rehydrate the tissues and to flush the kidneys. Without adequate fluid, treatment will not be successful. If vomiting is severe and continuous, use the suggestions under "Vomiting." Particularly, try the homeopathic remedy *Ipecac* 3X as described in that section.

LIVER PROBLEMS

The liver may be the most important organ of the body. It is involved in innumerable events, including: the manufacture of blood proteins, fats and the proteins responsible for the blood clotting; storage of energy (as glycogen) for production of blood sugar as needed by the body; storage of the fat-soluble vitamins and iron; the detoxification of drugs, chemicals and other unusable substances; the inactivation of hormones no longer needed and the secretion of bile and other factors necessary for proper digestion. As if these tasks were not enough to keep it busy, the liver also must filter blood coming from the digestive tract to keep potentially harmful bacteria from reaching other parts of the body. It is the organ that prepares toxic material and waste products for subsequent elimination by the kidneys.

Therefore, as you can imagine, inflammation of the liver (hepatitis) and other disturbances of this vital organ are very serious conditions. Symptoms of liver trouble include nausea, vomiting, loss of appetite, jaundice (yellowing of the tissues, best seen at the whites of the eyes in animals) and perhaps the passing of light-colored or "fatty"-looking bowel movements (from insufficient bile and poor digestion) and the swelling of the abdomen from fluid accumulation.

Liver malfunction is caused by many conditions. Some factors are viral infections or the swallowing of poisonous substances, but in most cases it's hard to tell just what initiated the problem.

TREATMENT

Because the liver is so central to the whole process of breaking down and using food, treatment includes minimizing the work it must do by fasting or feeding small, frequent, easily digested meals. In the early, acute stage of liver inflammation, fasting is best, especially if a fever is present. Follow the directions for fasting given in chapter 15. Keep your dog on a liquid diet for a few days until his temperature returns to normal or there is some improvement. During this period give the following treatments.

Vitamin C: 500 to 2,000 milligrams four times a day, depending on size. This is most easily given as sodium ascorbate powder dissolved in a small amount of water. (¼ teaspoon is about 1,000 milligrams.)

One of the following remedies can also be helpful.

Tissue Salt—*Natrum sulphuricum 6X (sodium sulfate):* Use "Homeopathic Schedule 1," page 348. If the Natrum sulphuricum doesn't help after 24 hours, try the following homeopathic remedy.

Homeopathic—*Bryonia 6X (wild hops):* Use "Homeopathic Schedule 1," page 348. Bryonia is indicated when the animal is very thirsty, is reluctant to move (because of pain) and vomits after drinking warm liquids.

Homeopathic—*Belladonna 6X (deadly nightshade):* This is most useful for the stage of fever, restless agitation, hot head and dilated pupils. Use "Homeopathic Schedule 1," page 348.

As the animal improves and the symptoms subside, ease it onto a diet similar to that for kidney failure. You should, however, reduce the fat content by sticking to lean meat and eliminating the added oil. Eggs usually are well-tolerated by the liver patient, as are grains. Feed small amounts at a time, dividing the day's ration into four servings, and warm the food to room temperature. Hold back on fats until the condition is normal. Then reintroduce them, starting in small amounts.

After a month or two of recovery, you can gradually and carefully move back to the basic recipes as outlined in chapter 4. During this time of healing, emphasize raw foods as much as possible (cottage cheese, eggs, meat and finely grated vegetables). Some foods, of course, must be well-cooked for digestion (like grains and beans). Combine the foods only after the cooked ingredients have cooled. This precaution will provide optimal amounts of unaltered nutrients needed for the quickest possible recovery. If these foods are accepted, try including raw grated beets (about one to three tablespoons) every day as a liver stimulant. One to two tablespoons of fresh minced parsley is also useful.

During recovery also continue the vitamin C. If after some improvement there is a relapse, go back to using the last remedy that was most useful. Usually the vitamin C can be discontinued after all symptoms are gone.

LYME DISEASE

This disease was first recognized (in people) in Europe in the early 1900s and has since been reported throughout Europe, Australia, Russia, China, Japan and Africa. It has been called Lyme disease in this country since 1975, when it was first found to cause arthritis in children in Old Lyme, Connecticut. Considerable research revealed that the condition was caused by a spirochete (a microbe related to syphilis, though not spread by sexual contact) and transmitted by tick bites.

In people Lyme disease causes a skin rash, tiredness, fever and chills, headache, backache, arthritis and other symptoms. The situation is very different for animals, however, and that makes it difficult to discuss. On the one hand, there is a lot of concern about this disease in dogs and a lot of press about it. On the other hand, there is almost no evidence that it is a real disease in animals.

By this, I mean that even though a lot of veterinarians are making this diagnosis and doing treatment, there is no research that shows it is actually a disease. Almost every attempt to reproduce this disease experimentally has ended in failure. Furthermore, there is no relationship between a positive blood test and the presence of symptoms. More than 50 percent of normal, healthy dogs test positive for the organism in their blood, yet have not had any illness. What this means is that dogs are frequently exposed to the Lyme disease organism (through tick bites) but rarely get sick from it. Some veterinarians have even suggested that there is not so much a "Lyme disease of dogs" as that a small percentage of dogs have an excessive reaction more like an allergy.

There is a vaccine for Lyme disease, but the company that produces it says that its testing methods are a trade secret and therefore other research labs cannot confirm their claims. Is it effective? Who knows. The only way they could test the vaccine was to first suppress each dog's immune system with cortisone. Considering how unnatural this is, it is difficult to say anything about the significance of the disease or the vaccine prepared against it.

What about the disease when it *does* seem to appear in dogs? Veterinarians who live in areas with high rates of Lyme disease report that some dogs will develop fever, depression and hot and painful joints (especially the "wrist" joints) with reluctance to move. About 85 percent of these ill dogs will permanently recover with antibiotic treatment (and probably also *without* antibiotics, though no studies have been done to determine this). The remaining 15 percent stay chronically ill—regardless of what antibiotics are used or how long they are used.

In any case, from the research available so far and from my personal experience over the last several years, it is my opinion that (in contrast to the situation for humans) Lyme disease is an insignificant condition for dogs and other animals.

PREVENTION

The best prevention is to keep your dog healthy. Following the nutritional and other advice in this book will achieve that goal. In addition, you can control ticks (which carry the disease) by use of repellents and frequent combing (see the discussion on ticks in "Skin Parasites").

TREATMENT

If your dog does show the symptoms of fever and joint inflammation, these treatments are helpful.

Homeopathic—*Aconitum napellus 30C (monkshood):* This remedy is often suitable for the very earliest stage of illness with high fever, especially if it is accompanied by a restless anxiety. Use "Homeopathic Schedule 3," page 348.

Homeopathic—*Bryonia alba 30C (wild hops):* Often dogs will lie very quietly, crying out at the slightest motion. Give this medicine to the dog that is reluctant to move because of the pain. Use "Homeopathic Schedule 3," page 348.

Homeopathic—*Rhus toxicodendron 30C (poison ivy and poison oak):* This is indicated for the dog that is stiff and sore, especially on first moving after lying for a while. As she moves around, however, the joints seem to limber up and the stiffness is not so noticeable. Use "Homeopathic Schedule 3," page 348.

Homeopathic—*Pulsatilla 30C (windflower):* Give this medicine to the dog that becomes submissive (when ill) and does not want to drink water. Use "Homeopathic Schedule 3," page 348.

Homeopathic—*Mercurius vivus (or solubilis) 30C (the element mercury)* is helpful to the sick dog that has, along with the other symptoms, red and inflamed gums, bad breath and a tendency to drool or salivate. Use "Homeopathic Schedule 3," page 348.

Remember that any time there is an acute illness with fever, it is also helpful to fast your dog for several days (see chapter 15).

MANGE

See "Skin Parasites."

MITES

See "Ear Problems" and "Skin Parasites."

NEUTERING

See "Spaying and Neutering."

NOSE PROBLEMS

See "Foxtails" and "Upper Respiratory Infections."

OBESITY

See "Weight Problems."

PANCREATITIS

Pancreatitis often first appears as a sudden, severe condition usually seen in overweight, middle-age dogs. Symptoms can include a complete loss of appetite, severe and frequent vomiting, diarrhea that may contain blood, reluctance to walk, weakness and abdominal pain (crying and restlessness). The severity of the attack can vary from a mild, almost unnoticeable condition to a severe shocklike collapse that can end in death.

The problem centers in the digestive tract, with a focus in the pancreas. The underlying cause is not known, but I think it will soon be apparent that pancreatitis is another of the immune diseases (like hyperthyroidism in cats). As an immediate trigger, attacks can come on after overindulgence in rich or fatty foods, especially after a raid on a garbage can or compost pile. Frequent attacks of pancreatitis can finally result in a lack of insulin, leading to diabetes (see "Diabetes").

PREVENTION

Prevention consists partly of a properly balanced natural diet coupled with regular and adequate exercise. Exercise is important because it improves digestion and peristaltic movements of the intestinal tract, thus regularizing the bowels and keeping this part of the body preventively more healthy. It also keeps weight under control.

Do not overfeed your dog, because obesity is a predisposing factor to pancreatitis (no one knows why). Many people end up with fat dogs because they enjoy watching the animal eat heartily. For more information, see "Weight Problems."

Realize that this condition can also be chronic in nature, persisting in a low-grade form for months or years unless corrected. If you have a dog with a tendency toward pancreatitis, be especially careful about setting off an attack through a change of diet. I also advise using vaccines minimally in these animals because the immune system becomes much more active after vaccination, possibly precipitating an immune-mediated crisis.

TREATMENT

Treatment usually requires hospitalization, with fluid replacement therapy in the case of extreme vomiting and diarrhea. If the condition is mild but recurrent, the following measures should help to restore a balance of health.

Feed the basic natural diet and supplements (chapters 3 and 4) except omit vegetable oils or butter as well as other fatty foods that may irritate the pancreas. It's okay to use cod-liver oil for the vitamin A, but it would be better to switch to vitamin A capsules. Be sure to use vitamin E to help prevent pancreatic scarring (100 to 400 IU, depending on size). For vegetables emphasize corn (preferably raw) and raw grated cabbage, but include a variety of others as well. Avoid fruits.

Feed small, frequent meals instead of one large one. Offer all food at room temperature for best digestive action.

Use **vitamin C and bioflavonoids regularly.** Depending on the dog's size, give 250 to 1,000 milligrams of vitamin C three times a day, if possible. Sodium ascorbate powder may be better tolerated than ascorbic acid. (A teaspoon of sodium ascorbate powder has about 4,000 milligrams of C.) Give 25 to 50 milligrams of bioflavonoids (vitamin P) to enhance the action of the ascorbate.

Eliminate any food or supplement that seems to upset the digestive tract or aggravate the symptoms. Find a substitute form for any supplement you need to discontinue, for instance, a B complex instead of nutritional yeast.

In addition to these nutritional steps, try one of the following as a supportive treatment.

Herbal—*Yarrow (Achillea millefolium):* Use "Herbal Schedule 1," page 346. Yarrow strengthens the pancreas and helps to control internal hemorrhages. It is indicated if there is dark, chocolate-colored or black diarrhea (perhaps containing blood) that is foul-smelling.

Homeopathic—*Iris versicolor 6X (blue flag):* This remedy is particularly suited to the pancreas and may be more effective than yarrow. Use "Homeopathic Schedule 1," page 348. It is very useful when the dog vomits repeatedly with much drooling of saliva.

Homeopathic—*Spongia tosta 6X (roasted sponge):* Indicated if the pancreatitis is associated with coughing or breathing difficulties. Use "Homeopathic Schedule 1," page 348.

Tissue Salt—*Ferrum phosphoricum 6X (iron phosphate):* Use "Homeopathic Schedule 1," page 348. This treatment is most useful during the inflammatory stage with pain and fever.

Homeopathic—*Pulsatilla 30C (windflower):* Very helpful if the dog shows no sign of thirst, seeks cool surfaces to lie on and becomes clingy (wanting to be close all the time) and whiny. Use "Homeopathic Schedule 2," page 348.

Homeopathic—*Nux vomica 30C (poison nut):* Indicated for the dog that becomes very irritable, withdraws to another room (away from company) and is chilly. Use "Homeopathic Schedule 2," page 348.

PANLEUKOPENIA

See "Distemper, Chorea and Feline Panleukopenia."

PARALYSIS

Causes of paralysis can range from accidents that damage the spine to blood clots that form in brain arteries to intervertebral disk disease ("slipped disk") as well as many others. Here we will consider the two most common causes, which are intervertebral disk disease and spondylitis (a buildup of calcium on the spine from arthritis). To some extent we can regard these two conditions similarly because both are degenerative processes involving the spine.

In intervertebral disk disease the soft gelatinous material between the vertebrae escapes its normal position. The apparent cause is a breakdown of the ligaments that keep this material in place. This puts pressure on the spinal cord. The condition is worst in breeds that have long backs in relation to their legs, such as dachshunds.

Spondylitis appears more often in large dogs like German shepherds. It involves a long-term inflammation of the vertebrae, which the body attempts to alleviate by immobilizing spinal movements with calcium deposits. Eventually, these deposits encroach on the nerves that branch out from the spinal cord, interfering with their functions. Symptoms are not obvious to the untrained eye. Be on the lookout for some rigidity of the back and some difficulty or pain on getting up. Usually a diagnosis is made only after an x-ray is taken. Spondylitis often is associated with hip dysplasia as well, so read about that topic also.

PREVENTION

My opinion is that both intervertebral disk disease and spondylitis are expressions of the same problem—a deterioration of the spine brought on after years of poor nutrition, inadequate exercise and stress. They are better prevented than treated. Your best insurance is to follow the natural diet recommendations in chapters 3 and 4 and the general care advice in chapter 7. Also, avoid selecting a breed that is prone to intervertebral disk disease (long-backed dogs) and breeds that have more trouble with hip dysplasia (such as German shepherds).

TREATMENT

Intervertebral disk problems, once they have developed, may be alleviated by this program.

Nutrition should be emphasized. Avoid commercial foods and treats, using only the natural diet and supplements advised in this book. Be sure to add 100 to 400 IU vitamin E (depending on your pet's size) and ¼ to 1 teaspoon lecithin granules to the daily ration. In addition, give 500 to 1,000 milligrams of vitamin C twice a day to strengthen the connective tissue involved and to counteract stress.

For specific treatment you can try:

Homeopathic—*Nux vomica 6X (poison nut)*: This is most effective for animals with pain in the back, muscle tightness or spasms along the lower back and weakness or paralysis of the rear legs. Give it 3 times daily, especially when symptoms first appear or during attacks. Taper off when improvement occurs. If constipation develops after using this treatment for a couple of weeks, discontinue it until needed again.

If you catch the problem early, Nux vomica may help to prevent the pain, tightness and rear leg symptoms for which it is indicated. The dog that has been paralyzed for a long time will not respond easily. In such a case use "Homeopathic Schedule 6(a)," page 349.

A paralyzed animal will benefit from massage of the back and legs and passive movement of the limbs to keep the muscles from shrinking away. If there is slight voluntary movement of the legs, exercise the animal by helping it to "swim" in a bathtub or pool. Support most of its weight with a towel. Acupuncture and chiropractic have also been helpful for intervertebral disk problems.

Spondylitis, on the other hand, can be difficult to treat once it has developed. The chance of improvement is much less for a dog already paralyzed than for one that is only weakened. A short fast (see chapter 15) may be helpful, followed by the basic natural diet given in this book. The further instructions given under "Arthritis" will be very helpful.

Besides exercise and massage, try a course of treatment with:

Tissue Salt—*Silicea 6X*: Use "Homeopathic Schedule 6(a)," page 349. If you see encouraging signs, gradually increase the amount of exercise to encourage redevelopment of the muscles.

POISONING

See "Handling Emergencies and Giving First Aid" on page 337.

PREGNANCY, BIRTH AND CARE OF NEWBORNS

Also see "Reproductive Organ Problems."

The key to a successful and easy pregnancy and delivery is good nutrition. During gestation (63 to 65 days for cats, 58 to 63 days for dogs) tremendous demands are made on the mother's tissues to supply all the nutrients needed to build several new bodies. The general rule is that kittens or puppies come first. That is, they get whatever is available nutritionally, and the mother gets what's left. If she doesn't consume enough food to supply complete nutrition, her body provides whatever is lacking.

A female that is not adequately fed, or that is bred again and again, accumulates a nutritional deficiency that becomes greater with each pregnancy. Eventually, the mother will become diseased or the young will be weak and susceptible to disease—perhaps during their entire lives. The special recipes in chapter 5 for pregnant and nursing females and for young animals are designed to meet their special needs and prevent this nutritional depletion. Let's look at the two most common problems—eclampsia and dystocia (difficult delivery).

Eclampsia

Eclampsia is a severe disturbance that appears most often at the end of a pregnancy,

right after birth or during nursing. That's because it stems from calcium depletion. As new skeletons are formed or milk is produced, the calcium demand from the mother's body is great. Symptoms include loss of appetite, a high fever (sometimes dangerously so), rapid panting and convulsions. During convulsions the muscles become rigid and the animal falls over with its head back. More typically, you may see a series of rapid contractions and relaxations of the muscles that looks like uncontrollable shaking.

Strenuous treatment is necessary, including intravenous injections of calcium by your veterinarian and ice baths (to bring down the temperature). Such treatment is usually successful, but the condition can recur if the young continue to nurse.

It is much better to prevent this problem in the first place by proper and bountiful nutrition rather than to try to patch up the animal once it has occurred. In the event that your female already suffers from eclampsia, however, put her on the diet in chapter 5 that is appropriate for her state of pregnancy or lactation. Be sure to include all the ingredients, especially bonemeal.

The treatment most likely to help during the crisis is:

Homeopathic—*Belladonna 6C (deadly nightshade)*: Give one pellet every 15 minutes until the symptoms are alleviated. Then use "Homeopathic Schedule 1," page 348, until all is well. This treatment can be used whenever symptoms reappear.

Dystocia (Difficult Delivery)

Cats and dogs with normal anatomy rarely have problems giving birth, particularly if they are adequately fed during pregnancy. Lack of certain essential nutrients like calcium, however, may weaken the uterine muscles and cause weak or short contractions, a somewhat uncommon problem that has been increasing in incidence. In addition, certain fetal deformities can cause obstruction of the birth canal during labor.

But the greatest birthing problems occur in dogs with an abnormal anatomy, usually from breeding trends in which the pelvis becomes too small for the size of the puppies. Other than the use of caesarean sections, little can be done about this problem except the obvious: Avoid breeding such animals and don't select them as pets (which creates a market for them).

Let's first review how delivery usually goes when all is normal. Two or three days before delivery, the mother may lose her appetite and show nesting behavior (carrying toys or other things to a particular area, tearing up paper to make a nest). There will be swelling of the vulva and a slight discharge. Twenty-four to 48 hours before birth, there will be a sudden drop in body temperature to below normal (usually below 101°F, but this varies according to the individual and is best determined by checking the temperature twice a day for several days before).

The next thing is for labor to begin. Stage One is characterized by restlessness, panting and shivering (perhaps also vomiting food once). This lasts 6 to 12 hours (but can be longer with the first birth). Stage Two is visible contractions with delivery of the puppy. Some mothers will start this stage by wanting to go outside to urinate. They will lie on the side as contractions become stronger, straining and licking the genitals. Some dogs will groan or even scream. Between contractions there is rapid panting. This stage lasts from 15 minutes to an hour.

Stage Three is the passing of the afterbirth, which is usually promptly eaten. It is important that all the afterbirths be passed, so each (one to a puppy) must be accounted for.

Problems can begin to occur at stage two, when contractions are not producing results. You will know that this is happening because straining goes on too long. If the mother goes more than four or five hours with the first puppy, or three hours with subsequent puppies, then it has gone too long. In this case, use:

Homeopathic—*Pulsatilla 30C (windflower)*: Give one pellet every 30 minutes. As soon as labor proceeds, stop using the remedy, even if you've only given one or two doses. Remember that the mother will often naturally rest between deliveries, even napping for an hour or two. So don't rush things too much. If there is no delivery by six doses (three hours), then the remedy will not help.

If a puppy or kitten is part way out and seems stuck (not immediately slipping out), pulling on it *very gently* may help. Hold the body, not the legs or head, and note that anything more vigorous than an extremely gentle touch can cause damage to either the mother or the unborn. Get professional help if the baby has been trapped in the birth canal for more than a half hour (it will be dead by then). A caesarean section will probably be needed. If your veterinarian thinks it advisable, this can also be a good time for spaying.

If all goes well at home and the delivery is complete, use:

Homeopathic—*Arnica montana 30C (mountain daisy)*: Use "Homeopathic Schedule 2," page 348. This is most helpful to strengthen the mother and prevent infection.

If an afterbirth stays inside, however, serious problems can result. If one is retained and there is fever or infection, use this treatment along with what your veterinarian prescribes.

Homeopathic—*Secale cornutum 30C (ergot):* Use "Homeopathic Schedule 2," page 348. This remedy will often prevent or successfully treat infection following a retained afterbirth.

Care of the Newborn

Fortunately for you, the mother will generally do everything needed to care for the newborn, and it's best not to interfere unless there's a problem. Right after birth she will clean the little ones, and, as long as necessary, she will also lick up all the urine and feces voided by her growing young. This is nature's way of keeping a clean nest. It's convenient for you, but if the infants should develop diarrhea, you may miss the evidence.

Diarrhea is one of the more common problems at this stage of life, and it's usually caused by consuming too much milk (sometimes a problem with hand-raised puppies or kittens), infection in the mother's uterus or mammary glands (check if her temperature is above 102°F) or giving antibiotics to the mother (they can get into the milk).

A puppy or kitten with diarrhea will get cold and dehydrated (the skin will be wrinkled and look too big for the body). It may crawl away from the nest and usually cries, even when returned to the mother.

If the problem is with the mother's milk, you'll need to feed the babies by hand with a pet nurser bottle sold at pet stores. Use the nursing formulas in chapter 5 or a commercial kitten or puppy formula. Dilute the formula half and half with pure water until the diarrhea is under control. The problem should correct itself after a few feedings. If not, try one of these two methods.

1. Use a mixture consisting of half formula (regular strength) and half warm chamomile tea (one teaspoon herb to a cup of boiling water). Feed on a regular schedule until the problem is controlled, usually by two or three feedings.
2. Use the half formula/half water mixture, but add to it a crushed tablet of the homeopathic preparation *Podophyllum 6X* (mayapple). Mix well. One such therapeutic feeding should be enough, but repeat this formula every four hours if necessary.

Examine the mother's breasts to see if there are hard lumps, hot areas or painful places (on pressure). If so, there may be an infection (mastitis) that will need treatment before the milk is safe for the puppies (see "Reproductive Organ Problems").

After the diarrhea is under control and there is no problem with the mother, you can return the puppy or kitten to the nest, but be watchful in case the diarrhea returns.

If, as sometimes happens, the mother does not care for the young—letting them cry and avoiding contact and not nursing—then you have a potentially serious problem as the young ones cannot go long without eating. It is possible that there is something physically wrong with the mother like an infection or retained puppy or kitten, so you will need to have your veterinarian check out this possibility. If the problem is emotional, however, then here is a treatment that is quite helpful.

Homeopathic—*Sepia 30C (cuttlefish ink):* Use "Homeopathic Schedule 2," page 348. If the mother does not accept the young within a few hours, then the puppies or kittens will have to be raised with a bottle. See chapter 5 for guidance on this.

RABIES

Rabies is a serious disease that affects many different types of animals, including human beings. Once the clinical signs develop, it is usually fatal. These symptoms often include very aggressive behavior and biting, which is how the disease gets spread (via saliva). Even if untreated, however, many people or pets bitten by a rabid animal do not develop the disease. The hitch is that once the condition develops, there is no orthodox treatment to save the patient. (I have heard occasional reports of recovery by a variety of alternative methods, including homeopathy—fortunately, I have never treated it myself.)

One of the most exciting and promising new treatments is the use of vitamin C. It sounds unbelievable, but as far back as 20 years ago research studies were finding that vitamin C injections into guinea pigs infected with rabies *decreased the death rate by 50 percent.* Considering how few treatments are available for rabies, this is a dramatic finding. One can only hope that such research continues.

Because of its well-known fatality rate, however, the public is justly very afraid of this disease. For that reason local governments have adopted great precautions, including a legal requirement for a periodic rabies vaccination for dogs (cats are still optional in most states, but not all).

Most of the danger to humans is not actually from dogs and cats but from wild animals such as skunks and raccoons that are captured for sale and/or adopted as pets. Unfortunately, rabies vaccines developed for dogs and cats may not be completely safe or effective in these species. (For example, it is not recommended that wolf hybrids be vaccinated with rabies vaccine because of the risk of infection.) Since the chance of getting rabies from wild animals is so high—in addition to the ethical and ecological considerations of wild-animal adoption—it is not wise to keep them as pets. (See chapter 11 for ways to protect yourself from the bite of a dog and what to do if you have been bitten.)

RADIATION TOXICITY

The most common sources of radiation exposure for the average animal are diagnostic x-rays and radiation therapy (I do not recommend the latter). Other possibilities are less obvious—such as leakage from a nuclear power plant or storage area. In any case, the body must repair a lot of cellular damage using cell functions that also may be affected by the exposure. Fortunately, there are ways to enhance this healing process. Use them after any known or suspected radiation exposure. (If there is leakage from a power plant or other atmospheric leakage, it would be best to keep your animal and yourself indoors for a while.)

Nutrition is the main aid. Emphasize rolled oats as your choice of grains for several weeks. It helps counteract nausea and other side effects. Be sure to include the normal supplements of nutritional yeast, cold-pressed unsaturated vegetable oil (for vitamin F) and kelp (contains alginate, which helps to remove strontium 90 from the body and to block absorption of radioactive iodine). In addition, give rutin (bioflavonoids), which has reduced the death rate in irradiated animals by 800 percent; vitamin C, which works with rutin to strengthen the circulatory system and counteract stress; and pantothenic acid, which helps to prevent radiation injuries and has increased the survival rate in irradiated animals by 200 percent. Depending on size, give daily: 100 to 400 milligrams rutin, 250 to 2,000 milligrams vitamin C and 5 to 20 milligrams pantothenic acid.

If your animal is more than mildly affected by radiation and needs greater treatment, a trained homeopath can provide an individualized prescription that may be of great help.

REPRODUCTIVE ORGAN PROBLEMS

The two most common reproductive problems affect female animals—pyometra and metritis. In both cases the uterus (womb) is the seat of the disorder, and prompt treatment is needed before the condition progresses too far. We'll look at each of these, and then at mastitis (mammary gland infection).

Pyometra

Coming on slowly over weeks or months, pyometra first appears as irregular heat periods and a discharge of reddish mucus from the vagina *between* heats. If unrecognized and untreated, it progresses to the point of severe depression, loss of appetite, vomiting, diarrhea, discolored vaginal discharge (not always present), excessive consumption of water and excessive urination. The large water intake mimics kidney failure, but the other symptoms help you tell the difference, particularly if there is a vaginal discharge and the animal is an unspayed dog or cat several years old that had many heats without being bred. A probable secondary cause is a high-hormone diet (from glandular meats or meat containing hormones used to fatten cattle). Concentrated in meat meal and other commercial pet food, hormones may predispose the uterus to malfunction.

Prevention, therefore, is simple—the spay operation for the young female.

TREATMENT

Dogs (and sometimes cats) with pyometra can suddenly develop a crisis that may require surgical removal of the uterus, which often has become quite large and distended with fluid. The process is basically the same as a spay operation but much more serious and difficult.

Those animals not so severely affected may be helped by:

Homeopathic—*Pulsatilla 30C (windflower)*: Use "Homeopathic Schedule 3," page 348. This remedy is best for the animal that is not very thirsty (which is unusual) and wants to be comforted (petted or held). If there is a vaginal discharge, it is usually thick and yellowish or greenish.

Homeopathic—*Sepia 30C (cuttlefish ink):* Use "Homeopathic Schedule 3," page 348. If there has been no improvement within 5 days of completing the Pulsatilla treatment (above), then use this remedy. It is often sufficient.

Metritis

Right after giving birth and occasionally right after breeding, the uterus is susceptible to bacterial infection. Should infection occur, symptoms can be severe. They include fever, depression, not caring for the young and a foul-smelling vaginal discharge.

Normal vaginal discharge following an uncomplicated delivery is dark green to brown and odorless. If all the young and all the afterbirths have come out properly, within 12 hours it becomes more like clear mucus (though possibly tinged with blood). But if a dark green to reddish-brown, thick and unusually foul-smelling discharge continues for 12 to 24 hours after the delivery, the uterus is probably infected.

TREATMENT

Once metritis has developed, it can become severe, so you should seek professional help. However, these remedies may also help.

Homeopathic—*Aconitum napellus 30C (monkshood):* Use "Homeopathic Schedule 2," page 348. This remedy is indicated for the animal that has a fever and is acting very frightened or anxious. It will startle easily and be very agitated.

Homeopathic—*Belladonna 30C (deadly nightshade):* Use "Homeopathic Schedule 2," page 348. This remedy is an alternative to Aconitum and is needed by the animal that has a fever and *feels* hot (especially the head) and has dilated pupils. Sometimes there is also an excitability similar to delirium with a tendency to bite or act aggressively.

See the section on "Pregnancy, Birth and Care of Newborns" for information on infection from retained afterbirths.

Mastitis

The mammary glands are most susceptible to infection when they are actively secreting milk. An infected breast will be hard, sensitive, painful and discolored (reddish-purple). There may be abscesses and drainage as well. Your veterinarian will usually prescribe antibiotics. Successful homeopathic treatments I have used are:

Homeopathic—*Aconitum napellus 30C (monkshood):* For the very first signs of infection with fever, restlessness and anxiety. Use "Homeopathic Schedule 2," page 348.

Homeopathic—*Belladonna 30C (deadly nightshade):* For the dog with fever, dilated pupils and excitability. Use "Homeopathic Schedule 2," page 348.

Homeopathic—*Phytolacca 6X (poke root):* For mastitis where the breast is *very* hard to the touch and extremely painful. Use "Homeopathic Schedule 1," page 348.

Homeopathic—*Lachesis muta 30C (bushmaster snake venom):* Use when the left breast is affected, especially if the skin over the area has turned bluish or black. Use "Homeopathic Schedule 2," page 348.

Homeopathic—*Pulsatilla 30C (windflower):* For the dog that is whining, shows no sign of thirst and wants comfort. Use "Homeopathic Schedule 2," page 348.

RINGWORM

See "Skin Parasites."

SINUSITIS

See "Upper Respiratory Infections."

SKIN PARASITES

See "Ear Problems" for a discussion of ear mites.

External parasites (such as ticks and fleas) seem to be most attracted to animals in poor health. I have seen many pets with fleas on the outside, worms on the inside and some other problem like a chronic skin disease. I've also observed that when an animal is placed on my natural diet and my other recommended lifestyle changes are made, the number of fleas and other parasites often decrease markedly. They don't completely disappear, but they no longer constitute a problem. Other measures of control, if needed, are then much easier and more effective.

When I'm trying to evaluate an animal's overall health, I find it useful to judge the seriousness of any skin parasites that may be present. From least serious to most serious, I rank them in this order: ticks, fleas, lice and, finally, mange mites or ringworm. By this scale I consider a cat with lice to be more seriously ill than one with fleas, and a dog with mange worse off than one with ticks, and so on.

Let's discuss each of these parasites in turn and consider ways to control them without poisonous chemicals. You must realize, however, that by themselves, neither these suggested measures nor chemical insecticides are effective in the long run. The best results occur when an animal is on a natural diet, lives in a good environment, gets enough sunlight and is exercised and groomed regularly, as discussed elsewhere in the book.

Ticks

Ticks are not permanent residents. Rather, they attach themselves, suck some blood and later fall off to lay eggs. The young ticks that hatch out crawl up to the ends of branches and grasses and patiently wait (for weeks, if necessary) for something warm-blooded and good tasting to come along and brush against the vegetation. Then they drop on and find a nice, cozy place to attach.

PREVENTION

Groom your pet thoroughly before you let it run in an area likely to contain ticks, such as woods or fields. Remove loose hair and mats so access to the skin is easier, and dust the coat with an herbal flea repellent. (Commercial formulas containing eucalyptus powder are particularly useful.) Work the repellent through the hair and into the skin.

TREATMENT

When you return home after the adventure, check for any stalwart ticks that may have made it aboard your pet despite precautions. A fine-toothed flea comb may help to locate them or even capture any that are not yet attached. This also is a good time to remove foxtails (see "Foxtails"). Look especially around the neck and head and under the ears.

If you find a tick already attached, remove it like this: With the nails of your thumb and forefinger (or a pair of tweezers—some are now available just for this purpose), reach around the tick and grasp it as close to the skin as possible; don't worry, it won't bite! You want to remove the whole thing, not just pull off the tick's body and leave the head still embedded. Use a slow, steady pull (10 to 20 seconds) and, with a slight twist, pull out the little bugger—head, body and all. You will have to pull strongly *but not quickly*. Look closely to see if you got the tick's tiny head; it will probably have a little shred of tissue still attached to it. Wash your hands when you are done with removal.

If the head is left behind despite your care, the area may fester for a while, much like a splinter under the skin. But this is minor and can be treated with the herbs echinacea or calendula as described under "Abscesses."

Sometimes small ticks crawl down inside the ear. If your dog is shaking its head a lot after a trip through tick land, have your veterinarian look down the ear canal with an instrument to check for this or for a possible foxtail.

Fleas

Ah! The bane of dog and cat alike. Once again, I have found that a healthy lifestyle is the best defense. Following are some additional specific measures that can also help.

- Add plenty of nutritional yeast and garlic to the daily ration. Use anywhere from one teaspoon to two tablespoons of yeast (depending on your pet's size) to each meal.
- Mix fresh garlic, ¼ to 1 raw clove, grated or minced, into each feeding.
- Wash the skin daily, if necessary, with a lemon rinse (see chapter 7). This makes it less attractive to the fleas.
- Have your carpets treated with a borax-like powder that dramatically reduces flea populations (see chapter 7).

If, in spite of all this commendable effort, your animal still has a serious problem with fleas (not just a few but dozens), check for roundworms and tapeworms (which can be carried by fleas) which may be sapping your pet of energy (see "Worms"). Also, try a specific homeopathic remedy to help strengthen the body so that it isn't so attractive to fleas. The one that usually works best is:

Homeopathic—*Sulphur 30C (the element sulphur)*: Use "Homeopathic Schedule 4," page 348. This is the treatment to try first; however, you must still continue all the flea-control measures suggested above. The remedy will only make your pet better able to resist flea infestation; it will not kill fleas directly.

Homeopathic—*Psorinum 30C*: Use "Homeopathic Schedule 4," page 348. Give this remedy if there is no change for the better after the month of using sulphur.

A note about flea collars: They don't work. They are toxic. Some cats even hang themselves on them or get the collars caught between their jaws, causing serious damage. Others get permanent hair loss around the neck from allergic reactions, particularly when the collar is too tight.

Also beware of flea tags that hang on the collar and release a toxic gas that affects the nervous system. Don't use them. They affect the animal, you, your family and anyone else that breathes in the gases.

Chemical insecticides in shampoos, soaps, powders and sprays also are dangerous, as discussed in chapter 7. Notice the label warnings about wearing gloves or avoiding contact with your skin and so forth. How can it be so dangerous for you and yet safe for your pet? Think about it.

Lice

These little varmints are rather uncommon, but occasionally infest a run-down dog or cat. You have to look very carefully to see them on the skin or to see their eggs, which are attached to the animal hairs. Lice are slightly smaller than fleas, and they have a lighter color—more tan or beige rather than dark brown. Also, they don't jump like fleas. Fortunately, dog and cat lice do not infest people.

Treatment starts with frequent, preferably daily, use of a good shampoo containing d-limonene (a natural insecticide extracted from citrus). Leave the lather on for ten minutes before rinsing. Then follow with the lemon rinse described in chapter 7. The eggs are not killed by this, only the adults. The eggs continue to hatch out over a period of time, so continued baths are necessary until all the eggs are gone.

Without delay, build up the animal's health with a natural diet. Start right off with some home-prepared food and emphasize nutritional yeast and garlic as previously prescribed for fleas.

Use the same basic steps outlined in the flea program (including grooming) to eliminate the young lice as they hatch. Building up your pet's health will make its skin less desirable to lice.

Note: We are used to quick results like those we get with chemicals that kill the lice almost immediately. They will not do anything for the animal's run-down health, however, which engendered the problem in the first place. Indeed, the toxic effect may weaken the animal even further. To work with nature is to be patient.

Mange

The most common form of mange is demodectic mange, which is caused by a microscopic mite that lives in hair follicles. The other type is called sarcoptic mange, caused by a scabies mite that burrows into the skin, making pets and people itch (see chapter 11).

Demodectic mange occurs most often in dogs (though it is also seen in rare instances in cats). It usually appears first as a small, hairless patch near the eye or chin. It doesn't itch much and may pass unnoticed. The mite that causes it is very widespread and is actually found on most "normal" dogs and also on peoples' faces (around the eyebrows and nose) without any sign of its presence.

Demodectic mange causes a minor problem for some young dogs, but usually clears up spontaneously without treatment by the age of 12 to 14 months. In a small percentage of those affected, however, the mite continues to spread. Eventually, it can cover much of the body and result in hair loss and skin irritation and thickening. Bacteria (staph) can also get established, causing further complications such as "pimples" and a pustular discharge, particularly around the feet. This form of the disease is called generalized demodectic mange.

Animals that have generalized mange are susceptible to other serious illnesses and must be treated very carefully for their health to be restored. It is also very important that they not be vaccinated, as their immune system cannot react properly to the vaccine and only becomes more disordered.

TREATMENT

The orthodox treatment is harsh, poisonous and generally futile. (Mild cases clear up on their own anyway.) The hair is clipped off the whole animal. Then strong insecticides are "painted" on the skin or the dog is completely immersed in them. They are sometimes so toxic that only a part of the body can be done at a time. Unfortunately, anti-toxic nutrition or vitamin supplements are seldom recommended, so the dog's underlying health goes from bad to worse. Even those dogs that apparently recover after weeks or months of treatment can have recurrences, or another, more serious, "unrelated" problem will develop. Cortisone-type drugs should not be used under any circumstances. They depress the immune system further and, therefore, just about guarantee nonrecovery (in the true sense) by *any* methods.

I have had good results using just nutrition and homeopathic remedies, though treatment must be individualized and requires close attention to progress. Here are some general guidelines for a natural approach.

Fast the dog (if its weight and health are good) for five to seven days as outlined in chapter 15. Afterwards, use the natural diet described in chapters 3 and 4. Also add zinc (feed ground pumpkin seeds or give a tablet of chelated zinc—10 to 30 milligrams, depending on size), vitamin C (250 to 1,000 milligrams of ascorbate twice a day), vitamin E (100 IU to 400 IU) and lecithin (½ to 3 teaspoons a day). All of these supplements are very helpful to the functions of the immune system.

Rub fresh lemon juice on the affected spot every day, or use the lemon rinse recipe in chapter 7.

A homeopathic preparation that suits many cases of mange (either demodectic or sarcoptic) is:

Homeopathic—*Sulphur 6X (the element sulphur):* Use "Homeopathic Schedule 6(a)," page 349. When the condition is obviously clearing, use the sulphur less frequently on a tapering-off program.

The dog with a staph infection of the skin occurring along with the mange will benefit from the use of:

Herbal—*Purple cone flower (Echinacea angustifolia):* Use "Herbal Schedule 1," page 346, for internal treatment and "Herbal Schedule 4," page 347, for treatment of the skin (both at the same time). You can use both this and the sulphur treatment if necessary, giving the sulphur about 10 minutes before the echinacea dose.

The dog or cat with sarcoptic mange (more irritating than other kinds of mange) responds best to this treatment.

Herbal—*Lavender (Lavendula vera or L. officinalis):* Paint on oil of lavender (the pure oil diluted 1:10 with almond oil or an already prepared formula that contains oil of lavender) once a day until the hair begins to grow back.

Ringworm

Though this disease sounds like it's caused by some kind of curly worm, it is actually the result of a fungus that's similar to athlete's foot. The growth starts at a central point and spreads out in a ring shape, much like a ripple forms around the place where a stone is tossed in a pond. As the fungus grows in the skin cells and hair, the skin may become irritated, thickened and reddened, and the hairs may break off and leave a coarse stubble behind.

In cats, which are more commonly affected, the condition often looks like circular gray patches of broken, short, thin hair without much sign of itching or irritation. Ringworm is contagious to people (especially children) and other animals; see the precautions in chapter 11. Like mange, widespread ringworm indicates the animal's health is not up to snuff, as it usually is the stressed, sick or weakened ones that get severe infestations. Like generalized mange, ringworm that covers most of the body is a very serious problem indicating a severely compromised immune system.

TREATMENT

Nutrition: Start with a fast of two or three days (see chapter 15); then follow with the basic natural diet program in this book. Also add 5 to 20 milligrams of zinc chelate and ½ to 2 teaspoons of granular lecithin to the food (depending on body size). Essential fatty acids are very important for the health of skin and hair. If possible, add ¼ to 1 teaspoon of cod-liver oil (depending on the animal's size) to the food once a day.

Direct treatment: First, clip the hair around the bare spot and about ½ inch beyond it, being careful not to injure the skin. If you clip the hair, ringworm is less likely to spread—and the local treatment is easier

to apply. Burn or carefully dispose of the infected hair that you remove, as it is contagious on contact. (In order to catch loose hairs, always be sure to vacuum carefully and frequently if you have a pet with ringworm. Also wash bedding and utensils often with hot water and soap.) Be sure to wash your hands.

Treating the sore spot will speed healing and help protect others from getting ringworm. Choose *one* of the following two herbs plus the homeopathic remedy.

Herbal—*Plantain (Plantago major):* Make a decoction of the whole plant by putting about ¼ cup of the plant (a common weed) per every cup of spring or distilled water into a glass or enameled pot. Boil about 5 minutes, then let the brew steep 3 minutes, covered. Strain and cool. Massage onto the skin once or twice a day until the condition clears.

Herbal—*Goldenseal (Hydrastis canadensis):* Make a strong infusion by adding 1 rounded teaspoon of the powdered rootstock to a cup of boiling water. Let stand till cold. Then carefully pour off the clear fluid and massage it onto the skin once or twice a day.

Homeopathic—*Sulphur 6X:* Use "Homeopathic Schedule 6(a)" on page 349.

SKIN PROBLEMS

Mange and ringworm are discussed under "Skin Parasites."

The poor skin gets dumped on from two sides. The rest of the body uses it to eliminate toxic material, especially if the kidneys aren't able to handle the job; at the same time, environmental pollutants or applied chemical products assault it from the outside. One thing is for sure—skin troubles are the number-one problem in dogs and cats.

On the positive side, if your animal's only health problem is a skin disorder, consider yourself lucky. It's much worse if a surface condition (such as a skin problem) has been suppressed with repeated drug use; a more serious condition would be likelier to arise in that case. If a skin condition is the only problem your pet has, you can help prevent deeper problems by addressing it in a more curative manner. (The problem of suppressing is discussed in chapter 14.)

The symptoms of skin disorder are among the easiest to detect. They usually include one or more of the following: very dry skin; flakiness or white scales resembling dandruff; large brown flakes, redness and irritation; itching (ranging from slight to so severe that blood is drawn); greasy hair and a foul odor to the skin and its secretions (which many people mistake as normal); pimples and blisters that form between the toes and discharge blood and pus; brown, black or gray skin discoloration; formation of scabs or crusts and hair loss. I also include chronic inflammation inside the ear canal (and under the ear flap), anal gland problems and underactive thyroid glands as related to skin disease.

Modern medicine tends to divide up these many symptoms and regard them as separate diseases. I think this only confuses the picture so that we don't perceive the problem as a whole. From a wider view these symptoms appear as one basic problem that manifests a little differently in individual animals depending on heredity, environment, nutrition, parasites and so on. Thus, one dog may have severely inflamed,

moist, itchy areas ("hot spots") near the base of its tail, while another may have thick, itchy skin along its back, with greasy, smelly secretions, but they are really the same health problem.

What are the causes of this overall disorder?

- ◆ Toxicity—probably most of it from poor-quality food and some of it from other sources, like environmental pollutants and deliberately applied pest-control chemicals.
- ◆ Vaccinations—inducing immune disorders in susceptible animals.
- ◆ Suppressed disease—remains of an inadequately treated condition that never was cured and that may periodically discharge through the skin.
- ◆ Psychological factors—boredom, frustration, anger and irritability. As I see it, these are nearly always secondary issues that simply aggravate an already-existing problem.

Thus, it is possible to alleviate or even eliminate skin problems simply through fasting, proper nutrition and the total health plan suggested in this book. It is surprising how much improvement can occur by these measures alone.

The homeopathic remedies listed below can also provide a real boost to healing. However, severe cases often require individualized treatment beyond the scope of this discussion; seek out a veterinarian who is skillful in the use of homeopathy, acupuncture or other alternative therapies.

The most difficult conditions to treat are those previously dosed with lots of cortisone or its synthetic forms (azium, depo, flucort, prednisone or prednisolone). Corticosteroids effectively suppress symptoms like inflammation and itching, but are in no sense curative. You may not know if your animal has received cortisone because your veterinarian may have used terms like *anti-itch shots* or *flea allergy pills.* They usually look like clear or milky-white injections or little pink or white tablets. If you have good communication with your veterinarian, ask if he or she is giving your pet steroids. Generally, a natural approach will not work well if you also continue cortisone therapy.

Another typical treatment is a series of allergy desensitization injections with solutions made from the common flea or other suspected allergens. Sometimes they help, but often as not the relief is partial and not as satisfactory as eliminating the problem entirely.

TREATMENT

For an animal with acutely inflamed, irritated skin ("hot spots"), that is otherwise in good condition, start with a fast. Use the directions in chapter 15, breaking the fast after five to seven days for a dog, and after three to five days for a cat. This fast mimics natural conditions in which wild predators' bodies have a chance to clean out between hunts. It also removes the demand on the system to both digest food and deal with the disorder at the same time.

Afterward, carefully introduce natural foods, as described in chapters 3 and 4. This healthier diet will supply needed nutrients and help to rebuild damaged tissue. Be sure all your ingredients are fresh and of high quality. Emphasize raw foods as much as possible.

The standard supplements in our diet are all helpful for skin problems, but the following will be especially useful. Be sure to include nutritional yeast and granular lecithin (both found in the Healthy Powder, page 39), cod-liver oil, cold-pressed unsaturated vegetable oil and vitamin E (or wheat-germ capsules). It would also be wise to include 5 to 20 milligrams daily of chelated zinc. In addition, vitamin C is very helpful—give 500 to 2,000 milligrams a day, depending on your dog's size (see page 226).

It helps to clip away the hair on severely inflamed areas and give a bath with nonirritating soap (*not* a medicated flea soap; use a natural organic soap as in chapter 7). After drying the skin, apply a poultice or wash the area frequently with a preparation of black or green tea. It supplies tannic acid, which helps to dry up the moist places. Two to three times a day, or as needed, you also can smear on some vitamin E oil or fresh aloe vera gel (from the living plant or in a liquid preparation found in a health food store).

Useful homeopathic remedies include:

Homeopathic—*Graphites 6X (a form of carbon):* Use "Homeopathic Schedule 1" on page 348. This remedy is indicated when the "hot spots" ooze a sticky, thick discharge, about the consistency of honey.

Homeopathic—*Mercurius vivus (or solubilis) 6X (mercury):* Use "Homeopathic Schedule 1" on page 348. Use this one if there's a puslike, yellowish or greenish discharge. Also, the hair will tend to fall out around the eruptions, leaving raw, bleeding areas. The condition is usually worse in hot weather or in very warm living quarters.

Homeopathic—*Rhus toxicodendron 6X (poison ivy, poison oak):* Use "Homeopathic Schedule 1" on page 348. Give this medicine to a dog that has very intense itching with redness and much swelling of the affected skin. Also, the animal may feel better from warmth, though this is not always the case.

Homeopathic—*Arsenicum album 30C:* This remedy suits dogs with skin eruptions that cause a great deal of restlessness and discomfort. They seem to be driven almost insane—constantly chewing, licking and scratching. The skin lesions are very red and dry with loss of hair and an "eating away" of the skin leaving angry red sores. Especially indicated if the dog becomes very thirsty as well. Use "Homeopathic Schedule 2" on page 348.

For the animal with a long-term, low-grade condition of itchy, greasy or dry and scaly skin (who may also have an underactive thyroid), start by fasting it one day every week, offering only broth (see chapter 15). The rest of the time feed only natural foods and supplements. It's important that you don't give any commercial foods or supplements with questionable ingredients (see chapter 2) because part of your pet's problem may be a hypersensitivity or allergy to artificial additives or processed ingredients. For example, many animals will have allergic reactions to cooked, but not raw, meat.

If the skin is greasy and foul-smelling, bathe your pet as often as once a week, as described in chapter 7. If the skin is dry, bathe less often. Also be sure to control fleas (see "Skin Parasites"), using the lemon rinse described in chapter 7.

Constipation or sluggish bowels may also be contributing to the problem. If they are, address that first. Use one of the following two remedies.

Herbal—*Garlic (Allium sativum):* Give daily ¼ to 1 whole clove (fresh grated or minced) or 1 to 3 small garlic capsules. You can continue giving garlic indefinitely, as it also discourages fleas.

Homeopathic—*Nux vomica 3X:* Give 1 tablet before each meal, as needed, until bowels are regular (see also "Constipation").

If constipation or "hot spots" are not the present problem, then try working with one of these treatments.

Homeopathic—*Sulphur 6X (the element sulphur):* Use "Homeopathic Schedule 6(b)" on page 349. This remedy is very helpful for the average case of dry, itchy skin, especially if your dog tends to be thin, "lazy" and not very clean, with red-looking eyes, nose or lips. These animals generally don't like a lot of heat but sometimes will seek out a warm stove in cooler weather.

Homeopathic—*Pulsatilla 6X:* Use "Homeopathic Schedule 6(b)" on page 349. Those animals needing this medicine will be easy-going, good natured and affectionate. Their symptoms tend to be worse when eating rich or fatty food, and it is noticed that they rarely drink water. Often there is a preference for lying on cool surfaces as well.

Homeopathic—*Graphites 6X (a form of carbon):* Use "Homeopathic Schedule 6(b)" on page 349. These dogs tend to be overweight, constipated and easily overheated. Eruptions ooze sticky fluid. The skin is easily inflamed, even by slight injuries like scratches, and it does not heal easily. The ears can be plagued with irritation, a bad smell and waxy discharge.

Homeopathic—*Thuya occidentalis 30C (arborvitae):* Use "Homeopathic Schedule 4" on page 348. This remedy is an antidote to illness following vaccinations. Many of the animals I treat developed their skin problems within a few weeks after being vaccinated. I find that giving this remedy occasionally during treatment really helps such dogs recover. Another time to consider Thuya is when other medicines have not done much good. If so, giving Thuya and then going back to one of the above remedies will sometimes result in progress.

Tissue Salt—*Silicea 6X (silicon dioxide):* Indicated for the animal that gets little pimples, discharges pus or has inflammations around the nails. Use "Homeopathic Schedule 6(b)" on page 349.

Note: In general, these deeply ingrained skin conditions require patience and persistence. You will usually see clear, beneficial effects from the program within six to eight weeks.

Because vaccines tend to aggravate the condition, it is very important to avoid them during the treatment period. Sometimes medicines like those used for heartworm prevention will set off an attack. In this case it is best to use the monthly type of heartworm medication and give it only every six weeks (or stop using it altogether in severe cases).

Some obstinate cases will not completely recover no matter how long you treat them (though they will generally improve). These need more individualized treatment with other homeopathic remedies or one of the holistic approaches described in chapter 14. If you can, find a skilled professional to help.

For the animal suffering hair loss, try a slightly different program. Sometimes a pet will just begin to lose hair without any other apparent problem. Or the hair loss could be the result of poisoning—not necessarily the intentional kind, but rather the accumulation of toxic substances that may affect sensitive individuals. Common agents to consider include fluoride (in some drinking water and commercial pet foods; see chapter 8) and aluminum (from use of aluminum bowls or cooking utensils). Sensitivity to aluminum seems to vary, and not all animals show this reaction. Those that are poisoned by aluminum tend to have constipation problems as well.

It is also possible for hair loss to reflect a disturbance in the endocrine glands or a deficiency of a certain nutrient. If your veterinarian has diagnosed either of these problems, then feed only the natural diet with added kelp powder. This is particularly important because the powder's iodine content will help to stimulate the thyroid. Give ½ to 2 teaspoons of kelp powder daily (amounts depend on your animal's size). In addition, give 250 to 1,000 milligrams of vitamin C twice a day to aid detoxification and 5 to 20 milligrams of chelated zinc once a day to enhance the elimination of heavy metals. Discontinue use of aluminum utensils and fluoridated water (call your water company to find out if your tap water is so treated; if it is, use bottled or spring water).

If you have addressed all these things—nutrition, toxicity, water pollution—and your animal still has hair loss (not caused by scratching or chewing it out), then try these homeopathic remedies.

Homeopathic—*Thuya occidentalis 30C (arborvitae):* Use "Homeopathic Schedule 5" on page 349. Try Thuya first because it is an antidote to the effects of vaccination, which is the primary reason for a persistently poor hair coat or for poor hair growth. (Sometimes the hair loss is at a normal level, but the real problem is that no new hair grows in to replace it; in such a case this remedy is especially suitable.)

Homeopathic—*Selenium 30C (the element selenium)*: Use "Homeopathic Schedule 5" on page 349. Indicated for excessive hair loss with no new growth, especially if there are no other symptoms of illness. Use it after trying Thuya (above) if that remedy has not been sufficient to resolve the problem.

If an animal develops the hair loss soon after giving birth, then use:

Homeopathic—*Sepia 30C (ink of the cuttlefish)*: Use "Homeopathic Schedule 4" on page 348.

SPAYING AND NEUTERING

Spaying is a surgery to remove a female's ovaries and uterus to prevent pregnancy and to eliminate her heats (periods of sexual receptivity). Neutering, or castration, removes a male's testes (leaving the scrotum, or sac) to prevent reproduction and to reduce aggression, wandering and territorial behaviors. Both operations are performed painlessly under anesthesia, and recovery is usually rapid and uneventful. Natural treatments can help ease the process.

If your pet is slow to wake up, groggy or nauseous after surgery, give:

Homeopathic—*Phosphorus 30C (the element phosphorus)*: Use "Homeopathic Schedule 4," page 348. Response is usually fast—from a few minutes to an hour.

If your pet has discomfort, pain or restless behavior on returning home, try:

Homeopathic—*Arnica 30C (mountain daisy)*: Use "Homeopathic Schedule 2," page 348. In addition to Arnica, I often use

Dr. Bach's rescue formula (see page 218), 2 drops 4 times a day for 2 to 3 days.

For any red irritation or a discharge of fluid or pus around the skin sutures give:

Homeopathic—*Apis mellifica 6C (honeybee venom)*: Use "Homeopathic Schedule 1," page 348. Also bathe the incision site in a mixture of 10 drops of Calendula tincture, ¼ teaspoon sea salt and 1 cup of pure water. Dip a warm washcloth in the solution and hold it against the incision for a few minutes 3 or 4 times a day.

Extra vitamins A, E and C are also useful after any surgery to help detoxify anesthetics and drugs. My standard regimen, regardless of size, is 10,000 IU of A, 100 IU of E and 250 milligrams of C, all given once a day for three days both before and after surgery.

DOES THIS SURGERY DO HARM?

Some people are concerned about the health effects of such a major surgical alteration. Although it is surely a major intervention, the best I can say at this point in time is that neutering does not seem to cause major health problems or increase incidence of such common problems as skin allergies or cystitis. Most neutered dogs and cats live long and healthy lives. Some do tend to become less active, to act less aggressively (a benefit) and perhaps to gain weight. Any obesity often follows indulgent feeding and lack of regular exercise.

On the other hand, I *have* seen more obvious harmful effects when neutering is used as a medical treatment for prolonged heats, cystic ovaries, infertility problems, spontaneous abortions, vaginitis, infections and the like. These reproductive problems are the result of chronic ill health. Simply removing the affected organs will not really cure the underlying state. So the animal later develops other symptoms that are really the same disease with a different focus.

When pets have reproductive health problems, I first recommend nutritional therapy and homeopathy, assuming that it's not an emergency and we still have some time. If this is not effective, surgery is still an option. However, if we are successful, as we often are, the chronic disease is cured. Then the animal can be neutered for the usual reasons without any long-term problem.

What *are* the reasons to neuter a healthy animal? A female dog or cat comes into heat two or more times a year. Preventing her from breeding is demanding, frustrating to your animal and a potential source of health problems (see "Pyometra," page 297). Allowing her to breed adds to the tremendous animal overpopulation problem. Repeated breeding can also drain her health (see pages 293-296). Spaying also reduces her risk for breast cancer.

Neutering reduces the havoc wreaked by intact males—property damage, fights, the smell and stain of territorial marking, accidents caused when they wander onto public roadways, and packs that attack or threaten other animals or even people. By contrast, a neutered male is typically more affectionate and gentle, making a better companion.

The best time for surgery is after a pet reaches sexual maturity, which insures the least effect on the neuro-endocrine system and allows full development of a normal adult body shape. Most females reach this point at age 6 to 8 months, most males at 9 to 12 months.

Some animals mature later, however, so you may want to wait until the signs are clear. For a female this means after her first heat (keep her carefully confined to prevent pregnancy). A male cat matures when his urine develops an odor and he begins to show signs of territorial spraying of urine. The male dog will begin to lift one leg to urinate (and mark territory), mount other dogs, fight, roam and become more aggressive. The risk of waiting, however, is contributing to the overwhelming surplus of puppies and kittens. In most cases plan to neuter females at six to seven months and males at nine to ten months.

There are really no safe alternatives to neutering surgically. Over the years, various hormones and drugs have been used to prevent females from coming into heat or to stimulate abortion if necessary. These drugs always cause some problems, however, and they are soon pulled off the market. Perhaps a safe alternative to neutering will be found someday, but there is nothing out there now that I can recommend.

So if you are vacillating over having your animal altered, my advice is to wait no longer. If you're worried about money, contact a nearby low-cost spay/neuter clinic or call your local humane society for information about special reduced-fee programs arranged with area veterinarians.

STOMACH PROBLEMS

The stomach has its share of upsets, usually from eating the wrong kind of food (spoiled, tainted, indigestible) or too much food. (Beware the greedy eater!) However, stomach problems also can indicate a wide variety of other disorders—such as infectious diseases, kidney failure, hepatitis, pancreatitis, colitis (inflammation of the lower bowel), something foreign that doesn't belong in the stomach (swallowed toys, string, hair) and problems like worms.

Be aware that problems in other areas of the body can also cause symptoms like vomiting, nausea and lack of appetite, fooling you into thinking that only the stomach is involved. Have your veterinarian make a diagnosis, especially if vomiting is persistent or severe, which may indicate a serious, even life-threatening, problem.

Here we will discuss three common problems that are centered in the stomach itself: acute gastritis (sudden upset), chronic gastritis (low-grade, persistent upset) and gastric dilation (swelling with gas, sometimes causing the stomach to twist shut). The suggestions offered are alternative treatments for those animals newly diagnosed as having these problems or animals that have them repeatedly so that ways to deal with this other than the usual drugs are needed.

Acute Gastritis

Gastritis is a term that means inflammation (not infection) of the stomach. *Acute* signifies that the attack is sudden, appearing in a few minutes or hours. The most common sufferer is the dog that likes to raid garbage cans or to eat dead animals found on roads or in the woods (cats, being more finicky, rarely have this as a cause). As partial scavengers, dogs often scrounge about in garbage cans and consume an extraordinary mixture of foods (often spoiled) that just don't sit well in the stomach. Compost piles are another common source of spoiled treasures.

The vomiting (and usually diarrhea) that follows is the body's attempt to right the wrong by getting rid of the noxious material. Some dogs instinctively try to remedy things by eating grass, which stimulates vomiting. This behavior also occurs in animals with low-grade stomach irritation.

Another cause of acute gastritis is eating indigestible material like large bone fragments. This is mostly a problem for dogs not used to eating bones or the result of their consuming *cooked* bones (which are more apt to splinter) or inedible materials such as cloth, plastic, metal, rubber toys, golf balls and the like. If bones are causing the problem, give your pet only large *raw* bones and give extra B vitamins to dogs to ensure adequate stomach acid. Supervise carefully. If your dog keeps trying to swallow large pieces, it's best not to trust him with bones.

Indigestible foreign objects often require surgical removal, though sometimes they can be retrieved by passing a tube into the stomach. Cats may swallow sewing thread or yarn; if there is a needle attached, it can get caught up in the mouth or tongue while the thread passes down into the intestine. The unpleasant result can be a "crawling" of the intestine up along the thread, which is often fatal unless corrected quickly.

To help prevent your pet from swallowing such objects, don't let them play by themselves with any toy or object that could cause problems.

TREATMENT

If you suspect that your animal has swallowed something dangerous, get professional help within a few hours or serious complications can arise. If you aren't sure what was swallowed, do not encourage vomiting. It would be too traumatic and dangerous for the object to come up if it is sharp, pointed or very large. Such objects must be removed surgically. Meanwhile, you can use the treatment below to discourage vomiting.

If you know, however, that the swallowed material is small and not sharp or irregular, vomiting may expel the object, so you can allow the vomiting to proceed while you are waiting to see the vet.

The remedy that is useful for discouraging vomiting because of objects in the stomach is:

Homeopathic—*Phosphorus 30C (the element phosphorus):* Use "Homeopathic Schedule 2," page 348. The vomiting is often associated with taking in water—occurring about 10 to 15 minutes after drinking. This remedy will relieve the vomiting for a while, but most likely the foreign material will need to be removed (see above).

The following treatments will help for a simple acute gastritis *not* caused by foreign bodies. The symptoms are: pain in the abdomen (it hurts the animal when you press its stomach, the animal doubles up with cramps, sits hunched and acts depressed), vomiting or attempts to vomit, vomiting after eating or drinking, salivation, excessive drinking of water and eating grass.

First, withhold all food for at least 24 hours and then reintroduce it slowly in small quantities. See the fasting instructions in chapter 15. Make fresh, pure water available at all times or, if vomiting is part of the problem, offer one or more ice cubes to lick every couple of hours. (You don't want to aggravate vomiting and stomach irritation by encouraging too much drinking.)

Many dogs and cats will also eat grass to make themselves vomit when the stomach is upset. This is a natural response and is appropriate behavior at the beginning of a stomach upset. If the problem is not quickly resolved, however, eating grass only makes the situation worse.

As a supplementary treatment make chamomile tea. Pour a cup of boiling water over a tablespoon of the flowers, steep 15 minutes, strain, and dilute with an equal quantity of water. If the tea isn't accepted, just make the ice available. This treatment will suffice for mild upsets.

For more serious upsets one of the following is useful:

Herbal—*Peppermint (Mentha piperira):* Use "Herbal Schedule 1" on page 346. This is a good herbal treatment for dogs (cats don't like mint) and is often readily available.

Herbal—*Goldenseal (hydrastis canadensis):* Use "Herbal Schedule 1" on page 346. This very useful herb is indicated when what is vomited up is thick, yellowish and "ropy" (for example, thick strands).

Homeopathic—*Nux vomica 6C (poison nut):* Use "Homeopathic Schedule 1," page 348. Especially indicated for the dog or cat that acts ill with the vomiting and wants to go off by itself rather than seek company. This remedy also suits the animal that is sick from overeating.

Homeopathic—*Pulsatilla 6C (windflower):* Use "Homeopathic Schedule 1," page 348. Indicated for the dog or cat that wants attention and comfort, especially if it is not interested in drinking. Animals requiring this remedy often are made ill by eating food that is rich or fatty.

Homeopathic—*Ipecac 6C (ipecac root):* Use "Homeopathic Schedule 1," page 348. Useful where there is almost constant nausea and vomiting, especially if the problem was brought on by indigestible food or if there is blood in the vomit.

Homeopathic—*Arsenicum album 6C (arsenic trioxide):* Use "Homeopathic Schedule 1," page 348. This remedy is par excellence for gastritis brought on by spoiled meat (or spoiled food in general).

Homeopathic—*Belladonna 6C (deadly nightshade):* Use "Homeopathic Schedule 1," page 348. This is good for the animal that is primarily feverish, with dilated pupils and excitability.

Tissue Salt—*Magnesia phosphorica 6X (magnesium phosphate):* Use "Homeopathic Schedule 1," page 348. Indicated where there seem to be cramps (doubling up) every few minutes.

Chronic Gastritis

Some animals develop a long-term tendency to have digestive upsets, often after eating and sometimes once every few days. This can follow inadequate recovery from a previous severe attack of acute gastritis or may result from emotional stress, poor-quality or disagreeable food, drug toxicity or infections like feline infectious peritonitis or hepatitis. It can also be a part of an allergy problem, and many dogs and cats with skin eruptions will also have inflammation of the stomach and intestines. Sometimes there is no apparent cause.

Symptoms are poor digestion, a tendency to vomit, pain, depression or hiding (either immediately after eating or an hour or so later), loss of appetite and gas. Many animals with chronic gastritis eat grass in an attempt to stimulate vomiting and cleansing of the stomach.

TREATMENT

The first and foremost treatment I recommend is to put the animal on a natural diet. I can't overemphasize the importance of a good diet because the illness may be the result of the very food your pet has been eating. Also, be sure to read the discussion under "Allergies" to understand this possible underlying cause and to see recipes that you could use.

A further treatment might include *one* of the following, as indicated.

Herbal—*Goldenseal (Hydrastis canadensis):* Good for weak digestion, poor appetite and weight loss. Use "Herbal Schedule 2" on page 347.

Herbal—*Garlic (Allium sativum):* Especially useful for an animal that has a good appetite but gets upset with changes in the diet or is prone to gas and constipation. Make a cold extract by soaking 4 to 6 chopped cloves in ½ cup of cold water for 8 hours. Strain. Give ½ teaspoon to 1 tablespoon 3 times a day until the problem is relieved.

Homeopathic—There are several homeopathic medicines that are helpful for acute gastritis (discussed above) that are also helpful for the chronic condition. Sometimes the acute episode is the beginning of an illness that will turn out to be long-lasting, though, of course, you can't know that at the beginning. Look over the remedies for acute gastritis, as any of them can be useful when the animal has the same indications as given there.

The main difference to understand is that with the chronic form of illness, the symptoms are often not as marked or as intense as in the acute stage, though the indications for the remedy are still there. For example,

Pulsatilla is a frequently needed medicine. As with the acute condition, you may notice that your pet has become more "clingy," wanting attention. In addition, he may drink a lesser amount of water, but still some. None of these symptoms, however, will stand out as strongly as when they are seen in the acute form.

Consider, in particular, the remedies Arsenicum album, Nux vomica and Pulsatilla.

An additional remedy that was not mentioned before is:

Tissue Salt—*Natrum muriaticum 6X (sodium chloride):* Useful for the cat that has excessive hunger, is thirsty and has discomfort after eating. Also good for stomach problems associated with worms. Use "Homeopathic Schedule 6(a)," page 349.

Gastric Dilation (Bloat)

This serious problem is seen mostly in the larger dog breeds (especially the Great Dane, St. Bernard and Borzoi). Its cause is unknown, though veterinarians have found it to be linked with the feeding of commercial foods (especially large meals of concentrated dry forms of food). It occurs most often in dogs between the ages of two and ten years, and most often at night.

The symptoms of the condition are that approximately two to six hours after eating, the stomach (upper abdominal area) gets enlarged with liquid and gas and sometimes feels like a tight drum. Most often, you will see excessive salivation, drooling, unsuccessful attempts to vomit, extreme restlessness and discomfort, desperate attempts to eat grass and, eventually, weakness and collapse.

This is an emergency situation because the increased pressure on the walls of the stomach causes fluids to leak in from the blood with consequent dehydration, shock and possible death in a few hours. Another complication is that the stomach can rotate on itself—in a condition called volvulus—and the twisting can completely block entry into or exit from the organ. Immediate surgery is required in this instance.

PREVENTION

Feeding a natural, home-prepared diet seems to be the best way to avert such problems. Feed two or three small meals a day instead of a single one.

Especially avoid feeding dry food or concentrated foods that will absorb water after they are eaten. The dog will eat more than its capacity, and when the food becomes distended with water, the total weight of the food is greatly increased. This can prevent the stomach from its natural emptying and also increase the chance of the stomach twisting around and blocking the movement of food out of it.

Regular exercise which strengthens the muscles and "massages" the stomach and bowels is extremely helpful.

TREATMENT

When gastric dilation first occurs it is rather sudden and can be shocking. Sometimes the only thing noticed is that the dog is restless and desperately eating grass. If you look closely, you may see that the animal's belly is larger than normal, distended with gas.

Get to your veterinarian as soon as possible. If the condition is one of just stomach dilation, it can be temporarily relieved at the hospital by passing a tube into the stomach.

However, the condition tends to recur. Each time the attack comes on sooner and with more severity. Eventually, the animal is put to sleep because of the apparent hopelessness of the situation and the high cost of repeated medical measures.

If there is also volvulus, then surgery must be done to straighten out the twisted stomach and allow open passages in and out. The stomach wall is also "tacked down" by suturing it to the inside of the abdominal wall to prevent it from twisting in the future.

Even though you must see your veterinarian immediately, it is still appropriate for me to give you some treatment suggestions because there will be times when you cannot get veterinary service immediately; further, the condition tends to recur and you will become aware of the early signs. If you can intervene with treatment soon enough, it is possible to head off an attack. But it's important to remember that these treatments should never be considered a substitute for veterinary attention.

One of the easiest and most available herbal treatments is one discovered by one of my clients, Betty Lewis of Amherst, New Hampshire. She breeds Great Danes and has found that freshly made raw cabbage juice is an effective treatment at the beginning of bloat and has used it successfully many times.

Herbal—*Cabbage (Brassica oleracea):* This plant is a member of the mustard family. Reduce fresh cabbage leaves to a liquid (with a juicer); do not add water. Give 1 to 2 ounces of this as a dose (to large breeds, less to smaller animals), repeating the treatment if symptoms return later.

Because of vomiting and the pressure closing off the opening to the stomach, I use primarily homeopathic preparations. The pellets or tablets will act especially quickly, even if not swallowed, if they are first crushed to a powder (between folded heavy paper) and placed on the tongue.

Of course, you will need to plan ahead and order these in advance since you will need them immediately. (See "Suppliers of Homeopathic Remedies," on page 354, for information on obtaining a homeopathic emergency kit.)

Homeopathic—*Nux moschata 30C (nutmeg):* This remedy is indicated for the dog with a greatly enlarged abdomen, belching or passing of gas, unsuccessful attempts to vomit, a dry mouth or thick saliva, legs that feel cool to the touch, disorientation, dizziness or sleepiness. Give a dose of 3 crushed pellets every 15 minutes for a total of 3 treatments.

Homeopathic—*Nux vomica 30C (poison nut):* Best for the dog that becomes withdrawn, irritable and chilly. This is the best treatment when the stomach has become twisted. Give a dose of 3 crushed pellets every 15 minutes for a total of 3 treatments.

Homeopathic—*Carbo vegetabilis 30C (charcoal):* Dogs needing this remedy will be greatly distended with gas and look very ill with cold legs and ears and bluish color to the tongue and gums. It is suitable for the state of shock that accompanies this condition. Give a dose of 3 crushed pellets every 15 minutes for a total of 3 treatments.

Other dogs that may benefit from this homeopathic remedy will have a less severe kind of attack. However, they will already have had at least one serious episode from which they have not fully recovered. Thus you'll see a pattern of recurring indigestion and gas, with periodic swelling of the animal's stomach that causes breathing difficulty. This state of chronic ill health will produce progressive weakening, low energy and a cold body. Use "Homeopathic Schedule 4," page 348, and, for this chronic condition, give the treatment at a time when there is no crisis.

Homeopathic—*Silicea 6X:* Use "Homeopathic Schedule 6(b)" on page 349. Here is another treatment to use between crises with the idea of preventing further attacks. It is indicated for the dog that has a history of skin or ear eruptions with itching and discomfort. Sometimes this history is not very apparent; the original skin problem may have been suppressed in the past and no longer be remembered. If this treatment is successful, the stomach will improve and the skin eruption will come back for a while. Further treatment may then be necessary to resolve this condition. (See "Skin Problems.")

Homeopathic—*Raphanus 30C (black garden radish):* This is most useful when there is tremendous bloating with an inability for the gas to come up (as "burps") or go down (flatulence). Give a dose of 3 crushed pellets every 15 minutes for a total of 3 treatments.

Note: If you see favorable results with one of these treatments, bear in mind that using drugs like tranquilizers, antibiotics, stimulants or depressants immediately after a positive homeopathic response will very likely cancel out the favorable response and lead to a return of the original condition.

For this reason, minimize or eliminate such treatment if the homeopathic remedies are doing the job.

STONES

See "Bladder Problems."

TEETH

See "Dental Problems."

TICKS

See "Skin Parasites."

TOXOPLASMOSIS

This disease deserves to be discussed in some detail, not so much because of its importance to cats (which usually recover from it without treatment, very often without any symptoms), but because of its importance to unborn children. If a woman is infected for the first time during pregnancy, the fetus may be born prematurely, born with serious damage to the brain, eyes or other parts of the body or stillborn. Such problems are estimated to occur in 2 to 6 out of every 1,000 births in the United States.

Before we consider this disease further, first let's put things in perspective. The toxoplasma protozoa infest almost all species of mammals and birds in the world. Infection ranges from 20 to 80 percent of all domestic animals, depending on geographical area. In the United States about 50 percent of the human population is also infected. But, despite the widespread occurrence of this little parasite, few infected individuals actually get sick from it. People who do get clinically ill are those whose immune systems have been suppressed as a response to drugs used with organ grafts or by cancer chemotherapy or x-ray therapy. People who have an immuno-suppressive disease like AIDS may also get clinically ill with toxoplasmosis.

Cats are unique in that they are natural hosts for the parasite—toxoplasmosis grows better in cats than in any other animal. Those who do show symptoms will have mucus or blood-tinged diarrhea, fever, hepatitis (liver inflammation) or pneumonia (difficult breathing). They usually get over it on their own, developing a strong immunity that protects against further infection.

Commonly, both cat and human can acquire the parasite and have no symptoms whatsoever. Here is where the danger lies: About one to three weeks after infection, the cat will often start passing oocysts, egglike structures that can infect other individuals after a day or so of further development in the warm feces or soil. The cat passes these oocysts until it develops immunity—in about two weeks. (If its immune system is depressed with cortisone-like drugs, however, the process can start up again.) These eggs can then be picked up by a pregnant woman who has not already had a chance to develop her own immunity. Thus, the disease spreads to the fetus, where it can cause the serious problems already mentioned.

Here are the ways this organism can infect pregnant women (and other people):

- ◆ A bit of cat feces is accidentally ingested during the two weeks of oocyst shedding.
- ◆ By some mischance, soil used as a bathroom within the previous year by an infected cat is consumed.
- ◆ Infected raw or undercooked meat is prepared or eaten. This is actually the most common route of entry for both people and cats. And though you may deny your cat raw meat as a protective measure, remember that freshly caught mice and birds ain't cooked!

If you think about it, the possibilities for the spreading of the disease are pretty great. For instance, while changing a litter box, digging in the garden or cleaning a sandbox you might wipe your mouth. Or, after doing one of these jobs, you might eat something before you've washed your hands. Does your cat walk from the litter box to your kitchen counter, table or your pillow? Do you fix salad on the same board used to trim raw meat? You can see why such a large proportion of the population is infected.

Now all this is not meant to scare you. If you are among the 25 to 45 percent of women in the United States aged 20 to 39 who are already exposed and therefore immune to problems from this organism, you needn't worry about it at all; you won't pass it on to your unborn child. Your doctor can perform a serum test to find out if you're in this group. Your cat can also be tested to see if it has developed an immunity from previous infection. If so, he won't pass oocysts in his stool anymore, and the danger to you is much less.

If neither you nor your mate has developed an immunity by the time you conceive, take special precautions for the next nine months. Don't feed your cat raw meat. If you eat meat yourself, be careful to prepare it separately from foods to be eaten raw, like salads. Wash your hands well after any meat preparation, cat-petting, gardening and the like.

Unless you know that your cat already is immune, use gloves when you clean the litter box and wash up afterward. Better yet, have someone else clean the litter box. Dispose of the contents in a sealed container (not on the ground). If you want to disinfect the pan, rinse it with boiling water. Also control flies and cockroaches, because they can carry oocysts from the cat's feces onto food.

If you wanted to keep your cat from getting toxoplasmosis in the first place (assuming he hasn't already had it), you would have to make some serious compromises. Raw meat, for example, is nutritionally superior to cooked, but to prevent toxoplasmosis, you'd always have to cook it. You also would have to keep your cat from hunting and keep him away from any soil possibly contaminated by other cats. Obviously, the only way you can manage these restrictions is by keeping him inside all the time, which is not such a healthy solution. The choice is yours, of course, but with reasonable precautions you will have a much better idea what risks you really face.

If your cat is diagnosed with this problem, in addition to what your veterinarian prescribes, you can use the advice given here. Go to the section of this Quick Reference guide that discusses the symptoms you see (for example, diarrhea), and follow those instructions.

UPPER RESPIRATORY INFECTIONS ("COLDS")

The upper respiratory tract, which includes the nose, throat, larynx (voice box) and trachea (windpipe), is one of the favorite highways for germs traveling inside the body. Many microorganisms and viruses dry out and masquerade as dust. Others are embedded in dried secretions and scabs, which break into small particles and get stirred up into inhaled air.

In animals these coldlike illnesses often start and remain in the upper respiratory tract, causing such symptoms as a runny nose or eyes, sneezing, a sore throat, coughing and, sometimes, inflammation of the mouth. These infections resemble the human cold in many ways but have some unique aspects for pets. The three most common upper respiratory diseases found in companion animals are canine infectious tracheobronchitis (often called kennel cough), feline viral rhinotracheitis (FVR—a viral attack on the cat's eyes and upper respiratory tract) and feline calicivirus (similar to FVR, but generally less involved with the eyes and nose). (Distemper is covered as a separate entry in this Quick Reference guide.)

Canine Infectious Tracheobronchitis

Also known as kennel cough or canine respiratory disease complex, canine infectious tracheobronchitis is thought to be caused by a variety of viruses and sometimes complicated by bacterial infection as well. It's common where many stressed dogs, especially young ones, are in close contact. It crops up in boarding kennels, animal shelters, grooming establishments, veterinary hospitals, dog shows and pet shops.

Symptoms, which usually appear about eight to ten days after exposure, are typically a dry, hacking, awful-sounding cough that ends with gagging or retching, and perhaps a clear, watery discharge from the eyes and nose or a partial loss of appetite. Though it sounds awful, it's not a serious condition. A minimal number of dogs may have complications because of their weak immune systems.

TREATMENT

Antibiotics are not recommended in most cases because the disease is viral. Often cough suppressants are used, but they do not help much and can have unpleasant side effects. The most effective thing to do is to place the affected dog in a steam-filled room (such as a bathroom with a tub full of hot water or after running a hot shower) or in a room with a cold-mist vaporizer. Veterinarians recognize this as a disease that just has to "run its course" (two or three weeks) before recovery. If possible, isolate your dog, since some of these viruses may also affect cats and people.

You can assist the healing process by putting your pet on a fast, giving vitamins and using an herbal cough treatment.

A liquid fast can be useful when the symptoms first appear and should be continued for three days. Follow the directions for fasting in chapter 15, taking care to reintroduce solid foods carefully and slowly.

Vitamins help in several ways. Vitamin C is a good antiviral agent. Depending on the size of your dog, you can give 500 to 1,000 milligrams three times a day. Vitamin E stimulates the immune response. Give 50 to 100 IU of fresh d-alpha tocopherol from a capsule three times a day. Puncture the capsule and squeeze the oil right into the dog's mouth. Taper off frequency at recovery. Vitamin A also boosts immunity, helps counteract stress and strengthens the mucous membranes of the respiratory tract. Use ¼ to 1 teaspoon of fresh cod-liver oil three times a day (depending on the animal's size) or give a 10,000 IU capsule of vitamin A once a day. Treat for a total of five days with vitamin A.

Herbal treatment can consist of an herbal cough syrup available at health food stores; adjust the recommended dose to your animal's size. Such preparations typically contain several of the following: wild cherry bark, licorice, comfrey root, coltsfoot, mullein, slippery elm and horehound.

Alternatively, you can make your own herbal treatments.

Herbal—*Peppermint (Mentha piperita):* This is best suited for the dog with a hoarse "voice" and with coughing made worse by barking. Touching his throat is irritating and may bring on the cough. Use "Herbal Schedule 1" on page 346.

Herbal—*Mullein (Verbascum thapsus):* Especially indicated where the cough is deep and hoarse and worse at night. It's also useful when the throat seems sore to the touch or there is trouble swallowing. Use "Herbal Schedule 1" on page 346.

After recovery your dog should be relatively immune for some time, perhaps a year or two. However, a different but similar virus could re-create the "same" condition. Remember, stress seems to be the necessary factor to allow the virus to get established.

Feline Viral Rhinotracheitis (FVR)

This viral disease primarily affects the eyes and upper respiratory tract of cats. Symptoms include sneezing attacks, coughing, drooling of thick saliva, fever and a watery discharge from the eyes. The condition ranges from mild and barely noticeable to severe and persistent. In the latter the nose gets plugged up with a thick discharge, ulcers form on the eye surface (cornea) and the eyelids stick together with heavy discharges. The cat becomes thoroughly miserable, refusing to eat and unable to care for itself.

There is no allopathic treatment which shortens the duration of the disease, but usually antibiotics, fluid therapy, forced feeding, eye ointments and other measures are used to provide the best possible support for the ailing body. These cats are so out of sorts, however, that they often resist handling and treatments. It can be a real challenge to provide adequate care.

TREATMENT

If you catch the condition early, this regimen may avert the more serious stage: Give no solid food the first two to three days or until the temperature is back to normal (less than 101.5°F). The cat usually will not eat anyway. Instead, provide liquids as described in the section on fasting in chapter 15. Give vitamin C (⅛ teaspoon sodium ascorbate powder dissolved in pure water, every four

hours), vitamin E (50 IU twice a day) and vitamin A (½ teaspoon cod-liver oil or 2,000 to 2,500 IU vitamin A from fish-liver oil sources, once a day). Treat with vitamin A a total of five days so as not to overdo it (too much vitamin A can be a problem).

Homeopathic—*Aconitum napellus 30C (monkshood):* This remedy corresponds to the early stages of illness, which are marked by fever and a general sense of not feeling well. If given when these symptoms first appear, it may avert any further development of the illness. Use "Homeopathic Schedule 2," page 348.

If the cold condition is already established, one of these remedies may help.

Homeopathic—*Nux vomica 30C (poison nut):* A remedy commonly suited to this condition, Nux vomica is a good choice for the cat that is grouchy and averse to being held or touched. Often it will retire to a quiet room so as not to be disturbed. Use "Homeopathic Schedule 2," page 348.

Homeopathic—*Natrum muriaticum 6C:* This remedy is most helpful when the cold starts with much sneezing. As it develops there may be thirstiness and a white discharge from the nose. Use "Homeopathic Schedule 1," page 348.

Homeopathic—*Pulsatilla 30C (windflower):* Cats needing this medicine are sleepy, sluggish and have a thick discharge from the nose or eyes. Often the discharge is greenish in color. Such a cat may want to be held or comforted. Use "Homeopathic Schedule 2," page 348.

Generally, at this stage it helps to clean the eyes and nose with a saline solution, which is similar to natural tears. Stir ¼ teaspoon of sea salt into one cup of pure water (without chlorine). Warm this to body temperature. Using a cotton ball, drip several drops into each nostril to stimulate sneezing and flushing of the nose. Also put some into each eye and carefully clean the discharge away with a tissue.

If the condition is very advanced when you start treatment, you'll need to take a different approach. Blend raw beef liver with enough water to make a soupy mix. Add two teaspoons of sodium ascorbate powder to every cup of this blend. Feed one teaspoon of this mixture every hour to provide health-boosting nutrients, including B vitamins from the liver and about 150 milligrams of vitamin C with each dose.

Clean the eyes and nose with a warm saline solution (as described above). If necessary, saturate a cloth with the solution and hold it against the nostrils briefly to soften and loosen the dried nasal discharge. Then carefully remove the discharge and continue with the saline nose flush. Put a drop of castor oil, cod-liver oil or almond oil in each eye; apply some to the nose, too (twice a day).

If your cat is not eating at this stage, you may need to force-feed it. Use the force-feeding recipe in chapter 15.

Useful treatments are:

Homeopathic—*Pulsatilla 6C (windflower):* This is useful for the cat with thick greenish or yellow discharge, an obstructed nose, loss of appetite, bad breath and a sleepy, sluggish demeanor. Often these cats will be attacked by other cats in the family when they are ill. Somehow the other cats sense a weakness. Use "Homeopathic Schedule 6(a)," page 349.

Homeopathic—*Causticum 6C (a mineral remedy):* Use this one if, along with the typical cold symptoms, the eyelids are actually stuck together from the discharge and have to be manually separated (with careful cleaning). Use "Homeopathic Schedule 6(a)," page 349.

Homeopathic—*Thuya 30C (arborvitae):* This remedy is sometimes needed if there is no response to other treatments or if the cold symptoms have come on within 3 to 4 weeks after receiving a vaccination. The nasal discharge can look very much like that described for Pulsatilla (above). Use "Homeopathic Schedule 3," page 348.

Herbal—*Goldenseal (Hydrastis canadensis):* This herb is very helpful if the nasal discharge (or discharge at the back of the throat) is very yellow and stringy. There may also be considerable loss of weight, even if the cat is still eating sufficiently. Use "Herbal Schedule 2" on page 347.

Once the cat is eating, encourage a variety of fresh and raw foods, especially meats, grated vegetables and brewer's yeast. Continue the vitamin C and eye treatment until recovery is complete.

Feline Calicivirus (FCV)

Sometimes FCV cannot be distinguished from FVR (above), but generally the nose and the eyes are not as involved. Typical signs include pneumonia and ulcers of the tongue, the roof of the mouth and the end of the nose (above the lip). This condition is very difficult to treat because the mouth is so sore that the cat resists having anything put in it. You may need to wrap the cat up in a towel during treatment to keep from getting scratched (see chapter 15).

TREATMENT

Use the same early treatment as described above for FVR. In practical terms, at this stage you may not really know which of these viruses your cat has, so don't worry about making any distinction; the treatments we are discussing are suitable for either disease.

If it is clear from the pneumonia or ulcers that you are dealing with feline calicivirus, there are a couple of other remedies that may be more suitable for this problem.

Homeopathic—*Phosphorus 30C (the element phosphorus):* Use this remedy if there is pneumonia (fever, rapid breathing, gasping, perhaps coughing). It's especially indicated if your cat desires *cold* water and vomits about 15 minutes after drinking or, with the pneumonia, prefers to lie on her right side. Use "Homeopathic Schedule 3," page 348.

Homeopathic—*Nitricum acidum 30C (nitric acid):* This remedy is indicated if the focus of the illness is ulcers in the mouth. The mouth odor is very bad, the saliva blood-tinged and the tongue red and "clean" looking (instead of heavily coated). These cats usually become very cranky and are difficult to handle or medicate. Use "Homeopathic Schedule 3," page 348.

Homeopathic—*Mercurius solubilis (or vivus) 30C (quicksilver):* Cats needing this medicine are very similar to those described just above for Nitricum acidum. The difference is that they are not so irritable, they produce more saliva and their tongues are coated with a yellow film and are often swollen, so that you can see indentations of the teeth on the edges. Use "Homeopathic Schedule 3," page 348.

Your cat is recovering from this illness once her appetite returns and she is eating well. This is the major turning point.

UREMIA

See "Kidney Failure."

VACCINATIONS

The prevention of communicable diseases by administering "weakened" forms of the germs that cause them is a very popular and strongly supported method of disease prevention. If a "live" vaccine is injected into the body, the organism will grow in the tissues and produce a sort of mini-disease that stimulates the immune response. This response is intended to protect the body against the real thing for a variable period of time—months or years. Sounds wonderful, doesn't it?

I must point out, however, that there are some problems with vaccinations that should be understood by anyone interested in a holistic health approach. There are two factors to consider: Vaccines are not always effective, and they may cause long-lasting health disturbances.

VACCINE INEFFECTIVENESS

Many people assume that vaccines are 100 percent effective. This belief can be so strong that even a veterinarian may tell you, "Your dog can't have distemper (parvovirus, hepatitis or whatever) because he was vaccinated for that disease. It must be something else." But one thing I learned from my doctoral studies in immunology is that vaccines are far from 100 percent effective. It is not just the injection of the vaccine that confers immunity; the response of the individual animal is the critical and necessary factor.

Several things can interfere with an ideal response (production of antibodies and immunity). These include vaccinating when the animal is too young; vaccinating when it is sick, weak or malnourished; using the wrong route or schedule of administration or, most important, giving the vaccine to an animal whose immune system has been depressed because of previous disease, bad inheritance or drug therapy.

For example, the routine practice of giving vaccinations at the same time a pet is undergoing anesthesia or surgery (for example, a spay operation) can introduce the vaccine organism at a time when the immune system is depressed for several weeks. It is equally unwise to use corticosteroids (to control skin itching, for instance) at the time of vaccination. The steroid acts to depress the immune response and disease resistance at the same time the vaccine challenges the body to respond vigorously to an introduced organism.

Even if your animal does have a good vaccine response and develops antibodies, there is no guarantee the disease will not occur. The immunity may be more against the vaccine organism than the natural disease. Or it may be that a mutant germ comes along that will not be susceptible to the antibodies formed. Or if something weakens the animal's immune system later, that system may lack the ability to respond fully, and the natural disease may be able to get a foothold. Such weakening factors include the kinds of things we've been discussing throughout this book—stress, malnutrition, lack of vitamins, toxicity, drug effects and so on.

So we see that the effectiveness of vaccination is a complex phenomenon depending on many factors, not the least of which is the overall level of health as determined by the total lifestyle.

It is interesting that retrospective studies of human vaccination practices now show that the actual protective effect falls far below previous estimates. At the same time, there is emerging evidence of much harm done—especially to children.

HARMFUL EFFECTS OF VACCINATION

Besides the possibility that they may not work, vaccines might also *cause* an acute disease or a chronic health problem. I have often noticed certain animals getting ill a few days to a few weeks after receiving vaccinations. Often the explanation given is that the dog or cat was already incubating the disease and was going to get it anyway. Granted that this may occasionally happen, in my opinion most of these instances are illness from the vaccine itself.

It is likely that the animal was in a weakened state and the vaccine virus therefore caused a more severe reaction than the "mini-disease" intended. Whatever the reason, I have seen this problem occur most often after canine distemper, canine parvovirus, feline rhinotracheitis or feline calicivirus vaccines were given (sometimes these latter two also cause a low-grade nose or eye inflammation in cats, which may last for months). Other vaccines, like the feline leukemia vaccine, do not seem to induce the illness they are supposed to prevent, but instead create conditions for another equally serious illness. The most frequent example of this, in my experience, is the occurrence of feline infectious peritonitis (FIP) a few weeks after administration of the feline leukemia vaccine. Sometimes the second virus was already in the cat, but the immune system was strong enough to withstand it until weakened by the vaccine disease (that is, the immune system was not able to cope with both diseases at the same time).

Long-term effects are the more serious possibility. Over the years doctors practicing homeopathic medicine have accumulated information on the more subtle but stubborn problems of vaccination. To quote a contemporary writer on the subject, George Vithoulkas, "The experience of astute homeopathic observers has shown conclusively that in a high percentage of cases, vaccination has a profoundly disturbing effect on the health of an individual, particularly in relation to chronic disease."

This disorder "engrafted" onto an individual by injection of a foreign disease is called vaccinosis and can be associated with a wide range of conditions. In many cases homeopaths have found it necessary to address the effects of vaccinations before full health can be restored. For example, Vithoulkas describes the case of a woman with terrible anxieties that were the result of a rabies vaccination she received as a child. She had experienced this condition for almost 40 years until cured by a method of homeopathic treatment chosen to antidote the ill effects of this vaccine.

Do these chronic effects occur in vaccinated animals? Very definitely. They are among the most common problems that I face in my practice. I believe this because I have learned that it's usually necessary to use a homeopathic remedy that removes the effects of prior vaccinations before I am able to make significant progress in the difficult, chronic cases often brought to me. I have had a number of cases in which the individual dog or cat invariably took a turn for the worse whenever it was vaccinated.

Based on the experience of over 17 years of homeopathic practice, it is my opinion that most animal skin allergies (and similar skin diseases) are the result of repeated annual vaccinations. I also suspect that the widespread increase in diseases caused by immune system disorders (such as hyperthyroidism, inflammatory bowel disease, lupus and pemphigus) is a result of increased use of vaccinations, especially of combination formulas. These vaccinations are highly unnatural to the body. Under natural conditions an animal is exposed to pathogens, but its body has ways to defend itself at the normal points of entry (the nose, mouth or other mucous membranes). When a combination vaccine is given, a massive invasion of several potent pathogens charges quickly into the bloodstream, bypassing the front-line defenses. Is it any wonder that the immune system gets confused, "panics" and begins attacking the body itself?

Fortunately, many other veterinarians are now recognizing this problem. Reports have appeared in journals over the last few years describing diseases that follow routine vaccinations—bleeding disorders, bone and joint inflammation, even tumors and cancers in some cats. At this point the attitude of most veterinarians is that these happenings are an anomaly. I think it will take many more years for the realization to dawn that some degree of adverse health effects occur in the majority of those vaccinated.

WHAT TO DO?

What you can do depends on your access to a qualified holistic veterinarian. As an example, we have not used vaccinations in our practice for 17 years. In their place we give homeopathic remedies called nosodes, which are made from natural disease products. *Distemperinum*, for example, is made from the secretions of a dog ill from canine distemper. It is sterilized, diluted and carefully prepared in accredited pharmacies. When properly used, this medicine can protect a dog from distemper even better than the vaccine can. In fact, this method of disease protection, first developed by a veterinarian in the 1920s, showed impressive results even before vaccines were developed.

Nosodes are also available for kennel cough, parvovirus, feline leukemia, feline infectious peritonitis and other common dog and cat diseases. We have been using this method of protection for several years now with very satisfactory results and without the side effects and illness associated with vaccine use.

What if you cannot find this service or you are afraid to not vaccinate? Let me suggest a modified plan that will at least minimize the chance of vaccine problems.

♦ *Use single or simple vaccines instead of complex vaccines.* Ideally, this means vaccinating for one disease at a time.

Most practitioners will balk at such a request, however, because they will have to buy each single-disease vaccine in quantity to serve only one client, suffering financial loss and wasting the unused vaccine. So you are generally offered the choice of getting a "simpler" combined vaccine, that is, fewer individual vaccines contained in a single shot. For dogs this will be a "DH" (distemper-hepatitis) and for cats a "3-in-1" (Panleukopenia, Rhinotracheitis and Calici virus). Though not perfect, these are *far* better than getting mega-mixes that might include Distemper, Hepatitis, Leptospirosis, Parvovirus, Parainfluenza, Bordetella, Rabies, Lyme Disease, Brucellosis and more (which may be given all at the same time to dogs) or Panleukopenia, Rhinotracheitis, Calici, Feline Leukemia, Rabies, Chlamydia, Feline Infectious Peritonitis and such (often given simultaneously to cats).

♦ *Where possible, use only "killed" or "inactivated" vaccines (as opposed to "modified live").* These "killed" vaccines cannot grow in the body and are generally safer to use.

♦ *Use a reduced vaccination schedule for young animals.* You do not have to give a lot of vaccinations to have as much protection as is possible. In most instances immunization of puppies or kittens is enough for several years or a lifetime of protection.

♦ *Don't vaccinate an animal too early.* Avoid the temptation to vaccinate before 16 weeks of age. Remember that the earlier your animal begins vaccinations, the more harm may be done to the immune system, and also the more vaccines received, the greater the chance for vaccine-induced illness.

- *Avoid annual boosters.* There has never been much justification for the yearly booster shots recommended by most veterinarians, even though they have become a popular practice. I advise against any further vaccinations after the initial series, as they are not necessary. Also, the latest official veterinary opinion states that annual revaccinations are neither required nor effective. Your veterinarian may not know of this or even agree with it. Rest assured, however, that experts in the field of veterinary immunology have taken this position and support your decision not to have your animal vaccinated every year.

DOGS

If you really want to play it safe, keep your new puppy isolated from contact with other dogs and just vaccinate once—at age 22 weeks or older. In my opinion, the only essential vaccines are distemper and parvo. Get the distemper vaccine at 22 weeks of age and the parvo a month later. (As I noted above, however, you'll probably have to get distemper–hepatitis together.)

This should be very safe if your puppy is not exposed to other sick animals, but if it seems too risky to you, I suggest getting two vaccinations (for each disease), starting at 16 weeks, using this schedule.

- First distemper (hepatitis): 16 weeks
- First parvo: 20 weeks
- Second distemper (hepatitis): 24 weeks
- Second parvo: 28 weeks

CATS

The distemper (feline panleukopenia) vaccine can be given once at age 16 weeks and is sufficient for the life of the cat. I do not recommend the rhinotracheitis and calici virus vaccines. Further, it has been my experience that the feline leukemia vaccines are the most harmful of all the cat vaccines available.

It is with cats that the danger is greatest of activating a latent virus infection by repeated administration of vaccines. Be careful of this.

THE RABIES PROBLEM

What about rabies vaccination? This is a difficult problem for many people to face. From my own experience I am convinced that some animals are made ill by this vaccine. Yet rabies is the only vaccine required by law for dogs (and for cats in some states). This requirement is really for the protection of human beings, regardless of its benefit or harm to pets.

DOGS

The most common disturbances following rabies vaccination are aggressiveness, suspicion, unfriendly behavior, hysteria, destructiveness (of blankets, towels), fear of being alone and howling or barking at imaginary objects. These can be treated with homeopathic medicine, but sometimes with difficulty. One of the saddest things in our practice is to restore a dog's health (sometimes after prolonged and careful work), only to have the animal suffer a relapse and go into a decline after we acquiesce to a required rabies vaccine. It would be far better if we didn't have to vaccinate these animals again, but our present legal situation requires it. We find that the best we can do is to have clients administer an appropriate homeopathic medicine to the dog within two hours of getting the vaccine. This seems to help in preventing subsequent problems.

At this point you have no legal alternative to getting rabies vaccinations for your dog. Many states require that you vaccinate your puppy at age 4 months (check your specific state requirements). How can we fit this into our recommended schedule? The best scenario is to have the rabies vaccine last, at least a month after completing all the others. However, this means waiting until your dog is 6 to 7½ months old (depending on the schedule you use). If this is not possible, then get the rabies vaccination first at age 4 months (16 weeks), wait until age 22 weeks and then carry on with the schedule I gave you above.

CATS

If the law requires that your cat be vaccinated for rabies, the best timing is one month after the distemper vaccine is received (age five months). If your state requires that you vaccinate your cat every year, specify to your veterinarian that your cat is to receive a one-year, killed virus vaccine. Some veterinarians will use the three-year rabies vaccine even when a one-year is called for. I do not recommend this practice.

VOMITING

Vomiting is one of those symptoms of underlying illness that rarely occurs just by itself. Most often it is associated with an upset stomach, but it also can occur in response to poisoning, failed kidneys, side effects of drugs, pain or inflammation in some other area (like the peritoneum, pancreas or brain), surgery, severe constipation and many other conditions. Therefore, it's always necessary to look beyond just the vomiting to understand what the underlying situation is and to treat that.

There are times, however, when nothing else seems to be wrong or when vomiting is by far the major problem. If not controlled, prolonged vomiting can lead to severe dehydration and the loss of certain vital salts, particularly sodium chloride and potassium chloride.

TREATMENT

The problem in treatment is that nothing given by mouth will remain in the stomach long enough to act, so the best way to administer medicine is to use crushed homeopathic pellets, which will act almost immediately through absorption in the mouth.

The best choice is:

Homeopathic—*Ipecac 6C (ipecac root):* Useful for persistent nausea and constant vomiting where much saliva is generated because of the nausea. Use "Homeopathic Schedule 1," page 348.

In addition, withhold all food and water during the vomiting period, allowing the animal to lick ice cubes occasionally. To replace fluids and salts (if there is dehydration), give a small enema every couple of hours as instructed in chapter 15. To each pint of enema water, add ¼ teaspoon of sea salt (or table salt as a second choice) and ¼ teaspoon potassium chloride (sold as a salt substitute in many markets). Given as an enema, this fluid will be retained and absorbed in a dehydrated animal.

WARTS

Dogs and older animals are the pets most likely to develop troublesome warts, which sometimes itch and bleed. Most often, these warts (and similar growths) are an expression of vaccinosis (see "Vaccinations"). Such animals may also tend to develop more serious types of growths in the future if not corrected at this point.

There is no simple formula for treating warts, as it is most necessary to address the underlying tendency with individualized treatment (called constitutional prescribing in homeopathy). There are, however, some general things to be done that may be quite helpful.

Homeopathic—*Thuya 30C (arborvitae):* This is appropriate for the tendency towards wart formation. Give Thuya first, using "Homeopathic Schedule 4," page 348. Let the stimulus of this medicine act for a month (though you may also be doing the local treatment described below). If the warts are not gone (or going), then use one of the next two remedies.

Homeopathic—*Causticum 30C (a mineral remedy):* This remedy is indicated for warts that tend to bleed easily. Use "Homeopathic Schedule 4," page 348.

Homeopathic—*Silicea 30C (silicon dioxide, quartz):* Useful when the wart is very large, especially if it occurs over the site of a prior vaccination. Use "Homeopathic Schedule 4," page 348.

During the time that these remedies are being used, you may do one of these local skin treatments.

Nutrition—*Vitamin E:* Regular application of vitamin E from a punctured capsule can sometimes greatly reduce the size of a wart. It must be continued for several weeks to be effective.

Herbal—*Castor oil:* This oil is quite helpful when applied directly to warts and growths to soften them and to reduce irritation. Apply it when the wart is itchy or in some way troublesome. Castor oil can be obtained at most pharmacies.

WEIGHT PROBLEMS

Obesity

Like people, a significant number of pets become overweight, especially if they are inactive and are fed fatty or sweet snacks by well-meaning owners. Such foods contain inadequate amounts of protein, vitamins, enzymes and other essential nutrients. Because of a lack in the nutrients it needs, the animal develops excessive cravings. The same thing can happen as a result of feeding poor-quality commercial diets.

In other animals the problem can result from a disturbance in the metabolism that causes an excessive and almost uncontrollable hunger that is very difficult to manage. In addition to the weight-loss program outlined below, such animals may need specific treatment (beyond the scope of this book) to correct the underlying imbalance.

In either case it's important to get excess fat off your pet because it can strain the heart, make the circulation sluggish, seriously complicate other disorders and probably shorten life span.

My basic weight-loss program for pets involves three principles.

1. *Increase activity levels.* Take your dog for daily walks and runs. Encourage

your cat to play. Increased activity raises the metabolic rate and burns calories faster.

2. *Resist the temptation to feed extra snacks and treats.* If your pet is really begging, you may feed modest amounts of the following: lean meat, carrots or other vegetables, apples, unsalted popcorn (preferably without oil) and raw bones.

3. *Feed a highly nutritious, low-fat, high-bulk diet that provides about two-thirds of the calories needed to maintain your animal's ideal weight.* While they are low in fat, the following diets are high in protein, enzymes, vitamins and minerals. They also include plenty of bran or vegetables to help fill your animal's stomach and minimize begging. This helps your animal to lose weight gradually and safely, while insuring enough of the basic nutrients it needs.

Be sure to include the daily vitamin-mineral pet supplements noted, which are available in pet supply outlets, in natural food stores or from many veterinarians.

DOG WEIGHT LOSS DIET #1

4   cups cooked vegetables (carrots, peas, green beans, corn and so on; use frozen or canned if you must for convenience)

2   cups oat or wheat bran

2   cups rolled oats

1   cup uncreamed cottage cheese

1   cup ground or chunky turkey, chicken, lean beef, heart, liver or lean hamburger

5,400 milligrams calcium (or 2 rounded tablespoons bonemeal or 1 tablespoon eggshell powder)

1   teaspoon vegetable oil

3   tablespoons nutritional yeast

Balanced dog vitamins

Cook the vegetables, using 3 to 4 cups water. When they are soft, add the bran and oats. Cover and let it sit for 10 minutes or until the oats are soft. Add the remaining ingredients, except the vitamins. Refrigerate extras. When serving a meal portion, add a balanced dog vitamin that supplies the minimum daily standards, as recommended on the label. (You may also add a bit of Healthy Powder, as described in chapter 3.)

The low-fat content of this diet will aid in weight loss. However, it's also best to restrict the quantities you feed. Decide what your dog's ideal weight should be and feed two meals a day, together totalling approximately the amount shown below—a little less if your dog is inactive, a little more if it's active. Make sure there is no access to other food, except low-calorie snacks like carrot sticks. Averages 150 kilocalories per cup.

Ideal Weight (lb.)	Feed (cups)
10	2
25	4
40	5½
60	7½
85	9¼

Variations: Instead of the oats you may substitute 2½ cups cooked brown rice (1 cup dry + 2 cups water) or 3+ cups cooked bulgur (1¼ cups dry + 2½ cups water). Instead of cooking the grains with the vegetables (as with the oats), cook them separately.

DOG WEIGHT LOSS DIET #2

This recipe is simpler and more palatable—but best suited for a smaller dog because it uses relatively higher amounts of meat.

>   2   cups (1 pound) ground or chunky turkey, chicken, lean beef heart, liver or lean hamburger
>
>   4   cups boiled or baked potatoes (or 3 cups cooked bulgur or rice)
>
>   ½   cup oat or wheat bran (or vegetables, such as peas, green beans, carrots or corn)
>
>   2   teaspoons vegetable oil
>
>   2,400 milligrams calcium (or 4 teaspoons bonemeal or 1⅓ teaspoons eggshell powder)
>
>   Balanced dog vitamins

Combine all ingredients except the vitamins. When serving, add a balanced dog vitamin supplying the minimum daily standards. (You may also add a bit of Healthy Powder, as described in chapter 3.) Feed about the same amounts as for diet #1. Immediately refrigerate extras.

CAT WEIGHT LOSS DIET

>   2   cups (1 pound) ground or chunky turkey, chicken, lean beef heart, liver or lean hamburger
>
>   1½   cups boiled or baked potatoes (or 1 cup cooked bulgur or rice)
>
>   ½   cup oat or wheat bran (or vegetables, such as peas, green beans, carrots or corn)
>
>   1   teaspoon vegetable oil (optional)
>
>   1,800 milligrams calcium (or 1 tablespoon bonemeal or 1 teaspoon eggshell powder)
>
>   Balanced cat vitamins

Combine all ingredients except the vitamins. When serving, add a balanced cat vitamin supplying the minimum daily standards, as recommended on the bottle label. (You may also add a bit of Healthy Powder, as described in chapter 3.) Averages 216 kilocalories per cup. Feed as follows:

Ideal Weight (lb.)	Feed (cups)
6	⅔
8	¾
10	1
12	1¼

Underweight

If your animal has the opposite problem and is underweight, obviously a different approach is needed. If the weight loss is sudden, it may be from an infection or some other problem that needs to be taken care of first. Have your veterinarian check out this possibility.

To help bring up the weight, use the basic natural foods diets in chapters 4 or 5 and also treat with:

Herbal—*Alfalfa (Medicago sativa):* Use "Herbal Schedule 2" on page 347. Continue treatment until the desired effect is achieved—increased hunger and weight gain.

Another treatment suitable for older, run-down animals is:

Tissue Salt—*Calcarea phosphorica 6X (calcium phosphate):* Especially good where there apparently is poor digestion or poor utilization of nutrients as evidenced by lack of weight gain in spite of good nutrition and adequate appetite. Use "Homeopathic Schedule 6(a)," page 349.

WORMS

Worms are internal parasites that live in the intestines of animals. They are commonly found in most animals (especially when the animals are young) and are usually not a serious problem.

We can consider worm-infested animals in three categories.

- Very young animals that acquired them from the mother before or after birth (roundworms)
- Young or mature animals infested with fleas or those that eat gophers or other wild creatures (tapeworms—carried by fleas and gophers, usually the latter)
- Mature but run-down animals that are in a toxic state and are susceptible to parasites, both inside (roundworms, hookworms, whipworms, tapeworms) and outside (fleas, lice, ticks)

The last category is beyond the scope of this discussion since treatments can vary considerably. I suggest that you work closely with your veterinarian for such problems. Here we will consider the first two categories, which are more common and less severe. First of all, let's talk a little about the worms themselves.

How to Identify Worms

Tapeworms grow in the small intestine. Each worm has a "head" that stays attached to the intestine as well as dozens of egg-filled segments that break off and pass out with the feces when ripe. These passed segments look like cream-colored maggots about $\frac{1}{4}$ to $\frac{1}{2}$ inch long and are visible in the fresh stool or around the anus. They do not crawl quickly, but move by forming a sort of "point" on one end. After drying out, they look a lot like a piece of white rice stuck to a hair near the anus.

Though chemical worming treatment can kill the worm, sometimes it just causes the sudden loss of most of the segments, leaving the head still attached. Unfortunately, the head that remains behind soon grows a new body that begins passing segments again. Another problem is that animals get reinfested through eating wild creatures (and occasionally from swallowing fleas).

Roundworms infest most young puppies and kittens and are acquired from their mother, both before and after birth. Usually the infestation is not apparent and must be diagnosed by a veterinarian through a microscopic exam of the feces. Be sure to ask if the infestation is light, medium or heavy and what kind of worms were found.

If the infestation is heavy, you can usually spot outer signs such as an enlarged belly, poor weight gain and, perhaps, diarrhea or vomiting. Sometimes whole worms are actually vomited or passed with the feces. They resemble white spaghetti several inches long and will often wiggle when first voided. Usually, only young animals a few weeks old to a few months of age will vomit roundworms.

Hookworms are generally less common than tapeworms and roundworms in this country; but they are still significant. They are more of a problem in the southern parts of the United States or in areas where crowded and unsanitary conditions prevail. Severe hookworm infestation is serious because the worms suck the animal's blood and cause severe anemia. In this kind of situation, it may be best to seek professional help. In young animals with severe infestation, the loss of blood into the intestine causes the stool to look black and tarlike. It may also become fluid and foul smelling. The gums will become pale, reflecting the developing anemia, and the youngster will appear weak and thin.

Whipworms are in a category of their own. They are quite common but usually cause no symptoms, often lying dormant for long periods. If there are symptoms—usually persistent, watery diarrhea—I believe it means something is wrong with the animal's immune system. If so, individualized treatment is required.

TREATMENT, CATEGORY 1

Early roundworm problems in young animals can be mild and insignificant or severe and life-threatening, depending on the health of the puppy or kitten at birth. At a certain stage of pregnancy, worms that have been sleeping dormant in the mother become active and migrate to the developing young in the uterus, infesting them even before birth. This can happen even if the mother tests negative.

It sounds awful, but it is seldom a serious problem because there are usually just a few of these worms. If the mother is not healthy, however, these worms take advantage of the situation and migrate in larger numbers than usual. Puppies or kittens born from these weak mothers can be heavily parasitized and never thrive.

It's important to understand that if the young animals are otherwise healthy and if they are fed a very good diet that's high in protein, the roundworm numbers will gradually decrease to almost nothing over the first few months of life without any treatment at all. After the age of six months, dogs are seldom infested with this worm (as detectable with stool exams). Cats, once they get over their initial worms, become immune for life and are never again reinfested. In both dogs and cats a few of the original worms may persist in a dormant state until pregnancy occurs (thus spreading to the next generation), but they do not cause any problem and are not detectable with stool tests.

One important factor in the continued resistance of mature animals to roundworms is that they have sufficient vitamin A. A long-term deficiency of vitamin A will allow worms to reinfest and grow in otherwise resistant animals.

My experience with the care of young animals is that they do not need worm treatment unless they have large numbers of worms or show visible signs of their effects (failure to thrive, pot-bellied, diarrhea or soft stools). Usually, it is enough to see that they have good nutrition. Therefore, I do not support the practice of routinely worming puppies and kittens without even checking to see if they do have a significant worm problem. Why give them these toxic chemicals needlessly? I have seen problems from routine worming treatments, such as poor growth, diarrhea and loss of appetite—ironically, these are just the problems you want to avoid.

What if you do need to treat young animals? I suggest the following measures (use all of them, if possible).

Homeopathic—*Cina 3X (Wormseed)*: Give 1 tablet 3 times a day for at least 3 weeks. Have the stool checked again in a microscopic evaluation at a lab to make sure the worms are gone.

Nutrition—Add ½ to 2 teaspoons (depending on the animal's size) of wheat or oat bran to the daily fare. This roughage will help to carry out the worms. Also, feed the same quantity of one of these vegetables—grated raw carrots, turnips or beets.

Herbal—*Garlic (Allium sativum):* Depending on the pet's size, mix ½ to 2 cloves of fresh, chopped or grated garlic into the daily ration.

Mineral—*Diatomaceous earth (skeletal remains of diatoms, a very small sea creature):* Can be purchased at natural food stores and some pet stores. This substance, which is sometimes used for the control of fleas, is also effective against roundworms. The action is the same—the shell remnants of the diatoms are irritating to the outside of worms (as they are to the fleas) and cause them to loosen their hold and be flushed out. Add ¼ to 1 teaspoon of natural (unrefined) diatomaceous earth to each meal.

Alternatively, there are several herbal wormers available now that are quite useful in treatment. If you purchase one at a health food store, follow the directions on the label.

I suggest that you give this nontoxic treatment a three-week trial and then check again for worms. If the worms are still there, then it is best for your pet to get the conventional drug treatment. If a young animal has gone through this program, even if the program was not completely effective, I find that it seems to withstand the drug treatment better.

Other Worm Problems

If your puppy or kitten has been diagnosed with hookworms (a problem in some southern states), go ahead with conventional treatment first. Hookworms can be a more serious problem, and I would rather you treat this parasite under supervision. You can, however, do my treatment after the usual worming as a way to "mop up" any remnants and to prevent further infestations.

Tapeworms are not usually a problem in young animals. They're more likely to appear after the animal is old enough to go hunting (see below).

TREATMENT, CATEGORY 2

After the animal equivalent of childhood, the most common problem is tapeworms. (If you do have a roundworm problem, however, just use the treatment outlined above for Category 1.) Tapeworms are always picked up from eating another creature (such as fleas, rodents or, usually, gophers). They are not directly passed from one dog or cat to another, even if the stool is eaten. The tapeworm must go through a developmental cycle inside another animal before it can grow into the infectious form. What this means is that parasites will recur as long as your animal continues to hunt and eat wild creatures.

Tapeworm parasites do not usually cause any detectable health problems and are not serious (though they are disgusting to see). There's no reason to panic, thinking they must be eradicated immediately. If you follow the natural health program in this book, particularly the fresh diet, you will find that parasite problems lessen as your pet's general health improves. As your animal detoxifies and builds up strength, many parasites will be sloughed off.

The idea in treating tapeworms is to use substances that annoy or irritate the worms and to use them over a long period of time. Eventually, the worms will give up and loosen their hold, passing on out.

Herbal—*Pumpkin seeds (Cucurbita pepo):* These seeds are a wonderfully safe treatment against tapeworms. Obtain the whole, raw seeds and keep them in a sealed container at room temperature. Grind them to a fine meal and give them to your pet to consume immediately. If, for some reason, you must grind the seeds ahead of time, store the ground seeds in a sealed container in your freezer. Take out the needed portion quickly each day and reseal the container before much moisture enters it. It's best, however, to grind the seeds fresh before use. An electric seed grinder (sold in health food stores) or a food processor can do the job. Add ¼ to 1 teaspoon (depending on the size of your animal) to each meal.

Nutritional—*Wheat-germ oil:* Buy a very good quality wheat-germ oil at a health food store, and you have an excellent natural tapeworm discourager as well as a good adjunct to other treatments. Add ¼ to 1 teaspoon, depending on the animal's size, to each meal.

Nutritional—*Vegetable enzymes:* The enzymes of many plant foods, especially those from figs and papaya, eat away at the outer coating of the worm. Dried figs can be chopped or ground and added to food (more accepted by dogs than cats). Use ¼ to 1 teaspoon, depending on your animal's size, to each meal.

Papaya is an excellent enzyme source, but it's not readily available everywhere. You can use enzyme supplements that contain papain (the papaya enzyme) and other digestive enzymes. Follow the instructions on the label.

Homeopathic—*Filix mas 3X (male fern):* A time-honored herb used against tapeworms, this remedy can be given as 1 tablet 3 times a day. (The remedy discussed under roundworm treatment, *Cina* 3X, can also be used if Filix mas is not available.)

Fasting once a week, allowing just a raw bone and water or broth, is an excellent practice generally. It's especially useful, however, if worms are a problem because it weakens them and makes them more vulnerable to the treatments being used. Since the worms get their food from the animal's food, they don't get to eat either.

If your pet has a stubborn problem in getting rid of any type of intestinal worm, also try an occasional dose of castor oil. Giving this after a day of fasting will flush out all the weakened worms. Use ½ teaspoon for puppies less than three months old and for all young cats; 1 teaspoon for puppies three to six months old and adult cats; 1½ tablespoons for medium-size dogs and 2 tablespoons for large dogs.

A Last Segment

In the above discussion I suggest some relatively simple things to do for worm problems. If they don't work, then I recommend using conventional drug treatment. However, I know some of you will not want to give up on a natural approach to this problem. So I am including this more complicated naturopathic approach as a backup. Though more involved, this is a highly effective method (adapted from the suggestions of herbalist Juliette de Bairacli-Levy).

The same program can be used for either tapeworms or roundworms. Basically, it consists of fasting and the use of repellent herbs, along with castor oil (to flush out the intestinal tract).

1. *Start by feeding a special diet for three to four days that will help weaken the worms by eliminating foods they prefer (fats, sugars, eggs, whole milk).* Give two small meals a day, consisting of rolled oats (softened with water or skim milk), lightly boiled fish and a liberal sprinkling of nutritional yeast.

2. *Next, fast the animal for two days primarily on water.* If the animal is younger than six months, fast it for just a day on water with a bit of honey added for energy. On the first night of this fast, give some castor oil to act as a purgative to help clear the bowels. Use ½ teaspoon for puppies less than three months old and for all young cats; 1 teaspoon for puppies three to six months old and adult cats; 1½ tablespoons for medium-size dogs and 2 tablespoons for large dogs (see page 226).

On the second day of the fast, give herbal deworming tablets (available at many health food stores or by mail; see "Pet Supplies"). Alternatively, make your own formula by combining equal parts of fresh grated garlic with powdered rue and wormwood (herbs) in No. 2 gelatin capsules (sold at drugstores). Make this fresh each day or refrigerate it because of the garlic. Dose according to product instructions or as follows (for the homemade mix): three to five capsules for small or young animals; six to eight capsules for medium or large dogs.

About 30 minutes after giving the herbs, administer another dose of castor oil (same amount as before). Then wait another 30 minutes and feed a small amount (about a cup for a medium dog) of a warm, laxative, semiliquid mixture of raw milk thickened with slippery elm powder, honey and rolled oats. If this is vomited, try again in 30 minutes. The slippery elm forms a smoothing jelly that helps to remove the worms and eggs from the intestines.

3. *For the next three days continue feeding this same mixture of milk, elm, honey and oats in three small meals a day.* Each morning, at least 30 minutes before feeding, give the herbs again, but cut the dose in half. Each evening it helps to give a mild, cleansing laxative, such as ⅛ to ½ teaspoon (depending on body size) of powdered senna with a pinch of ginger. Give it in a capsule or mix into water or food.

4. *Slowly return to a normal natural-foods diet over the next few days.* Stop giving the evening laxative once the animal is eating solid food and having bowel movements. For some time afterward include in the daily diet the foods recommended earlier (carrots, pumpkin seeds, beets and so on).

During this period and for about three weeks after the fast, use fresh garlic regularly on the food or give it in gelatin capsules at about half the dose used in the worming capsules. Also, feed an occasional charcoal tablet (once every two or three days, but for no more than a month afterward) to absorb and remove any remaining impurities in the intestines.

With careful application of either of these programs, you should meet with success in nearly all cases. Just to be certain all the worms are gone, have your veterinarian check the stool about six to eight weeks after treatment and periodically thereafter until you are sure the problem is resolved.

Note: Your parasitized animal can be a

source of health problems for other animals or for children. Especially with roundworms and hookworms, people can become exposed by contact with contaminated soil. Though these parasites do not really grow well in people and do not usually cause serious problems, they can be troublesome and annoying (primarily causing skin irritation). Until the problem is cleared up, it makes sense to take special care to prevent contamination of the environment. Collect all fecal material to bury (deeply) in one place, flush down the toilet or package carefully to dispose of through your sanitary service.

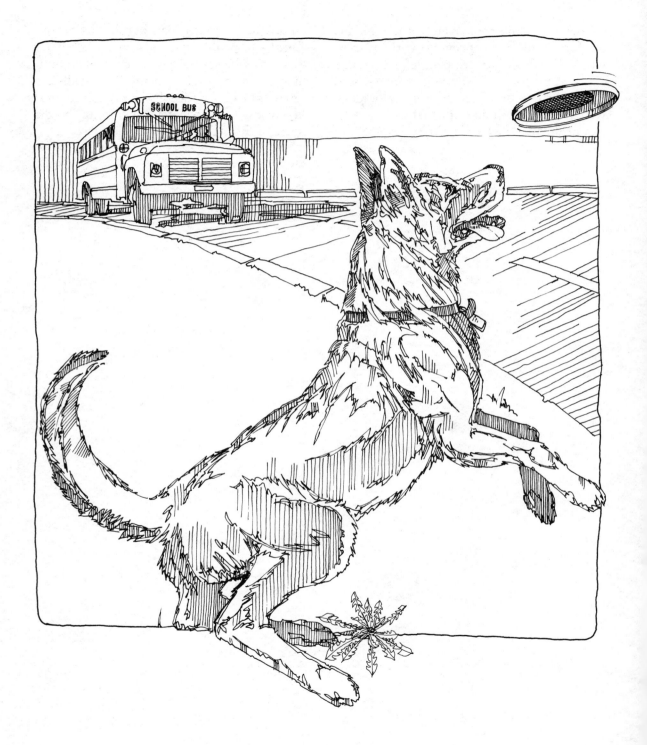

HANDLING EMERGENCIES AND GIVING FIRST AID

Important. Read This First! The care you give an animal in the first few minutes of an emergency can make the difference between life and death. The first-aid remedies I suggest definitely work and will be tremendously helpful in that time between the beginning of the emergency and arrival at your veterinarian's office. But they are meant as temporary lifesaving procedures to use while contacting the doctor and readying transportation. Do not use these methods as a way of delaying needed professional help. Instructions for more prolonged treatment apply only if you *cannot* reach medical care.

For this information to serve you, plan ahead and have supplies on hand in a convenient place. An emergency is not the time to begin assembling these tools and remedies or to start reading "how to do it." The information that follows is given in brief outline form, alphabetically, for ready reference when needed. But you should study all the categories ahead of time so you can find the right heading in a hurry during a time of crisis.

Here is a list of supplies you should have on hand in order to make full use of my suggestions. See "Suppliers of Homeopathic Remedies" on page 354 for suppliers of the homeopathic remedies and Dr. Bach's stress-relieving rescue formula. The tissue salts are sold at many health food stores, and the other supplies are found in drug stores.

HOMEOPATHIC REMEDIES

- *Aconitum* 30C—a bottle of 250 tablets or a two-dram vial of #35 pellets
- *Arnica montana* 30C—a bottle of 250 tablets or a two-dram vial of #35 pellets
- *Calendula* 6X—a bottle of 250 tablets or a two-dram vial of #35 pellets
- Calendula tincture—one-ounce dropper bottle
- Calendula-Hypericum ointment—can be purchased as such from homeopathic pharmacies. Sometimes called Hyper-Cal.
- *Carbo vegetabilis* 30C—a bottle of 250 tablets or a two-dram vial of #35 pellets
- *Ferrum phosphoricum* 6X (tissue salt)—a bottle of 250 tablets
- *Glonoine* 30C—a bottle of 250 tablets or a two-dram vial of #35 pellets
- *Hypericum* 30C—a bottle of 250 tablets or a two-dram vial of #35 pellets
- *Ledum* 30C—a bottle of 250 tablets or a two-dram vial of #35 pellets
- *Nux vomica* 30C—a bottle of 250 tablets or a two-dram vial of #35 pellets
- *Phosphorus* 30C—a bottle of 250 tablets or a two-dram vial of #35 pellets
- Urtica urens tincture—one-ounce dropper bottle

OTHER REMEDIES

- Activated charcoal granules
- Ammonia water

- Fresh warm coffee (caffeinated)
- Raw onion
- Dr. Bach's stress-relieving rescue formula—10½-milliliter dropper bottle of the stock. Use this purchased stock by preparing a solution made in this manner: Add four drops of stock to a one-ounce dropper bottle filled a third of the way with brandy as a preservative. Add enough spring water to fill the bottle and mix well. Make this diluted solution in advance and use it as recommended for treatment. It will keep for at least a year if kept out of the sun and away from heat.

MATERIALS

- (2) blankets—thick and strong
- Adhesive tape—one-inch-wide roll
- Elastic bandage—three inches wide
- Enema bag
- Gauze pads—one package
- Natural soap—like Dr. Bronner's or Basic-H
- Plastic bowl—for preparing dilutions
- Water—for dilution (spring or distilled water is best; tap water is okay)

WHAT TO DO IN EMERGENCIES

Breathing Stopped

Follow these steps to apply Artificial Respiration Technique.

1. *Open the mouth,* pull out the tongue, check back into the throat to make sure no obstructions are present. Clear away mucus and blood if necessary. Replace the tongue.
2. *Give one dose of Carbo vegetabilis 30C.* Place two pellets on the tongue.
3. *Close the mouth and place your mouth over the nostrils.* Exhale as you fill the animal's lungs, allowing it to exhale after. Do this 6 times a minute for dogs, 12 times a minute for cats. Inflate the chest until you can see it rise.
4. *Administer Dr. Bach's rescue formula* starting after 5 minutes. Place two drops on the gums or tongue and continue every 5 minutes until breathing is restored. Then every 30 minutes (if you can't reach help) for four treatments.

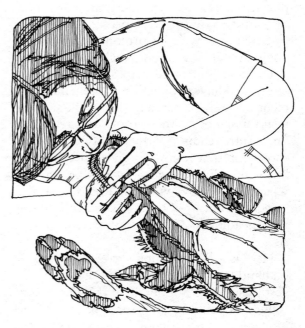

Artificial Respiration: Holding the mouth closed, breathe into the animal's nostrils. Allow it to exhale. Pace the breathing at 6 times a minute for dogs, 12 times a minute for cats.

Breathing and Heart Both Stopped

(Listen at chest.)
Follow these steps.

1. *Apply Cardiopulmonary Resuscitation Technique.* Use the Artificial Respiration Technique including use of one dose of *Carbo vegetabilis* 30C (see "Breathing Stopped") and the External Heart Massage Technique (see "Heart Stopped"), step one, at the same time. This is easiest for two people.
2. *Apply acupressure.* Use the edge of your thumbnail or the pointed cap of a pen to put strong pressure over the center of the large pad of each rear foot. After a few seconds, release and apply pressure to the point on the nose shown in the diagram. Alternate between acupressure and cardiopulmonary resuscitation. If two people are working, have each one apply one of the techniques continuously.
3. *After five minutes, give one dose of Arnica montana 30C.* Place two pellets on the tongue.
4. *After 5 more minutes, administer Dr. Bach's rescue formula.* Place two drops on the gums or tongue and continue every 5 minutes until breathing is restored. Repeat every 30 minutes (if you can't reach help) for four treatments.

Burns

("White" skin or scorched hair)
Use one technique.

1. *Apply Urtica urens tincture.* Add six drops of the tincture to one ounce (two

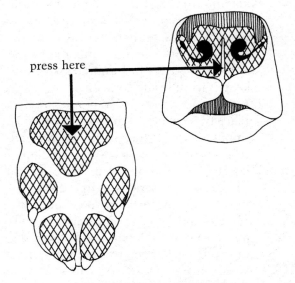

press here

Acupressure: Use the acupuncture points for resuscitation.

full tablespoons) water. Saturate gauze with the solution and place over the burn. Do not remove the gauze, but keep it moistened with more of the solution. If necessary, hold in place with a bandage.
2. *Administer Dr. Bach's rescue formula.* Give internally, two drops on the tongue every 30 minutes.

Car Accidents

(Obvious injury; greasy or very dirty coat)
Follow these steps.

1. *Move the animal to a safe place.* If the animal is found on the road, without bending its spine or changing its position, slide it onto a board or taut blan-

ket and transport it to a better location. You may need to tie a strip of cloth or wrap a pressure bandage around the mouth temporarily (as a muzzle) or put a blanket over the animal's head to keep it from biting someone.

2. *Give a dose of Arnica montana 30C.* Place two pellets on the tongue every 15 minutes, for a total of three doses. Do this only if it is safe to do so. An injured animal will bite without restraint and can cause very serious injury. If it seems unsafe to administer a medicine, dissolve two pellets in some water or milk and drip it onto the lips from a safe distance. If you happen to have a syringe with a needle on it, you can squirt the diluted medicine fairly accurately between the lips and into the mouth.

3. *Keep the animal warm and watch for shock* (see "Shock" in this section).

Cardiopulmonary Resuscitation

(See "Breathing and Heart Both Stopped" in this section.)

Convulsions

(Stiffening or alternate rapid contraction/relaxation of muscles; thrashing about; frothing at the mouth)

1. *Do not interfere with or try to restrain the animal during the convulsion.* It is too dangerous to you and does not help the animal.

2. *If breathing stops after the convulsion, use artificial respiration* (see "Breathing Stopped" in this section). If the heart stops too, use cardiopulmonary resusci-

tation (see "Breathing and Heart Both Stopped").

3. *Give Aconitum 30C.* If possible, put two pellets on the tongue (see warning about being bitten in "Car Accidents" section).

4. *After 5 minutes, administer Dr. Bach's rescue formula,* two drops every 15 minutes, if the animal is frightened or disoriented.

5. *Consider poisoning as a possible cause* (see "Poisoning" in this section).

Cuts

(Lacerations, tears)
Follow these steps.

1. *Flush out the cut with clean water.* Remove obvious debris like sticks, hair and gravel.

2. *Apply calendula lotion.* Add six drops calendula tincture to one ounce (two full tablespoons) water; saturate gauze pads and tape them in place.

3. *Wash minor wounds that do not need professional care with soap and water and dry carefully.* Clip hair from the edges of the wound. Apply calendula-hypericum ointment twice a day until healed. Leave unbandaged.

Also give *Calendula* 6X twice a day (one pellet) until the wound is clearly on its way to recovery.

Fractures

(Leg "bends" at sharp angle; animal won't use leg.)

◆ *If the lower leg is obviously broken,* very

carefully wrap a roll of clean newspaper or magazine around it and tape it to prevent unrolling. Do not try to set the leg yourself; just keep the lower end from swinging back and forth.

- *If a wound is present at the fracture site,* cover it with clean gauze before applying a temporary splint.
- *If the fracture is not apparent or is high up,* do not attempt to splint. Let the animal assume the posture most comfortable to it. A padded box may be best for transporting small animals to the veterinarian. Walking on three legs may be best for a larger dog.
- *Give Arnica 30C,* two pellets every hour for as many as four doses (if needed because of delayed help). If administration causes struggling and possible further injury, discontinue treatment.

Gunshot Wounds

(Look for two holes opposite each other on the body, much pain and anxiety.)

1. *Give Arnica 30C,* two pellets every 15 minutes for a total of three doses.
2. *Apply hand pressure* with dry gauze over the wound, if necessary, until bleeding stops. Or temporarily use the Pressure Bandage Technique (see "Pressure Bandage Technique").
3. *Give Hypericum 30C if there is no relief from the three doses of Arnica.* Give two pellets every 15 minutes for three doses.
4. *Continue treatment with Arnica 30C or Hypericum 30C, whichever was most useful.* Give a dose of two pellets every hour as long as it seems needed to control pain.

Heart Stopped

(No heartbeat felt or heard at chest)
Follow these steps:

1. *Apply External Heart Massage Technique.* Place the animal with its right side down on a firm surface. Place one or both hands (depending on animal's size) over the lower chest directly behind the elbow. Press firmly and release at the rate of once every second (see the illustration on page 342). *Caution:* Excessive pressure can fracture ribs.
2. *Give one dose of Carbo vegetabilis 30C.* As soon as you can get it, place two pellets on the tongue.
3. *Administer Dr. Bach's rescue formula.* Put two drops in the side of the mouth, repeating every 5 minutes until there is a response. Then every 30 minutes (if no help is available) for four doses.
4. *Apply artificial respiration if the heart does not start within a minute* (see "Breathing Stopped" in this section).
5. *Successful heart massage (and respiration) can be estimated* by the return of normal "pink" color to the gums.

Heat Stroke

(Animal found unconscious in hot car)
Follow these steps.

1. *Remove the animal immediately* to a cool, shady area. Use the car's shadow if necessary.
2. *Wet the animal with water.* Apply continuously to cool the body as much as possible. Place ice packs around the body and head during transport to the veterinarian.

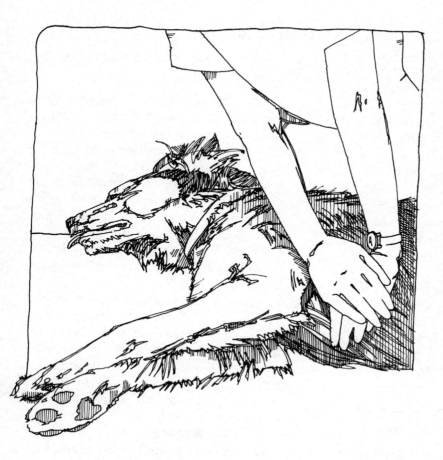

Heart Massage: Using both hands, press firmly and release 60 times a minute.

3. *If you have it, give a dose of Glonoine 30C.* Place two pellets on the tongue.
4. *Administer Dr. Bach's rescue formula.* Put two drops in the mouth every ten minutes until you arrive at the veterinarian's.
5. *If breathing has stopped,* follow instructions for "Breathing Stopped" in this section.

Hemorrhage

(Bleeding from a wound or body opening) For skin wounds, use these treatments.

1. *Give Arnica 30C,* a dose every 15 minutes for a total of three treatments.
2. *Give Phosphorus 30C,* a dose every 15 minutes for three treatments, if *Arnica 30C* is not sufficient.
3. *Locally apply calendula lotion* (six drops in one ounce of water).
4. *If necessary, use the pressure bandage* (as described under its own heading in this section).

For internal bleeding use these treatments.

1. *Give Arnica 30C* as described in step one (above).

2. *Use Ferrum phosphoricum 6X,* one tablet every hour for four treatments, if *Arnica* 30C is not sufficient.
3. *Keep the animal calm.* If hysteria is a problem, begin treatment by placing two drops of Dr. Bach's rescue formula in the mouth every five minutes for three treatments. Then follow with Arnica.

Insect Bites

(Bee, hornet and wasp stings; centipede, scorpion and spider bites; red, painful swellings)

For local use: For bee, hornet or wasp stings, apply a freshly sliced onion. Alternatively, rub in one drop of ammonia water (can be purchased for cleaning floors and windows—in a pinch, you can use ammonia detergent or an ammonia-based window cleaner).

An effective herbal treatment is to rub in a drop of nettle extract (Urtica urens tincture or glycerine extract) directly on the sting.

Using a *dull* knife and holding it perpendicularly to the skin, scrape across the area of the sting a few times. This will grab the stinger and pull it out without pain. Do not try to grab a stinger with your fingers or with tweezers as it will squeeze more poison into the wound.

Internally, for all insect bites give *Ledum* 30C, one pellet every 15 minutes for a total of three treatments.

Poisoning

(Symptoms appear in three major forms: excess salivation, tears and frequent urination and defecation; muscle twitching, trembling and convulsions; severe vomiting.)

Follow these steps.

1. *Give granular activated charcoal.* Mix five heaping teaspoons of granules in 1 cup of water. Depending on the animal's size, give about ¼ to 1 cup by spoonfuls in the cheek pouch. If this causes excess struggle or worsens symptoms, discontinue. Your veterinarian will be able to apply treatment under sedation or anesthesia.
2. *Give Nux vomica 30C,* two pellets (whole or crushed) on the tongue every 15 minutes for a total of three doses. Do not continue treatment if the symptoms worsen.
3. *Keep the animal warm and as quiet as possible.* Stress has a very negative influence.
4. *Call the National Animal Poison Control Center if you know where the poison came from.* Call 1-800-548-2423 ($30 credit card charge per case) for specific advice on treatment or antidotes.

Otherwise, bring the suspected poisons and container (if known) as well as any vomited material to the doctor for possible identification of the poison.

Pressure Bandage Technique

(To control hemorrhage, excessive bleeding; to keep gauze and medication in place)

Follow these steps.

1. *Place dry or medicated gauze (calendula-hypericum ointment is a good choice) over the wound and wrap an overlapping elastic bandage around it. Apply only slight tension to the wrap*

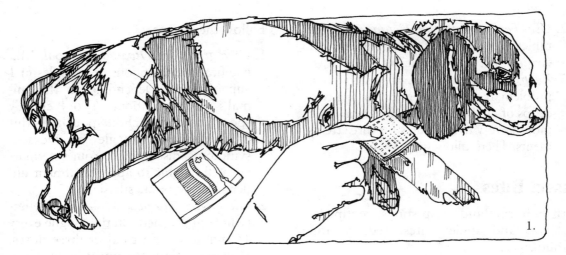

To Control Bleeding: Step 1: Place medicated gauze over the wound.

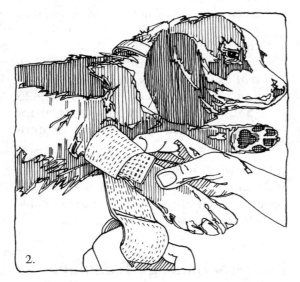

Step 2: Wind an elastic bandage around the wound to hold the gauze in place.

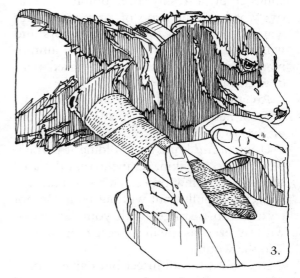

Step 3: Cover the bandage with adhesive tape to hold it securely.

because excessive pressure (especially on a leg) can cut off blood flow like a tourniquet. If the wound is on the lower half of the leg, wrap all the way to and including the foot (to prevent swelling).

2. *Apply adhesive tape to the end of the bandage* to keep it from unwinding.
3. *Remove the bandage at once if swelling occurs below the wrap* (as on a leg). If you can reach to feel the foot pads, periodically check that they remain warm; if

they're cold, then the bandage is too tight. Remember, bandaging is a temporary measure; use it until bleeding stops or you can reach the veterinarian.

Punctures

(From teeth, claws, sharp objects)
Follow these steps.

1. *Wash wound* with soap and water. Use a natural soap, not a strong detergent.
2. *Pull out* any embedded hair you see in the hole.
3. *Apply direct pressure* over the wound with gauze only if bleeding is excessive (see "Pressure Bandage Technique"). Moderate bleeding will flush out the wound.
4. *Give Ledum 30C,* two pellets every two hours for four doses.

Shock

(Accompanies serious injuries. Symptoms are white gums, rapid breathing, unconsciousness.)

◆ *If much bruising or trauma is evident or internal hemorrhage is suspected,* use *Arnica* 30C, one pellet every ten minutes until a response is seen. Then treat every two hours until the gums are once again pink and your pet seems to be normally alert.
◆ *If the animal is unconscious,* give *Aconitum* 30C, one pellet every ten minutes until consciousness returns. If there is no response within four doses, switch over to *Arnica* 30C and do the same schedule.
◆ *If the animal appears to be dying* (cold, blue, lifeless), give *Carbo vegetabilis* 30C, one pellet every five minutes for three doses. If he rallies, follow with *Arnica* 30C as described in the first step of this section.

Note: Keep the animal warm with a blanket and in a horizontal position.

Sudden Collapse

(Sudden unconsciousness without warning; fainting)
Follow these steps.

1. *First check to see if breathing or the heart has stopped.* If so, use the treatment described under "Breathing Stopped" or "Breathing and Heart Both Stopped."
2. *Use Dr. Bach's rescue formula,* two drops every 5 minutes until a response, and then every 30 minutes.
3. *Give a warm coffee enema* (for caffeine). Depending on the animal's size, use ¼ to 1 cup. Press gauze against the anus for 15 minutes to prevent the fluid from coming out.
4. *Count out the heart rate* for a minute, if possible. This will be useful information for your veterinarian as an abnormal heart rate (too fast or too slow) is a frequent cause of fainting.

SCHEDULE FOR HERBAL TREATMENT

General Directions: Use freshly harvested and dried herbs if possible, preferably this year's crop. After a few years herbs lose potency from exposure to air. Alcoholic extracts of herbs, called tinctures, are an especially useful form because they are more stable, maintaining potency for at least two years and sometimes longer. Available in one-ounce dropper bottles, they are easily added to water for dilution. Gelatin capsules are also useful for preserving powdered herbs. They help the herbs stay fresh by excluding the oxygen, which degrades them.

SCHEDULE 1: INTERNAL

In this schedule you give the herbs *three times a day* until there are no more symptoms or for a maximum of seven days. Depending on the form of herb you use, they're prepared a little differently (see chapter 15 for more information on herbs and on techniques for giving medications to pets). Here are the options.

(a) *Infusions*. Make an infusion by first bringing one cup of pure water (filtered or distilled) to a boil. Pour it over one rounded teaspoon of dried herb or one rounded tablespoon of fresh herb. Cover and steep for 15 minutes. Then extract the liquid by straining it through a cheesecloth or sieve.

Here's how much to give your pet three times a day (morning, mid-afternoon and at night before bed): ½ teaspoon (about two cubic centimeters) for cats or small dogs (less than 20 pounds); 1 teaspoon (about five cubic centimeters) for medium dogs (20 to 40 pounds); or one tablespoon for large dogs (40 pounds and over).

(b) *Cold extracts*. Add two rounded teaspoons of dried herb or two rounded tablespoons of fresh herb to one cup of cold water. Cover it and let it sit for 12 hours. Strain out the solids and administer the liquid extract three times a day in the same quantities listed above for infusions (a).

(c) *Decoctions*. In some cases the instructions specify that you should prepare a decoction, which is the way to prepare certain dried roots, rhizomes and barks. To do so, add one rounded teaspoon of the herb to one cup of pure water. Bring to a boil and simmer uncovered for 15 to 20 minutes. Strain out the solids and administer the liquid three times a day in the same quantities listed above for infusions (a).

(d) *Tinctures*. If you have the tincture form of the herb, dilute it, three drops to one teaspoon (nine drops to one tablespoon) of pure water. Administer this solution three times a day in the same quantities listed above for infusions (a).

(e) *Gelatin capsules*. Herb capsules that are prepared for human consumption can also be taken by animals, but in smaller doses. Small dogs and cats will get half of a capsule as a dose; medium dogs will get one as a dose; large dogs will receive two capsules each dose. Remember that one dose is given three times a day with this schedule.

SCHEDULE 2: INTERNAL

Here you give the herbs *twice a day*, on about a 12-hour schedule. Use the same procedures and quantities described in Schedule 1. Likewise, continue treating until symptoms are gone or a week has passed.

SCHEDULE 3: INTERNAL

With this program you'll give the herbs *only once a day* (every 24 hours). Again, follow the same procedures and quantities outlined in Schedule 1, treating until the symptoms are gone or for a maximum of one week.

SCHEDULE 4: EXTERNAL

This program calls for an herbal compress. First make a hot infusion, decoction or tincture dilution of the herb (or herbs), as in Schedule 1. Let it cool a bit so that it's hot but not so hot that it will burn or cause discomfort. If you can stand it, then it's likely your pet can also. Next, immerse a washcloth or small hand towel in the solution, wring it out and apply it to the affected area on your pet's body. Put a dry towel over this

moist compress to keep the heat in. After five minutes refresh the compress by dipping it back in the hot solution, wringing it out again and re-applying.

If you can, treat for 15 minutes, though your pet may only allow you 5 minutes or so. You can use this compress twice a day for up to two weeks.

SCHEDULE 5: EXTERNAL

Prepare a hot compress, as in Schedule 4, but alternate it a couple of times with a cold compress (a second cloth dipped in tap water). This method is more stimulating, encouraging a good blood supply to the area. First use the hot herbal compress for 5 minutes, and then follow it with 2 minutes of the cold water compress. Repeat one more time, using the same sequence. The whole treatment lasts about 15 minutes. This can be performed twice daily for a period up to two weeks.

SCHEDULE 6: EXTERNAL

In this approach you make a warm to hot infusion, decoction or tincture dilution of the herb (or herbs), as in Schedule 1. When the temperature is acceptable, immerse your animal's foot, leg or tail (the affected part) directly into the solution. If your pet will put up with it, soak the part for at least five minutes and then towel dry. Do this soak twice a day, as needed, for up to two weeks.

Schedule for Homeopathic Treatment

General Directions: Give the remedy by first dispensing one pellet or tablet into the vial cap or a clean spoon, or by crushing three of them in a small folded paper. (Pellets come in different sizes; we are assuming the standard #35 size.) Then pour them directly into your pet's mouth or throat (see chapter 15).

Homeopathic remedies do not work as effectively if they are added to food. Each of the schedules below indicates how long you should withhold food before and after giving the remedy.

Water is less of a problem, but it is a good practice to prevent your pet from drinking for five minutes before and after giving the medicine.

Schedule 1: Acute Disease Treatment

Give one pellet or tablet every 4 hours until the symptoms are gone. Provide no food for ten minutes before and after treatment.

If your animal shows signs of improvement, continue giving the treatment for five days, discontinuing it as soon as (before five days) the symptoms are gone. If you do not see a response within 24 hours, however, you should try one of the other suggested remedies.

Schedule 2: Acute Disease Treatment

Give one pellet or tablet every 4 hours for a total of three treatments. Provide no food for ten minutes before and after treatment. No further homeopathic treatment will be needed for the next 24 hours. If your animal is not noticeably improved by then, try another remedy or go to one of the other treatment choices.

Schedule 3: Acute Disease Treatment

Over the course of three days, give one pellet or tablet every 12 hours. Provide no food for ten minutes before and after treatment. If there is no improvement after these six doses, choose another remedy. If a definite improvement has occurred, then no further homeopathic treatment will be needed.

Schedule 4

In this method you give only one treatment. Give two whole pellets or three pellets crushed to a powder. Place on the tongue. Give no food for 60 minutes before and after the treatment. Wait for a full month before any further treatment; it would be a mistake to repeat the remedy in a few days. If at the end of that month no improvement is seen, then you will need to choose a new medicine.

SCHEDULE 5

Here you will give just three doses, 12 hours apart, and then wait for a month. For each of the three treatments, give two whole pellets or three pellets crushed to a powder. Place on the tongue. Provide no food for 30 minutes before and after each treatment. Do not give any further treatment for a month. If you have not seen any improvement by then, choose a new treatment.

SCHEDULE 6

Here you will repeat doses over a total period of four weeks. Depending on the recommended option, you will give it (a) once every day (b) once every two days or (c) once every three days. At each treatment time, place just one pellet or tablet on the tongue or down the throat. Provide no food for ten minutes before and after giving the medicine.

The timing for a treatment every two days or every three days is determined by counting forward from the day of treatment. For example, if you are on a three-day schedule and give a treatment on a Monday, then count three more days—Tuesday, Wednesday, Thursday—which gives you Thursday as the next treatment day. The next treat-ment after this is on Sunday, and so on.

If you see some evidence of improvement (but not a complete cure) after four weeks on this schedule, then continue the treatment as long as it keeps helping—up to several months duration.

Response to medication: Deciding whether a given treatment has helped so far is an important part of your overall success with homeopathic medicines. It determines your next move: whether to continue, stop or try another treatment.

The first and best sign that a treatment is helping is that your animal appears to feel better overall, with improved energy, spirits, activity level and moods. Secondarily, you will see specific improvements in its physical condition, though these will occur more slowly.

Another good sign that you could easily misinterpret is that the body may produce a temporary discharge as part of the healing process. Depending on the illness, this may take the form of brief diarrhea (one day), vomiting (once) or eruption and discharge from the skin. Or in the case of a virus infection, for instance, the body may produce a fever for a few days as it mobilizes its defenses. None of these reactions, however, should be severe or long-lasting. And, again, if the program is working, your animal will be feeling better in an overall sense.

Many health problems are complex and difficult to treat, and you will greatly benefit if you can work with a skilled veterinary homeopathic practitioner. If you are in doubt or your animal is getting worse, it is best to consult such a veterinarian.

ADDITIONAL RECIPES

WHEAT OR RYE CRISPS FOR DOGS

Here's one of Joan Harper's (The Healthy Dog and Cat Cookbook) simplest recipes for dog biscuits. (Commercial products often include meat meal, with all its disadvantages.) They're good for occasional treats or rewards and to exercise teeth and gums, but too low in protein and other nutrients for regular chow.

1	cup whole-wheat or rye flour
¼	cup soy flour
3	tablespoons lard, bacon fat or oil
½	teaspoon bonemeal
1	clove garlic, grated, or ¼ teaspoon garlic powder (optional)
⅓	cup water or broth
1 to 2	teaspoons nutritional yeast (optional)

Combine the dry ingredients. Add the water or broth and mix well. Roll out on a cookie sheet and bake at 350°F until golden brown. Break into bite-size chunks. Sprinkle with nutritional yeast if your dog is fond of it.

KITTY OR DOGGIE CRUNCHIES

This recipe, an adaptation of a tried-and-true kibble created by Joan Harper, is nice for an occasional treat or to help a confirmed kibble-eater make the transition to home cooking. It is nutritionally complete for both cats and dogs, with 35 percent protein, 14 to 15 percent fat and a calcium/phosphorus ratio of 1.3:1.

1	pound chicken necks and gizzards or other poultry, ground
1	(16-ounce) can of mackerel, chopped
2	cups full-fat soy flour
1	cup wheat germ
1	cup powdered skim milk
1	cup cornmeal (dry)
2	cups whole-wheat flour
1	cup rye flour (or another cup of wheat flour)
3	tablespoons bonemeal (or 5,400 to 6,000 milligrams calcium)
½	teaspoon iodized salt or 3 tablespoons kelp
4	tablespoons vegetable oil (half can be meat drippings or butter)
1	tablespoon cod-liver oil (or up to 25,000 IU vitamin A)
¼	cup alfalfa powder or trace mineral powder
3	cloves garlic, minced
½	cup chopped onions (optional)
	400 IU vitamin E
1	quart water
½	cup nutritional yeast

Mix all the ingredients except the yeast and knead into a firm dough. Roll it out on a cookie sheet about ½- to ¼-inch thick. (Using a pastry cutter to divide it into strips will make it easier to break into small bits later.) Bake at 350°F for 30 to 45 minutes. Cool and break into bite-size chunks. Sprinkle with the yeast and store in airtight containers. Refrigerate whatever amount will not be consumed in 3 days.

DOG BISCUITS DELUXE

2   cups whole-wheat flour
½   cup soy flour
¼   cup cornmeal
1   teaspoon bonemeal
½   cup sunflower or pumpkin seeds
1 to 2 cloves garlic, minced, or ½ teaspoon garlic powder (optional)
1   tablespoon nutritional yeast (optional)
2   tablespoons butter (melted), fat or oil
¼   cup unsulfured molasses
1   teaspoon salt
2   eggs mixed with ¼ cup milk

Mix the flours, cornmeal, bonemeal and seeds together. Add the garlic and yeast, if desired. Combine the butter, fat or oil, molasses, salt and egg mixture; set aside 1 tablespoon of this liquid mixture and combine the rest with the dry ingredients. Add more milk, if necessary, to make a firm dough. Knead together for a few minutes and let the dough rest ½ hour or more. Roll out to ½-inch thick. Cut into crescents, rounds or sticks and brush with the remainder of the egg mixture. Bake at 350°F for 30 minutes or until lightly toasted. To make harder biscuits, leave them in the oven with the heat turned off for an hour or more. Biscuits keep longer if you use oil instead of butter. These biscuits contain 18 percent protein, 19 percent fat and 63 percent carbohydrates.

KITTY CATNIP COOKIES

1   cup whole-wheat flour
2   tablespoons wheat germ
¼   cup soy flour
⅓   cup powdered milk
1   tablespoon kelp
½   teaspoon bonemeal
1   teaspoon crushed dried catnip leaves
1   tablespoon unsulfured molasses
1   egg
2   tablespoons oil, butter or fat
⅓   cup milk or water

Mix the dry ingredients together. Add the molasses, egg, oil, butter or fat and milk or water. Roll out flat on an oiled cookie sheet and cut into narrow strips or ribbons. Bake at 350°F for 20 minutes or until lightly toasted. Break into pea-size pieces, suitable for cats. Good for treats, exercising gums and cleaning teeth, but too low in protein to use for regular fare.

SOURCES OF NATURAL PET PRODUCTS

I am often asked to recommend specific pet foods among the many that claim to use better ingredients and to exclude artificial preservatives, colors and flavors, such as Nature's Recipe, Pet Guard, Natural Life, Abady, Sojourner Farms, Wysong, Lick Your Chops, Health Valley, Cornucopia and others. It is difficult to know which of these are best. Companies and ingredient quality can change over time, and it's almost impossible to verify product claims. In any case, no processed food can have the same quality as fresh, raw food. The convenience of these processed products is indisputable, however, and they have a definite place for many busy owners. Your best bet is to do a little research: Read labels and ask questions about the pet foods carried by natural food stores, quality pet outlets or any alternative-minded veterinarians in your area. Talk to local breeders. As with any product, quality usually costs more. If your local retailers do not carry any of the brands listed above, ask that they do. Several brands are also available through mail order (below).

PET SUPPLIES

Avena Botanicals, 20 Mill Street, Rockland, ME 04841, sells the following organically grown or wildcrafted herbal products for dogs and cats: a food supplement, calendula oil, ear mite oil, daily tonic, salves, flea-repelling powder and liquid castile soap with pure pine oil and herbal extracts. Send $2 for catalog.

Cedar-Al Products, 8353 Hoko-Ozette Road, Clallam Bay, WA 98326, sells several products that use cedar as a natural flea repellent. Some of these are cotton-covered pet pillows filled with cedar shavings, and carpet spray and freshener (good to reduce both fleas and pet odors). This company also sells a castile pet shampoo.

Color and Herbal Company, P.O. Box 5370, Newport Beach, CA 92662, produces and sells a line of natural pet items, including a cloth-covered herbal flea collar with reactivating herbal oils, flea-repelling herbal spray, an aloe-herbal pet shampoo and a tablet that is composed of yeast and garlic.

Dr. Bronner's Eucalyptus Castile Soap, sold in most natural food stores, makes a nice flea-repelling shampoo for pets and a good all-purpose soap for people. If unavailable locally, you can order it from Real Goods Trading Company, 555 Leslie Street, Ukiah, CA 95482. Please mail your envelope to the attention of the mail-order department.

Earthwise Animal Catalog, P.O. Box 654, Millwood, NY 10546, offers pet foods, supplements, furnishings, herbal products, homeopathic remedies and toys. All are selected by Anitra Frazier, author of *The New Natural Cat*, as pure, safe and earth friendly.

Fleabusters Rx for Fleas, 10801 National Boulevard, Suite 200, Los Angeles, CA 90064, has many licensed dealers around the country who can safely eliminate fleas from your home environment with a nontoxic natural mineral compound (orthoboric acid) that safely dehydrates developing fleas. The patented compound is EPA-registered, odorless and nonstaining. It's reported to be very effective by many clients. Neutral pH product does not damage your household furnishings. Money-back, one-year guarantee.

Halo, Purely for Pets, 3438 East Lake Road, Suite 14, Palm Harbor, FL 34685, sells several excellent products to veterinarians, including an herbal ear wash that reduces earwax buildup and a soothing herbal dip that can either be diluted with water or mixed with shampoo. They also sell a supplement that helps to ease flea-bite irritations, Dream Coat (contains essential fatty acids, garlic and Evening Primrose Oil), which may be used for all or for part of the vegetable oil called for in our recipes.

Harmony Farm Supply, P.O. Box 460, Graton, CA 95444, sells several excellent brands of alternative pest-control products, including Green Ban, Natural Animal (below) and Safer, a widely carried line of soaps, shampoos and sprays (for both pet and premises) that use pyrethrins and natural soaps to kill fleas.

Morrill's New Directions, P.O. Box 30, Orient, ME 04471, carries a variety of holistic pet-care products such as nutritional supplements, natural flea- and pest-control products, shampoos, homeopathic remedies, flower essences, training aids and books.

Natural Animal, 7000 U.S. 1 North, St. Augustine, FL 32095, makes and sells a variety of alternative pet products, including herbal powders, collars, shampoos, dips, and skin and coat enhancers. They also sell diatomaceous earth (to dehydrate fleas developing in cracks and crevices of the home), cedar spray for odors, catnip, cat litter made with peanut shells, pet snacks and all-natural supplements.

Nature Pet Care Company, 8050 Lake City Way, Seattle, WA 98115, is a good mail-order source for several brands of natural pet foods, supplements and flea-control products.

Pet Guard, 165 Industrial Loop South, Orange Park, FL 32073, produces a fine line of natural pet products: dry and canned foods using USDA-approved ingredients (passable for human consumption—unusual in the industry), vitamin-mineral supplements, a yeast-garlic powder mix, skin and coat supplements and natural shampoos good for skin irritations.

Vetri-Science, makes some nicely formulated supplements for dogs and cats, called NuCat and Canine Plus, both of which seem to be palatable to animals. They also supply Glycoflex and Vetri-Disk, two nutritional products that are helpful with arthritis and hip dysplasia. Sold through veterinarians only; you can ask yours to carry them.

Whiskers: Holistic Products for Pets, 235 East 9th Street, New York, NY 10003, is one of the most complete sources for mail-order natural pet foods, shampoos, flea products, herbs, natural remedies, treats, supplements, books, videos, toys and other pet-care products. Send for their free catalog.

Whole Animal Resource Store, 911 Cedar Street, Santa Cruz, CA 95060, is a mail-order source for several brands of natural pet foods, herbal flea products and shampoos and supplements.

Wysong Corporation, 1880 North Eastman Street, Midland, MI 48640, sells a natural, biodegradable litter-box filler (Wysong Litter Lite) and a concentrated source of natural pyrethrins (Wysong Py^2). This company also sells a wide variety of natural dog and cat foods.

OTHER USEFUL PET SUPPLIES

The Felix Company, 3623 Fremont Avenue, Seattle, WA 98103, makes high-quality sisal-covered scratching posts and platforms for cats, along with other feline specialty items.

The Dog's Outfitter, Humboldt Industrial Park, 1 Maplewood Drive, P.O. Box 2010, Hazleton, PA 18201-0676, is a wholesale catalog for pet professionals. They carry the "Doggie Dooley" and other in-ground mini-septic tanks to safely digest animal waste in your backyard. Many other useful items, including beds, scratching posts and cat furniture, pet doors, breakaway collars, tangle-free dog tie outs, flea combs, flea traps and a padded "kitty window perch." $50 minimum order.

SUPPLIERS OF PRODUCTS FOR NONTOXIC HOME ENVIRONMENTS

Real Goods Trading Company, 555 Leslie Street, Ukiah, CA 95482, sells water filters and products to test your home for electric fields, lead, radon and other household hazards as well as many resource-saving and nontoxic products.

Seventh Generation: Products for a Healthy Planet, 49 Hercules Drive, Colchester, VT 05446-1672, sells nontoxic household cleansers as well as many Earth-friendly products.

Nontoxic Environments: Products for Aware and Chemically Sensitive Individuals, 9392 South Gribble Road, Canby, OR 97013, sells natural and nontoxic building materials (paints, sealants, adhesives and such), fibers, bedding and flooring as well as full-spectrum lights, water and air filters and electromagnetic detection and shielding devices (see chapter 8).

SUPPLIERS OF HOMEOPATHIC REMEDIES

Boiron Borneman, 6 Campus Boulevard, Building A, Newtown Square, PA 19073.

Boericke & Tafel, 2381 Circadian Way, Santa Rosa, CA 95407.

Hahnemann Clinic Pharmacy, 828 San Pablo, Albany, CA 94706.

Standard Homeopathic Company, P.O. Box 61067, Los Angeles, CA 90061.

The Natural Pharmacy, 612 Calle de Valdes, Santa Fe, NM 87501.

Animal Natural Health Center, 1283 Lincoln Street, Eugene, OR 97401. Supplies a homeopathic remedy kit based on the remedies mentioned in this book, an emergency kit and tapes of Dr. Pitcairn's seminars. Please send a self-addressed, stamped envelope for information.

SUPPLIER OF BACH FLOWER REMEDIES

Nelson Bach USA, Wilmington Technology Park, 100 Research Drive, Wilmington, MA 01887.

SUPPLIERS OF HERBS

(Emphasizes organically grown or wildcrafted herbs where possible.)

Ambrican Enterprises, P.O. Box 1436, Jacksonville, OR 97530. Supplier of Juliette de Bairacli-Levy's original herbal formulas imported from England. Many other items are also available, including nutritional supplements, homeopathics and a complete herbal wormer. Publishes the Natural Rearing Newsletter.

Blessed Herbs, 109 Barre Plains Road, Oakham, MA 01068 (both dried herbs and tinctures).

Dial Herbs, P.O. Box 39, Fairview, UT 84629 (tinctures only).

Gaia Herbs, 12 Lancaster County Road, Harvard, MA 01451 (tinctures, oils, formulas).

Nature's Herbs Company, 1010 46th Street, Emeryville, CA 94608 (dried herbs; send 50¢ for catalog).

Mountain Rose Herbs, P.O. Box 2000, Redway, CA 95560 (send $1 for catalog).

HOLISTIC ANIMAL CARE MAGAZINES

Tiger Tribe: Holistic Health and More for Cats, 1407 East College Street, Iowa City, IA 52245-4410. Six issues per year, $18.

Natural Pet: Alternative Lifestyles for All Companion Animals, National Animal Health Alliance, P.O. Box 351, Trilby, FL 33593-0351. Six issues per year, $20.

HOLISTIC VETERINARY TRAINING AND ORGANIZATIONS

The following organizations provide holistic veterinary training. In this list the following key codes are used:

T = Provides professional veterinary training.

S = Seminars or conferences in holistic animal care open to the general public.

R = Provides referrals to veterinarians trained in their approach. Please send a self-addressed, stamped envelope and include your name, address and phone number.

J = Journal for members.

Academy of Veterinary Homeopathy, Richard Pitcairn, D.V.M., Ph.D., Director, 1283 Lincoln Street, Eugene, OR 97401, TSR.

American Holistic Veterinary Medical Association, 2214 Old Emmorton Road, Bel Air, MD 21014, SRJ.

American Veterinary Chiropractic Association, Sharon Willoughby, D.V.M., D.C., P.O. Box 249, Port Byron, IL 61275, TR.

East-West Animal Care Center, Training Program in Traditional Chinese Medicine, Cheryl Schwartz, D.V.M., 1201 East 12th Street, Oakland, CA 94606, T.

International Veterinary Acupuncture Society, Dr. Meredith Snader, Executive Director, 2140 Conestoga Road, Chester Springs, PA 19425, TR.

National Center for Homeopathy, 801 North Fairfax Street, Suite 306, Alexandria, VA 22314, TSRJ. In addition, this organization has local study groups that are open to laypeople.

Many lines of natural pet products have been developed and/or expanded, too many to mention here. There are many worthy products and, no doubt, many more to come. We use and recommend many of these products in our office; however, the inclusion or exclusion of any particular product does not imply an endorsement or lack of endorsement. Many are widely available in natural food stores and pet and feed supply outlets; however, mail-order sources are given in case you cannot find such products locally.

RECOMMENDED READING AND TAPES

CHAPTERS 3 TO 5

Harper, Joan. *Feed the Kitty—Naturally: Natural Recipes for Healthy Cats and Kittens* ($5.95) and *The Healthy Dog and Cat Cookbook* ($6.95). Creative, healthy fresh-food recipes for pets. Order from Pet Press, Box 328, Route 3, Richland Center, WI 53581. Include $1.20 for shipping and handling.

CHAPTER 8

Dadd, Debra Lynn. *Nontoxic, Natural and Earthwise: How to Protect Yourself and Your Family from Harmful Products and Live in Harmony with the Earth* (Los Angeles: Jeremy P. Tarcher, Inc., 1990). Excellent, comprehensive source book of information about the dangers of common household products, with more than 400 inexpensive do-it-yourself formulas and over 600 mail-order sources of nontoxic and Earth-friendly substitutes.

Pearson, David. *The Natural House Book: Creating a Healthy, Harmonious and Ecologically Sound Home Environment* (New York: Simon and Schuster, 1989). Beautifully illustrated classic with much information about why and how to use natural materials in homes.

Winter, Ruth. *A Consumer's Dictionary of Household, Yard and Office Chemicals* (New York: Crown, 1992). Lists hundreds of chemical ingredients in common products, with their derivations, uses, hazards and possible substitutes.

CHAPTER 9

Hart, Benjamin L., D.V.M., and Lynette A. Hart. *The Perfect Puppy: How to Choose Your Dog by Its Behavior* (New York: W. H. Freeman and Co., 1988). A helpful guide for anyone selecting a puppy, especially for the first time.

Pugnetti, Gino, and Elizabeth M. Schuler. (U.S. ed.), *Simon and Schuster's Guide to Dogs* (New York: Simon and Schuster, 1980). A well-illustrated guide to dog breeds.

Pugnetti, Gino, and Mordecai Siegal. (U.S. ed.), *Simon and Schuster's Guide to Cats* (New York: Simon and Schuster, 1983). A well-illustrated guide to cat breeds.

CHAPTERS 10 AND 13

Boone, J. Allen. *Kinship with All Life* (San Francisco: Harper San Francisco, 1976). This is a delightful true story of how one man came to understand animals and to respect and to communicate with them at a deeper level.

Minneapolis Institute of Mental Health, 1409 Willow Street, Suite 500, Minneapolis, MN 55403, sells a number of excellent, insightful books and tapes on reducing stress, anxiety, worry, depression, relationship conflict, grief and other common issues that can impact not only on you and your family, but also your pet. Order their free catalog.

CHAPTER 11

Benjamin, Carol Lea. *Second-Hand Dog: How to Turn Yours into a First-Rate Pet* (New York: Howell Book House, 1988). Witty, concise, loving book about rehabilitating dogs that have either never had a home or have been shuffled from one owner to the next, losing confidence, trust and self-esteem along the way.

Carlson, Jean. *Good Puppy* (Sound Dog Productions, P.O. Box 27488, Seattle, WA 98125-2488). A very useful videotape to help you train your dog and deal with behavioral issues. Phone consultations also available.

Kilcommons, Brian, with Sarah Wilson. *Good Owners, Great Dogs: A Training Manual for Humans and Their Canine Companions* (New York: Warner, 1992). We recommend this book to clients when they have canine behavior problems. As the author says, it's usually the owner that needs training—to learn how to effectively change unwanted dog behavior, prevent bad habits and create a warm, loyal dog.

McLennan, Bardi. *Dogs and Kids: Parenting Tips* (New York: Howell Book House, 1993). Unique focus on combining the principles of raising both dogs and children, especially useful for families with both.

McMains, Joel M. *Dog Logic—Companion Obedience: Rapport-Based Training* (New York: Howell Book House, 1992). A positive, in-depth guide that helps you train your dog to want to please you, by establishing a strong rapport between you.

CHAPTERS 14 AND 15

Day, Christopher. *The Homeopathic Treatment of Small Animals* (London: Wigmore Publications Limited, 1984). Good introduction to homeopathic treatment of animals by a highly respected English veterinarian.

Frazier, Anitra, with Norma Eckroate. *The New Natural Cat: A Complete Guide for Finicky Owners* (New York: Plume, Penguin Books, 1990). Sensitive, informative and insightful guide to natural cat care—a classic.

Kaslof, Leslie J. *The Traditional Flower Remedies of Dr. Edward Bach: A Self-Help Guide* (New Canaan, Conn.: Keats, 1988, 1993). A concisely written self-help guide for the beginner as well as the professional. In addition to outlining details on clinical and double-blind studies, this easy-to-understand reference contains a detailed self-help questionnaire specifically designed to assist readers in choosing the appropriate flower remedies for their needs.

Kruzel, Thomas, N.D. *The Homeopathic Emergency Guide* (Berkeley, Calif.: North Atlantic Books, 1992). A detailed reference guide to using homeopathic remedies in acute conditions.

Lazarus, Pat. *Keep Your Pet Healthy the Natural Way* (New York: Bobbs-Merrill, 1983). Interesting overview based on case studies and interviews with several veterinarians who treat pets with nutrition and other natural methods.

Levy, Juliette de Bairacli. *The Complete Herbal Handbook for the Dog and Cat* (New York: Arco Publishing, 1986). This book is full of useful tips drawn from herbal folk medicine and the author's lifetime of experience in using natural nutrition and remedies to treat animals.

Lust, John. *The Herb Book* (New York: Bantam, 1974). One of the best and most comprehensive guides to using, collecting and preparing herbs.

Panos, Maesimund B., and Jane Heimlich. *Homeopathic Medicine at Home* (Canada: Thomas Nelson & Sons, 1980). A very good introductory book with natural remedies for everyday ailments and minor injuries.

Schoen, Allen, D.V.M., M.S. (ed.), *Veterinary Acupuncture: Ancient Art to Modern Medicine* (Goleta, Calif.: American Veterinary Publications, 1994). Professional-level text on the modern practice of veterinary acupuncture, presenting research and practical guidance on its use.

Vithoulkas, George. *Homeopathy—Medicine for the New Man* (New York: Arco Publishing Company, 1980). The best introduction to the subject by an experienced practitioner. Highly recommended.

Vithoulkas, George. *The Science of Homeopathy* (New York: Grove Widefeld, 1980). Engaging, whole-picture insights into the nature of disease and healing, regardless of treatment methods used. Also an excellent foundation in the principles and use of homeopathy.

Vlamis, Gregory. *Flowers to the Rescue: The Healing Vision of Dr. Edward Bach* (New York: Thorsons Publishing Group, 1986). Interesting, readable introduction to the use of the Bach Flower Remedies, emphasizing Dr. Bach's stress-relieving rescue formula. Contains animal stories.

MAIL-ORDER SUPPLIERS

(Catalogs or information free unless stated otherwise)

Homeopathic Educational Services, 2124 Kittredge Street, Berkeley, CA 94704, carries books, tapes and computer software on the use of homeopathic medicines as well as introductory kits.

Homeopathic Informational Resources, Oneida River Park Drive, Clay, NY 13041, sells educational material on homeopathy.

Kent Homeopathic Associates, 828 Mission Avenue, Suite A, San Rafael, CA 94901, produces several computer software programs specially designed to assist in the selection of homeopathic remedies. The computerized "Acute Repertory" is especially useful for laypeople.

The Minimum Price Homeopathic Books, 250 H Street, P.O. Box 2187, Blaine, WA 98231. Many common and hard-to-find titles on homeopathy, from beginning to advanced levels.

NORMAL VALUES OF VITAL SIGNS

DOGS

Body temperature: 100.5 to 101.5°F (if taken at home when at rest, slightly higher in a veterinarian's office, but not over 101.8°). This range for normal temperature is more restricted than most veterinarians use, but is a more accurate guide based on considerable experience with "fever" cases.

Pulse: 70 to 120 beats per minute (at rest, higher if after physical exertion or if excited or frightened). The lower rate is seen in large dogs; higher rate in small dogs.

Respiratory rate: 10 to 30 breaths per minute (at rest, higher if after physical exertion or if excited or frightened). Generally faster in smaller animals.

CATS

Body temperature: 100.5 to 101.5°F (see qualifications as given for dog values, above).

Pulse: 110 to 130 beats per minute (same qualifications as for dogs, above).

Respiratory rate: 20 to 30 breaths per minute.

Parts of a Dog

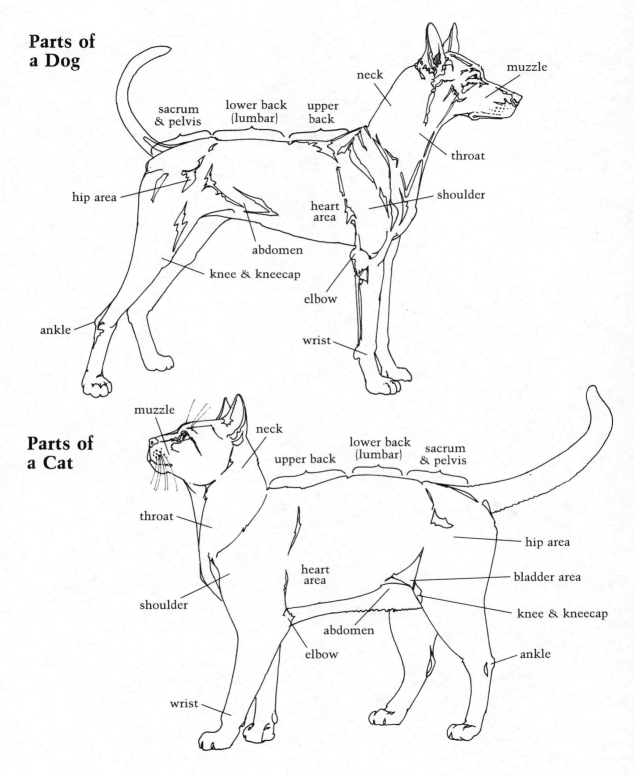

Parts of a Cat

INDEX

Note: <u>Underscored</u> page references indicate boxed text. **Boldface** references indicate illustrations.

A

AAFCO, 37, 58

Abscesses, 227–28, 232–33

Accidents. *See also* Emergencies, procedures
  car, 339–40
  dental problems from, 250
  paralysis from, 291

Acid, in commercial pet food, 240

Aconitum napellus, in alleviating fear, 178, 186–87

Acupressure, in treating breathing or heart cessation, 339, **339**

Acupuncture, 198–200, 203, 205

Additives, in commercial pet food, 17–18. *See also specific types*

Adoption, 179–80

Aggression
  in cats, 164–66
  in dogs, 151, 159

AIDS, 269, 272

Ailments. *See* Diseases; *specific types*

Airplane travel, 178

Air pollution, indoor, 108–9

Alfalfa, in easing change to natural diet, 87

Allergy problems
  desensitization injections and, 305
  diet and, 229
  drug treatments and, 96
  ear problems and, 261–62
  environment and, 231
  identifying, 231–32
  incidence of, 229
  natural diet in preventing, 229–31, 232
  recipes, for identifying food allergens and, 230–31
  skin problems and, 229
  symptoms of, 229
  urination problems and, 163
  vaccinations and, 232

Allium sativum. See Garlic

Aloe vera juice, for treating ear problems, 214

American Veterinary Medical Association, 199

Ammoniated glycyrrhizin, in commercial pet food, 17

Anal gland problems, 232–33

Anemia, 233–34

Antibiotics, birth defects and, 118–19

Antifreeze poisoning, 110

Antioxidants. *See specific types*

Ants, flea control and, 102

Anus, caring for, 214, 232–33

Appetite problems, 82, 210–11, 234–35

Arctium lappa (burdock), in easing change to natural diet, 87

Arnica (leopard's bane), in treating septicemia, 202

Arsenicum album, in treating sick or dying pets, 188, 203

Arthritis, 235–37

Artificial coloring, in commercial pet food, 18

Artificial flavorings, in commercial pet food, 18

Artificial respiration, 338–39, **338**, 341
Ash, in commercial pet food, 240
Association of American Feed Control Officials (AAFCO), 37, 58
Avena sativa (oats), in easing change to natural diet, 87–88

B

Barking, excessive, 158–59
Bathing
    conditioner for, 95
    flea control and, 94, 97
    grooming and, 94–95
    shampoos for, 94, 97
    sick pets, 211–12
    soaps for, 94
Beans. *See* Legumes
Bedding, 92, 97
Behavior. *See also specific types*
    aggressive
        in cats, 164–66
        in dogs, 151, 159
    appropriate, 150–52
    of cats
        aggressive, 164–66
        biting, 164–66
        by breed, 138–43
        controlling, 161–62
        correcting inappropriate, 162–66
        problems in, 162–66
        training and, 161–62
    diseases and problems with, 163, 166
    of dogs
        aggressive, 151, 159
        barking, excessive, 158–59
        biting, 151, 159–61
        by breed, 124–37
        controlling, 152–53

        correcting inappropriate, 155–56
        problems in, 158–61
        training and, 154–58
    inappropriate, 150
    problems, 236–39
        cat, 162–66
        diseases and, 163, 166
        dog, 158–61
Belching, 255
BHT, in commercial pet food, 18
Biological value of protein, 10
Biotin deficiency, 27
Birth. *See* Pregnancy
Birth control. *See* Neutering; Spaying
Birth defects
    antibiotics and, 118–19
    breeding and, preventing, 121–22
    cats
        brachycephalic head, 120
        brain and skull problems, 120
        by breed, 138–43
        cancer of ear, 120
        cardiovascular defects, 120
        cleft palate, 120
        cryptorchidism, 120
        deafness, 120
        eye and eyelid defects, 120
        hair abnormalities, 120
        hair balls, 120
        kidney missing, 120
        limb defects, 120
        mammary gland abnormalities, 120
        spina bifida, 120–21
        tail abnormalities, 121
        umbilical hernias, 121
    dental, 250–51
    dogs
        by breed, 124–37
        epilepsy, 119

eye problems, 119
 hernias, 119
 hip dysplasia, 119
 nervous system disorders, 119
drug treatments and, 118–19
environment and, 118–19
human vs. pet, rate of, 117
pregnancy and, avoiding, 118–19, 122
rate of, 117
Biscuits, as snacks, 35
Biting
 by cats, 164–66
 diseases caused by, 170–71, 296
 by dogs, 151, 159–61
Bladder problems
 in cats, 240–42
 commercial pet food and, 240
 common, 239–40
 in dogs, 242–44
Bleeding, 233–34, 342
Bloating, 313–15
Blood loss, 233–34, 342
Body openings, caring for, 212
Bone diseases
 arthritis, 235–37
 hip dysplasia, 119, 235, 280–81, 292
 invertebral disk disease, 291
 spondylitis, 291–92
Bonemeal
 in commercial pet food, 20
 as nutritional supplement, 38
Bones, as snacks, 34–35
Booster mixes, for dog kibble, 44–45
Bowel contractions, 255
Brachycephalic head in cats, 120
Brain and skull problems in cats, 120
Brain swelling in cats, 120
Breast tumors, 244–45

Breathing cessation, emergency procedures for, 338–39, **338**
Breeding
 birth defects and, preventing, 121–22
 effects of, 115–17
 ethical issues of, 117
 genetic weaknesses caused by, 117–18
 inbreeding and, 116–17
 for market demand, 117, 173
 neoteny and, 116
 population problems and, 151, 171–73
 safe methods of, 121–22
 selective, 116
 spaying and neutering vs., 171–72
Brewer's yeast, flea control and, 102
Brushes, for cleaning of coat, 94
Burdock, in easing change to natural diet, 87
Burns, emergency procedures for, 339
Butylated hydroxytoluene (BHT), in commercial pet food, 18

C

Calcarea fluorica (Calc. fluor.) therapy, 204
Calcarea phosphorica (Calc. phos.) therapy, 204
Calcarea sulphurica (Calc. sulph.) therapy, 204
Calcium
 chemical contamination and, counteracting, 111
 depletion, 293
 phosphorus ratio to, 37
 powder, 38
 requirements for cats and dogs, 28, 34
 supplements, 37, 38
 tablets, 38
Calculus buildup on teeth, 251

Calendula oil, for treating ear problems, 214
Cancer
    breast tumors, 244–45
    causes of, 245–46
    ear, in cats, 120
    preventing
        general methods of, 246
        natural diet in, 245–46
    treating, 246–48
Canine distemper, 257–59
Canine infectious tracheobronchitis, 175,
    317–19
Canine respiratory disease complex, 175,
    317–19
Capsules, administering to pets, 216, **218**
Car accidents, emergency procedures for,
    339–40
Carbohydrates, in commercial pet food, 11
Carcinogens, 70, 246
Cardiopulmonary resuscitation, 339
Cardiovascular defects in cats, 120
Carpet cleaning, flea control and, 97, 102–3
Car rides, 177
Carriers, pet, 178
Carrots, as vegetables in natural diet, 31
Castration, 162, 171, 172, 244, 308–9
Cataracts, 267
Cats. *See also* Recipes for pet food; *specific
        diseases*
    aggression in, 164–66
    bedding for, 92
    behavior of
        aggressive, 164–66
        biting, 164–66
        by breed, 138–43
        controlling, 161–62
        correcting inappropriate, 162–66
        problems in, 162–66
        training, 161–62

birth defects in
    brachycephalic head, 120
    brain and skull problems, 120
    by breed, 138–43
    cancer of ear, 120
    cardiovascular defects, 120
    cleft palate, 120
    cryptorchidism, 120
    deafness, 120
    eye and eyelid defects, 120
    hair abnormalities, 120
    hair balls, 120
    kidney missing, 120
    limb defects, 120
    mammary gland abnormalities, 120
    spina bifida, 120–21
    tail abnormalities, 121
    umbilical hernias, 121
body parts of, **361**
breeding and, effects of, 116
calcium requirement for, 28, 34
caloric needs for adult, 59
car rides with, 177
declawing, dangers of, 165
defecation problems in, 162–64
diet of
    bones in, 35
    changes in, 5
    extra needs, 66–67
    growth, 63–66, 74–75
    meat in, 20
    milk products in, 27
    nutrition in, 74–75
    raw foods in, 14–15
    taurine in, 15
    vegetables in, 31
    vegetarian, 74–75, 76–77
ear care for, 212, **213**, 214
eating cycles of, 59, 82

exercise for, 90–91, **91**
fights between, 162
housebreaking, 167
litter boxes for, 162–63, 167, 177
neutering or spaying, 162, 171, 172, 308–9
taurine requirement for, 15, 41, 76
toys for, 91, **91**
training, 161–62
trimming claws of, 165
urination problems in, 162–63, 240–42
vaccinations for, 325, 326
vital signs of, normal, 360
vitamin A requirement for, 39, 76
Checkup, health, <u>84</u>, 93
Chemical additives, in commercial pet food,
17–18. *See also specific types*
Chemical contamination
calcium in counteracting, 111
in commercial pet food, 18–20, 110–11
in environment, 93, 105–8, 231
in food, 18–20, 70, 110–11
grooming for removal of, 93–94
in meat, 20
minerals in counteracting, 111
skin problems and, 93
vitamins in counteracting, 111
waste products and, 195
Chemical pollution, in environment, 93,
105–8, 231
Chinese medicine, 195, 198–200, 203, 205
Chiropractic therapies, 195, 197–98, 204
Choosing healthy pets
checklist for, 122–23
importance of, 114–15
personal lifestyles and preferences and, 123
Chorea, 257, 259–60
Cleanliness
health of pet and, 92–93
sick pets and, 211–12

Cleansing reactions to natural diet, 83–84
Cleft palate in cats, 120
Cod-liver oil, as supplement, 39–40
Colds, 317. *See also* Upper respiratory
infections
Collapse, emergency procedures for sudden,
345
Coloring, in commercial pet food, 18
Combs, for cleaning of coat, 94, 97, 100
Commercial pet food
acid added to, 240
additives in, 17–18
ammoniated glycyrrhizin in, 17
artificial coloring in, 18
artificial flavorings in, 18
ash in, 240
bladder problems and, 240
bonemeal in, 20
butylated hydroxytoluene in, 8, 18
carbohydrates in, 11
chemical contamination in, 18–20, 110–11
color of, 18
concept of, 7–9
corn syrup in, 17
ethoxyquin in, 17
fats in, dietary, 11
fiber in, 11
4-D sources of, 16
gastric dilation and, 313
hormone levels in, 16
labels on, 9, 10–11
lead contamination in, 20
life energy concept and, 13
minerals in, 12–13
moisture content of, 12
nutrition of, evaluating, 9–10, 12
odor of, 16
propylene glycol in, 17
propyl gallate in, 17

Commercial pet food *(continued)*
  protein in, 9–11
  shortcomings of, 3, 9
    protecting pets from, 20–21
  sodium nitrate in, 18
  soft-moist, 16, 17–18
  sucrose in, 17
  synthetic flavorings in, 18
  during travel, 177
  trend in types of, 16
  unsavory ingredients in, 15–16
  vitamins in, 12–13
Conditioner, for coat, 95
Congenital problems. *See* Birth defects
Constipation, 177, 248–50
Conventional health-care therapies, 3–4, 191
Convulsions, emergency procedures for, 340
Corneal ulcers, 267–68
Corn syrup, in commercial pet food, 17
Coronaviruses, 270
Corticosteroids, in treating skin problems,
    304–5
Crude protein, 10–11, 12
Cryptorchidism in cats, 120
Cutaneous larva migrans (hookworms), 168,
    330–31
Cuts, emergency procedures for, 340
Cystitis, 241, 242, 282

D

Dairy products, 27–28, <u>33</u>. *See also specific
    types*
Dates, folic acid in, 35
Deafness in cats, 120
Death
  complexity of, 185
  euthanasia and, 186–87
  grief over, 185–86

home care and, 187–88
  hospital care and, 187
  significance of, 183–85
Declawing cats, dangers of, 165
Defecation problems in cats, 162–64
Dehydration, 211
Delivery, difficult, 293–95
Demodectic mange, 301
Dental problems, 250–53
Dermacentor andersoni (wood tick), 169
Dermacentor variabilis (dog tick), 169
Dermatitis, 229. *See also* Skin problems
Diabetes, 253–54
Diarrhea, 255–57, 295
Diatomaceous earth, flea control and, 103
Di-calcium phosphate supplement, 38
Diet. *See also* Fasts; Natural diet; Nutrition;
    Special diets
  allergy problems and, 229
  of cats
    bones in, 35
    changes in, 5
    meat in, 20
    milk products in, 27
    raw foods in, 14–15
    taurine in, 15
    vegetables in, 31
  changes, 5
  of dogs
    bones in, 34–35
    meat in, 20
    skin problems and, 3
    vegetables in, 31
  lacto-ovo vegetarian, 75
  new foods in, introducing, 81–84
  for sick pets, 210–11
  skin problems and, 3
  vegetarian
    for cats, <u>74–75</u>, 76–77
    for dogs, <u>72–73</u>, 77–79

health and, 69–70
issues in, 68–69
nutrition in, 72–75
recipes for, 76–79
Diethylcarbamazine, in heartworm
    treatment, 277–78
Dipylidium caninum (tapeworms), 168,
    330
Discharge, as sign of disease, 225–26
Diseases. *See also specific types*
    behavior problems and, 163, 166
    from bites, 170–71, 296
    discharge as sign of, 225–26
    healing of, 223–24
        body's role in, 224, 225–26
    holistic approach to treating, 222, 226
    homeopathic medications in treating, 222
    preventing, 222
    recovery from, 223
    relapses of, 224–25
    responsibility of owner in preventing,
        167–68, 169, 170, 171
    from scratches, 170–71
    from skin and hair contact, 169–70
    from wastes, 168–69
Distemper
    canine, 257–59
    feline, 257, 260–61
Doggie Dooley (mini-septic tank), 167
Dogs. *See also* Recipes for pet food; *specific*
        diseases
    aggression in, 151, 159
    attention and, providing, 152–53
    barking by, excessive, 158–59
    bedding for, 92
    behavior of
        aggressive, 151, 159
        barking, excessive, 158–59
        biting, 151–59, 161
        by breed, 124–37

controlling, 152–53
correcting inappropriate, 155–56
problems in, 158–61
training, 154–58
birth defects in
    by breed, 124–37
    epilepsy, 119
    eye problems, 119
    hernias, 119
    hip dysplasia, 119
    nervous system disorders, 119
bites from, 151, 159–61
body parts of, **361**
breeding and, effects of, 116
calcium requirement for, 28, 34
caloric needs for adult, 59
culture of, 153–54
diet of
    bones in, 34–35
    extra needs, 64–65
    growth, 72–73
    high-energy, 61–63
    meat in, 20
    nutrition in, 72–73
    skin problems and, 3
    vegetables in, 31
    vegetarian, 72–73, 77–79
distemper in, 257–59
ear care for, 212, **213**, 214
exercise for, 90, 91–92, 152
fights between, 160–61
housebreaking, 166–67
leadership role and, 153–54
lifestyle of city, 90
medications for, administering, 216, **217**,
    218
neutering or spaying, 162, 171, 172, 308–9
protein requirements for, 59
scent glands of, 232
sizes of, 63, 226

Dogs *(continued)*
  skin problems in, 2–3, 190
  toys for, 91
  training, 154–58
  vaccinations for, 325–26
  vital signs of, normal, 360
  vitamin A requirement for, 39, 76
Dog tick, transmission of Rocky Mountain
      spotted fever and, 169
Dr. Bach's 38 flower preparations. *See*
      Flower essences
Drug treatments
  allergy problems and, 96
  birth defects and, 118–19
  complications from, 191–92
  for cystitis, 282
  healing crisis and, interference with, 85–86
  heartworms and, 277–78
Dyes, food, 18
Dysentery, 255–57
Dystocia, 293–95

E

Ear cancer in cats, 120
Ear care, 212, **213**, 214
Ear mites, 264–65
Ear problems
  allergy problems and, 261–62
  anatomical problems, 262–63
  common, 261
  foxtails trapped in ear, 263–64
  mites, 264–65
  treating, 214
  water in ear canal, 263
Eclampsia, 293
E. coli poisoning, 26
Eczema, 93

Eggs, nutrition in, 27
Eggshell powder supplement, 38
Elbow, arthritis of, 235
Electromagnetic effects in environment,
      112–13
ELF energies, 112
Emergencies
  homeopathic remedies and, 337
  procedures
    artificial respiration, 338–39, **338**, 341
    for breathing cessation, 338–39, **338**
    for burns, 339
    for car accidents, 339–40
    cardiopulmonary resuscitation, 339
    for collapse, sudden, 345
    for convulsions, 340
    for cuts, 340
    for fractures, 340–41
    for gunshot wounds, 341
    for heart cessation, **338**, 339, 341
    heart massage, 341, **342**
    for heat stroke, 341–42
    for hemorrhage, 342–43
    for insect bites, 343
    for poisonings, 343
    pressure bandage technique, 343–45,
      346
    for punctures, 345
    for shock, 345
  supplies for use during, 337–38
Emotions
  health and, 144–48
  human, pet and, 147–48
  losses experienced by pets and, 145–47
  relocating of owner and, 174–75
  responding to, 146–47
  travel and, 174–75
Encephalitis, 159, 257–58, 265
Enemas, for sick pets, 211
Entropion, 268–69

Environment
    allergy problems and, 231
    birth defects and, 118–19
    chemical contamination in, 93, 105–8, 231
    correcting problems in, 113
    electromagnetic effects in, 112–13
    epilepsy caused by, 266
    food toxins in, 110–11
    home hazards in, 181–82
    microwave exposure in, 112
    nontoxic home products and, 108, 110,
        354
    poisonings in, pet, 110
    pollution in
        air, indoor, 108–9
        chemical, 93, 105–8, 231
        houseplants in reducing indoor, 108
        pesticides, house and garden, 109–10
        protecting pet from, 106–7, 113
        water, 111–12
    ultraviolet radiation in, 112–13
Environmental Protection Agency (EPA), 109
Epilepsy, 119, 265–67
Escherichia coli poisoning, 26
Ethoxyquin, in commercial pet food, 17
Euphrasia officinalis, in treating eye
        problems, 178, 212
Euthanasia, for dying pet, 186–87
Exercise
    for cats, 90–91, **91**
    for dogs, 90, 91–92, 152
    importance of, 90–92
    nutrition and, 89–90
    for traveling pets, 177
    waste products in body and, cleaning out,
        93
Extremely Low Frequency (ELF) energies,
        112
Eyebright, in treating eye problems, 178, 212
Eye care, 212

Eyelids, ingrowing, 268–69
Eye problems
    birth defects in cats and dogs and, 119,
        120
    cataracts, 267
    in cats, 120
    corneal ulcers, 267–68
    in dogs, 119, 178
    eyelids, ingrowing, 268–69
    inflammation, 268
    injuries, 267, 268
    treating, 178, 212

F

Fasts
    bone, 35
    breaking, 209–10
    break-in period of, 209
    digestive tract and, 93
    liquid, 209
    natural diet and, changing pets to, 82–83
    for sick pets, 208–9
    waste products in body and, cleaning out,
        93, 195
Fats, dietary
    animal, 11
    in commercial pet food, 11
    protein and, 59
    rancid, 11
FCV, 317, 320–21
FDA, 11, 17, 18
Fear in pets, alleviating, 178, 186–87
Feeding schedules for kittens, 68
Feline AIDS, 269
Feline calicivirus (FCV), 317, 320–21
Feline distemper, 257, 260–61
Feline immunodeficiency virus (FIV),
        269–70, 272

Feline infectious peritonitis (FIP), 203, 270–72
Feline leukemia (FeLV), 272–74
Feline panleukopenia, 257, 260–61
Feline viral rhinotracheitis (FVR), 317, 319–20
FeLV, 272–74
Ferrum phosphoricum (Ferr. phos.) therapy, 204
Fiber, in commercial pet food, 11
Fights
    cat, 162
    dog, 160–61
FIP, 203, 270–72
Fistulas, 227
FIV, 269–70, 272
Flatulence, 255
Flavorings, food, 18, 36
Flea control
    ants and, 102
    bathing and, 94, 97
    bedding and, laundering, 97
    brewer's yeast and, 102
    carpet cleaning and, 97, 102–3
    combs and, 94, 97, 100
    commercial products for
        ingredients in, 96, 98–101, 103
        labels on, 95–96, 96
    diatomaceous earth and, 103
    garlic and, 102
    herbs and, 102
    lawn care and, 101, 102
    lemon skin tonic and, 102
    mineral salts and, 102–3
    safe methods of, 96–97, 100–103
    sprays for, 103
Fleas, 96–97, 299, 300–301
Flower essences
    in health care, 205–6
    preparing, 219

suppliers of, 355
    in treating
        collapse, sudden, 345
        dying pets, 188
        nausea, 177
Fluoride, in water, 111
Folic acid, dates as source of, 35
Food. See Commercial pet food; Diet;
        Recipes for pet food; specific types
Food and Drug Administration (FDA), 11,
        17, 18
Food dyes, 18
Food groups, basic, 24–29. See also specific
        types
Food toxins, 18–20, 70, 110–11
Foxtails, 115, 263–64, 274–75
Fractures, emergency procedures for, 340–41
Fruit, as snacks, 35
FVR, 317, 319–20

G

Garlic
    flea control and, 102
    as food flavoring, 36–37
    natural diet and, easing change to, 87
Gas, buildup of stomach, 255
Gastric dilation, 313–15
Gastritis
    acute, 310–12
    chronic, 312–13
Goldenseal, in treating
    eye problems, 212
    human fever, 6
Grains
    in natural diet, 28–29
    protein in, 28
    recommended, 28–29, 28
    selecting, 32
Grief, from pet's death, 185–86

Grooming, 89–90, 93–95
Gum disease, 251–52
Gunshot wounds, emergency procedures for, 341

H

Hair abnormalities in cats, 120
Hair balls in cats, frequent, 120
Hair loss, 275, 307
Healing crisis, 85–86, 223–24
Health care. *See also* Holistic therapies
  acupuncture in, 198–200, 203, 205
  Chinese medicine in, 195, 198–200, 203, 205
  chiropractic therapies in, 195, 197–98
  complexity of health problems and, 189–90
  conventional therapies in, 3–4, 191
  drug treatments in, 191–92
  emotional connection in, 144–48
  flower essences in, 205–6
  herbs in, 195–97
  homeopathy in, 196, 200–203, <u>201</u>
  manual therapies in, 195, 197–98, 204
  naturopathy in, 194–95
  nutrition and, 3–4, 5, 6
  Oriental medicine in, 198–200, 203, 205
  physics in, 193–94
  reading and tapes about, 357–59
  tissue salts in, 203–5
  views of medicine and, 192
Healthy Powder, 37, 38–39
Heart cessation, emergency procedures for, 339, **339**, 341
Heart massage, 341, **342**
Heart problems, 275–77
Heartworms, 277–79
Heats (periods of sexual receptivity), 297, 308

Heat stroke, emergency procedures for, 341–42
Hemorrhage, emergency procedures for, 342–43
Hepatitis, 287
Herbology. *See* Herbs
Herbs. *See also specific types*
  dried, 215
  flea control and, 102
  fresh, 214–15
  in health care, 195–97
  homeopathic medications with, 203
  minerals in, 34
  modern drugs from, 196
  natural diet and, changing pets to, 87–88
  naturopathy with, 195
  preparing medicinal, 215
  as rinse for pets, 95
  schedules for treatment with, 346–47
  suppliers of, 355
  tinctures of, 215
  tissue salts with, 204
  in treating
    dying pets at home, 188
    eye problems, 178, 212
    human illness, 6
    motion sickness, 177–78
    sick pets, 214–15
Hering's Law of Cure, 224
Hernias, 119, 121
Hip dysplasia, 119, 235, 280–81, 292
Holistic therapies
  diseases and, treating, 222, 226
  magazines about, 355
  nutrition in, 6
  philosophy of, 4–5, 190
  use of, 4–5, 192–93
  veterinary training and organizations involved in, 355–56

Home care
    for dying pets, 187–88
    for sick pets, 207
    during travel by owner, 175–76
Home hazards, 181–82
Homemade diet. *See* Natural diet
Homeopathic medications
    acupuncture with, avoiding, 203
    administering, 216, 219
    benefits of, 196
    diseases and, treating, 222
    emergencies and first aid and, 337
    herbs with, 203
    naturopathy with, 195
    Oriental medicine with, avoiding, 203
    preparation of, 201
    schedules for treatment with, 348–49
    suppliers of, 354–55
Homeopathy, 196, 200–203, 201
Home remedy kit, 219
Hookworms, 168, 330–31
Hormone levels, in commercial pet food, 16
Hospital care
    for dying pets, 187–88
    for sick pets, 207–8
Hot spots, on skin, 93
Hot treatments, in naturopathy, 195
Housebreaking
    cats, 167
    dogs, 166–67
Human AIDS, 269, 272
Hydrastis canadensis. See Goldenseal
Hydrocephalus in cats, 120
Hygiene, 89–90, 92–93. *See also* Cleanliness
Hyperthyroidism, 223, 229

I

Identification, pet, 152, 162, 177, 180
Immune disorders, 229

Impaction, of anal glands, 232, 233
Inbreeding, 116–17
Infectious enteritis, 257, 260–61
Inflammation, of eye, 268
Inflammatory bowel disease, 229
Injuries, 267, 268. *See also* Emergencies,
    procedures
Insect bites, emergency procedures for, 343
Insecticides, 96, 98–101, 103
Insulin, lack of, 253
Intravenous fluid administration, 286
Invertebral disk disease, 291
Ion levels, in humans and pets, 113
Iron phosphate therapy, 204
Iron supplements, 40–41
Ivermectin, in heartworm treatment, 277,
    278

J

Jaundice, 281–82
Joints, degeneration of, 235

K

Kal bonemeal, 38
Kali muriaticum (Kali mur.) therapy, 204
Kali phosphoricum (Kali phos.) therapy, 204
Kali sulphuricum (Kali sulph.) therapy, 204
Kelp, in radiation toxicity treatment, 297
Kennel cough, 175, 317–19
Kennel stays, during travel by owner, 175
Kidney problems
    in cats, 120
    failure, 223, 282–86
    stones, 243
Kittens, feeding, 66–68, 69
Kneecap, dislocation of, 235

L

Labels
    on commercial pet food products, 9, 10–11
    on flea-control commercial products, 95–96, <u>96</u>
Labor, difficult, 293–95
Lacerations, emergency procedures for, 340
Lacto-ovo vegetarian diet, 75
Larch flower essence, in treating sick pets, 205
Lawn care, flea control and, 101, 102
Lead food contamination, 20, 110
Legumes
    in natural diet, 29
    protein in, <u>30</u>
    quick-cooking, 29
    selecting, <u>32–33</u>
Lemon skin tonic, flea control and, 102
Leopard's bane, in treating septicemia, 202
Leptospirosis, 168
Lice, 301
Licenses, dog, 152, 180
Life energy, concept of, 13
Limb defects in cats, 120
Linoleic acid, in vegetable oil, 39
Liquid medications, administering to pets, 216, **217**
Litter boxes, 162–63, 167, 177
Liver, limiting consumption of, 25
Liver problems, 281–82, 286–88
Losses experienced by pets, 145–47
Lost pets, 180–81, **181**
Lyme disease, 288–89

M

Magnesia phosphorica (Mag. phos.) therapy, 204
Magnesium phosphate therapy, 204

Mammary gland abnormalities in cats, 120
Mange, 170, 301–2
Manual therapies, 195, 197–98, 204
Mastitis, 295, 297, 298–99
McCarrison study of rats, 14
Meat. *See also specific types*
    in cat's diet, 20
    chemical contamination in, 20
    concerns about, environmental, 71–76
    in dog's diet, 20
    fatty, 25
    freezing, 26–27
    ground, 26
    lean, 25
    in natural diet, 25–27
    protein in, 25
    purer sources of, 25–26
    raw, 26, 168–69, 232
    selecting, 25–26, <u>33</u>
    in special diets, 70–71
    storing, 27
    varying feedings of, 25
Meatless burgers, as snacks, 36
Meat meal, digestion of, 11
Medicago sativa (alfalfa), in easing change to natural diet, 87
Mercury food contamination, 110–11
Metabolism disturbances, 327
Metritis, 297, 298
Microfilaria, 277
Microsporum canis (ringworm), 169, 170, 302–3
Microwave exposure, in environment, 112
Miliary dermatitis, 229
Milk products, digestion of, 27
Minerals. *See also specific types*
    chemical contamination and, counteracting, 111
    in commercial pet food, 12–13

Minerals *(continued)*
   in herbs, 34
   in raw foods, 13–14
Mineral salts, flea control and, 102–3
Mites, ear, 264–65
Motion sickness, 177–78
Moving of owner, response to, 174–75, 179

N

National Academy of Sciences, 109
National Cancer Institute, 109
Natrum muriaticum (Nat. mur.) therapy,
   204
Natrum phosphoricum (Nat. phos.) therapy,
   204
Natrum sulphuricum (Nat. sulph.) therapy,
   204
Natural diet. *See also* Recipes for pet food
   basic food groups in, 24–29
   carrots in, 31
   changing pets to
      body responses to, 85–86
      cleansing reactions to, 83–84
      fasts and, 82–83
      herbs in easing, 87–88
      interpreting reactions to, 86–87
      methods of introducing new food and,
         81–84
      problems in, common, 80–81
      results of, 22–23
   dairy products in, 27–28
   effects of, vs. processed diet, 14
   financial cost of, 30, _32–33_
   flavorings for, 36
   food selection for, 24, _32–33_
   grains in, 28–29
   legumes in, 29
   meat in, 25–27

nutrient balance in, 23–24
potatoes in, 31
in preventing
   allergy problems, 229–31, 232
   cancer, 245–46
   epilepsy, 266
snacks in, 34–37
supplements in, nutritional, 37–42
vegetables in, 31, 34
Natural pet products, suppliers of, 352–56
Naturopathy, 194–95
Nausea, 177–78, 310, 312
Neoteny, 116
Nephritis, 93
Net usable protein, 10
Neutering, 162, 171, 172, 308–9
Newborn animal, caring for, 295–96
Nitrogen balance index, 10
Nontoxic home products, suppliers of, 108,
   110, 354
Nose care, 212
Nose problems, 274, 317
Nutrition. *See also* Diet
   Association of American Feed Control
      Officials and, 58
   cleanliness and, 89–90
   in commercial pet food, evaluating, 9–10,
      12
   in eggs, 27
   exercise and, 89–90
   grooming and, 89–90
   health care and, 3–4, 5, 6
   in holistic approach to health care, 6
   in naturopathy, 195
   pregnancy and, 5, 293
   radiation toxicity and, treating, 297
   in raw foods, 13–15
   in recipes for pet food, 58–59
      for cats, _56–57_
      for dogs, _54–55_

rest and, 89–90
in sprouts, 34
vegetable oil and, 39, 297
in vegetarian diet, 72–75
Nutritional yeast supplements, 36, 297
Nuts, as snacks, 36
Nux vomica, for treating personality
    problems, 203

O

Oats, in easing change to natural diet, 87–88
Obesity, 327–29
Oriental medicine, 198–200, 203, 205
Orifices, caring for, 212, **213**
Orphaned animals, special diets for, 66–68
Overweight, 327–29
Owners of pets
  adoption of pet and, 179–80
  appropriate pet behavior and, 150–52
  cat behavior and
    controlling, 161–62
    problems with, 162–66
  disease prevention and, 167–68, 169, 170,
    171
  dog behavior and
    controlling, 152–53
    culture of dogs and, 153–54
    problems with, 158–61
    training, 154–58
  moving of, 174–75, 179
  population problems and, pet, 151,
    171–73
  relocating of, 174–75, 179
  responsibility of, 149–50
  travel by
    home care of pets during, 175–76
    kennel stays for pets during, 175
    pet's response to, 175–76
    preparing pets for, 176

P

Pancreatitis, 290–91
Panleukopenia, 257, 260–61
Paralysis, 291–92
Parasites
  ear mites, 264–65
  fleas, 96–97, 299, 300–301
  heartworms, 277–79
  hookworms, 168, 330–31
  lice, 301
  mange mite, 169–70, 301–2
  ringworm, 169, 170, 302–3
  roundworms, 168, 330
  tapeworms, 168, 330
  ticks, 169, 288, 289, 299–300
  toxoplasma protozoa, 315–16
Pasteurization, of milk, 27
Peke face in cats, 120
Peppermint, for treating nausea, 177
Periodontal disease, 251–52
Peristalsis, 255
Personality problems, 203
Pesticides, house and garden, 109–10
Pet food. *See* Commercial pet food; Recipes
    for pet food
Pet Food Institute, 11
Pets. *See* Cats; Dogs
Pet supplies, suppliers of natural, 352–54
Phenols, contamination from, 109
Phosphorus/calcium ratio, 37
Physics, in health care, 193–94
Pills, administering, 216, **218**
Poisonings, 110, 182, 343
Population problems, 151, 171–73
Potassium chloride therapy, 204, 211
Potassium phosphate therapy, 204
Potassium sorbate, in commercial pet food,
    17
Potassium sources, 35

Potassium sulphate therapy, 204
Potatoes, in natural diet, 31
Pottenger Cat Studies, 14–15
Pregnancy
  birth defects and, avoiding, 118–19, 122
  dystocia and, 293–95
  eclampsia and, 293
  newborn care and, 295–96
  nutrition and, 5, 293
Preservatives. *See specific types*
Pressure bandage technique, 343–45, **346**
Produce. *See specific types*
Propylene glycol, in commercial pet food, 17
Propyl gallate, in commercial pet food, 17
Protein
  biological value of, 10
  in commercial pet food, 9–11
  crude, 10–11, 12
  in dairy products, 27
  digestibility of, 10
  fats and, dietary, 59
  in grains, 28
  in legumes, 30
  in meat, 25
  net usable, 10
  requirements for dogs, 59
Psyche. *See* Emotions
Public Health Service, 105
Pulsatilla, in treating dying pets, 188
Punctures, emergency procedures for, 345
Puppies, feeding, 66–68
Pyometra, 297–98

Q

Quartz therapy, 204
Quiet time, 89–90, 92, 195

R

Rabies, 170–71, 296, 325–26
Radiation therapy, avoiding, 296
Radiation toxicity, 296–97
Radon contamination, 109
Rats, raw foods in diet of, 14
Raw foods
  cat study using, 14–15
  meat, 26, 168–69, 232
  minerals in, 13–14
  nutrition in, 13–15
  rat study using, 14
  vitamins in, 13–14
Reading and tapes about health care of pets,
    357–59
Recipes for pet food
  allergy problems and, 230–31
  cat
    basic, 50–53
    Beefy Oats, 50–51
    Cat Allergy Diet #1, 236
    Cat Allergy Diet #2, 236
    Cat Growth Diet, 63–65
    Cat Weight Loss Diet, 329
    fast and fresh, 53, 58
    Fatty Feline Fare, 53
    Feline Diet for Kidney Problems, 284–85
    Feline Feast, 51–52
    Healthy Powder, 39
    Kitten Formula, 67–68
    Kitty Catnip Cookies, 351
    Kitty Crunchies, 350
    Mackerel Loaf, 52–53
    meat, 50–53, 58
    meatless, 53, 76–77
    nutrition in, 56–57
    Pet Puree, 210–11
    Polenta for Cats, 76–77

Poultry Delight, 51
Quick Feline Eggfest, 53
Quick Feline Meatfest, 58
dog
  basic, 49–50
  Beans 'n' Millet, 79
  booster mixes, 44–45
  Canine Diet for Kidney Problems, 284
  Cottage Cheese Supplement for Dog
    Kibble, 45
  Dog Allergy Diet #1, 230–31
  Dog Allergy Diet #2, 231
  Dog Biscuits Deluxe, 351
  Doggie Crunchies, 350
  Doggie Oats, 46
  Dog Growth Diet A, 61–62
  Dog Growth Diet B, 62
  Dog Growth Diet C, 62–63
  Dog Loaf, 47–48
  Dog Weight Loss Diet #1, 328
  Dog Weight Loss Diet #2, 329
  Easy Eggs and Grain, 78–79
  fast and fresh, 49–50
  Fresh Egg Supplement for Dog Kibble,
    45
  Fresh Meat Supplement for Dog Kibble,
    45
  Healthy Powder, 39
  meat, 45, 47–48, 50
  meatless, 45–47, 49, 77–79
  Mexi-Dog Casserole, 78
  Mini Doggie Oats, 47
  nutrition in, _54–55_
  One-on-One, 48
  Pet Puree, 210–11
  Polenta for Dogs, 77–78
  Puppy Formula, 68
  Quick Canine Hash, 50
  Quick Canine Oatmeal, 49

  Quick Canine Oats and Eggs, 49
  Wheat or Rye Crisps for Dogs, 350
following suggested, 43
kidney problems and, 284
nutrition in, 58–59
  for cats, _56–57_
  for dogs, _54–55_
preparation for, streamlining, _44_
serving portions and, 43–44, 59, 63
Relocating of owner, pet's response to,
  174–75, 179
Renal failure, 223, 282–86
Reproductive organ problems, 297–99
Rest, 89–90, 92, 195
Retroviruses, 269
Rickettsia rickettsii (Rocky Mountain
  spotted fever), 169–70
Ringworms, 169, 170, 302–3
Rocky Mountain spotted fever, 169–70
Rosemary Conditioner, for coat, 95
Roundworms, 168, 330

S

SAD, 113
Salmonella poisoning, 26, 27
Salt-replacement fluid therapy, 211
Sanitation, 166–67. _See also_ Hygiene
Sarcoptic mange, 170, 301
Scabies, 170, 301
Scent gland problems, 232–33
Schiff Bone-all bonemeal, 38
Scratching
  by cats, preventing, 164–66
  diseases caused by, 170–71
Scratching posts, 164–65
Seasonal Affective Disorder (SAD), 113

Seeds, as snacks, 36
Seizures, 265–67
Selective breeding, 116
Selenium, in combating radiation, 111
Septicemia, 202
Serving portions, of pet food, 43–44, 59, 63
Shampoos, 94, 97
Shock, emergency procedures for, 345
Sick pets
    bathing, 211–12
    cleanliness and, 211–12
    diet for, 210–11
    home care for, 207
    hospital care for, 207–8
    treating
        Arsenicum album and, 188, 203
        bathing/cleaning and, 211–12
        body orifices and, 212, **213**, 214
        diet for, 210–11
        enemas and, 211
        fasts and, 208–9
        herbs and, 214–15
        homeopathic medications and, 216, 218
        home remedy kit for, 219
        Larch flower essence and, 205
        liquid medication and, 216, **217**
        pills/capsules and, 216, **218**
        Pulsatilla and, 188
        Tarentula cubensis and, 188
Silicea therapy, 204
Silicon dioxide therapy, 204
Skin care, 89–90, 93–95
Skin problems. *See also* Parasites
    allergy problems and, 229
    causes of, 303–4
    chemical contamination and, 93
    corticosteroids in treating, 304–5
    diet and, 3
    in dogs, 2–3, 190

eczema, 93
hair loss and, 275, 307
hot spots, 93
mange, 170, 301–2
miliary dermatitis, 229
ringworms, 169, 170, 302–3
Rocky Mountain spotted fever, 169–70
scabies, 170, 301
supplements and, nutritional, 3
symptoms of, 304
treating, 304–8
vaccinations and, 307
Sleep, 89–90, 92
"Slipped disk," 291
Snacks, in natural diet, 34–37
Soaps, 94
Sodium benzoate, avoiding consumption of, 40
Sodium chloride therapy, 204
Sodium nitrate, in commercial pet food, 18
Sodium phosphate therapy, 204
Sodium sulphate therapy, 204
Spaying, 162, 171, 172, 244, 308–9
Special diets, 60–61. *See also* Vegetarian diet
    for cats
        extra needs, 66–67
        growth, 63–66, 74–75
        nutrition in, 74–75
        vegetarian, 74–75, 76–77
    for dogs
        extra needs, 64–65
        growth, 72–73
        high-energy, 61–63
        nutrition in, 72–73
        vegetarian, 72–73, 77–79
    meat in, 70–71
    nutrition in, 72–75
    for orphaned animals, 66–68
Spina bifida in cats, 120–21

Spondylitis, 291–92
Spraying by cats, 167
Sprouts, nutrition in, 34
Star of Bethlehem flower essence, 205
Stomach problems
    acute gastritis, 310–12
    chronic gastritis, 312–13
    gastric dilation, 313–15
    indications of, 309–10
Stramonium (thorn apple), in treating
    personality problems, 203
Sucrose, in commercial pet food, 17
Supplements, nutritional
    benefits of, 37
    bonemeal, 38
    calcium, 37, 38
    cod-liver oil, 39–40
    di-calcium phosphate, 38
    eggshell powder, 38
    Healthy Powder, 37, 38–39
    iron, 40–41
    in natural diet, 37–42
    nutritional yeast, 36, 297
    skin problems and, 3
    with sodium benzoate, avoiding, 40
    taurine, 41–42
    vegetable oil, 39, 297
    vitamin, 39–40
    wheat-germ oil, 40
Surgery, 223, 308–9. *See also* Neutering;
    Spaying
Synthetic flavorings, in commercial pet food,
    18

T

Tail defects in cats, 121
Tapeworms, 168, 330

Tarentula cubensis, in treating dying pets,
    188
Taurine
    requirement for cats, 15, 41, 76
    supplements, 41–42
Thorn apple, in treating personality
    problems, 203
Ticks, 169, 288, 289, 299–300
Tissue salts, 203–5
Tooth decay, 253. *See also* Dental
    problems
Toxic contamination, from chemicals in
    food, 18–20, 70, 110–11
Toxins. *See* Chemical contamination; Food
    toxins
Toxocara canis (roundworms), 168, 330
Toxocara cati (roundworms), 168, 330
Toxoplasma protozoa, 315–16
Toxoplasmosis, 168–69, 315–17
Toys, 91, **91**
Training
    aids, 157
    cats, 161–62
    dogs, 154–58
Traumatic conditions, 205
Travel
    owner's
        home care of pets during, 175–76
        kennel stays for pets during, 175
        pet's response to, 175–76
        preparing pets for, 176
    pet's
        on airplane, 178
        commercial pet food during, 177
        emotions of pet and, 174–75
        exercise during, 177
        health problems related to, 177–78
Treatments, for diseases. *See specific diseases*
Trimming claws of cats, 165

U

Ulcers, corneal, 267–68
Ultraviolet radiation, in environment, 112–13
Underweight, 329
United States Department of Agriculture (USDA), 15–16, 20
Unsaturated fatty acids, in vegetable oil, 39
Upper respiratory infections. *See also* Distemper
  canine infectious tracheobronchitis, 175, 317–19
  colds, 317
  feline calicivirus, 317, 320–21
  feline viral rhinotracheitis, 317, 319–20
  symptoms of, 317
Urination problems in cats, 162–63, 240–42
USDA, 15–16, 20

V

Vacations. *See* Travel
Vaccinations
  allergy problems and, 232
  alternatives to, 324–25
  breast tumors and, 244
  cat, 325, 326
  dog, 325–26
  encephalitis and, 159
  epilepsy and, 265
  functions of, 321
  harmful effects of, 322–24
  ineffectiveness of, 321–22
  for Lyme disease, 288
  for rabies, 325–26
  skin problems and, 307

Vegetable broth, in liquid fasts, 209
Vegetable juice, in liquid fasts, 209
Vegetable oil, nutrition and, 39, 297
Vegetables. *See also specific types*
  in cat's diet, 31
  caution in using fresh, 31
  in dog's diet, 31
  in natural diet, 31, 34
  organic, 31, 34
Vegetarian diet
  for cats, 74–75, 76–77
  for dogs, 72–73, 77–79
  health and, 69–70
  issues in, 68–69
  nutrition in, 72–75
  recipes for, 76–79
Vegetarian Society of the United Kingdom, 75
Veggie burgers, as snacks, 36
Veterinary school training, 3–4, 5, 355–56
Vital force (underlying intelligence in body), 224
Vital signs, normal, 360
Vitamin A
  chemical contamination and, counteracting, 111
  in eggs, 27
  importance of, 12
  from liver, overdose of, 25
  requirement, for cats and dogs, 39, 76
  supplements, 39–40
Vitamin B_1, loss through heat processing, 12
Vitamin B_6, loss through heat processing, 13
Vitamin C, in combating chemical contamination, 111
Vitamin D supplements, 40
Vitamin E
  chemical contamination and, counteracting, 111

importance of, 12
supplements, 40
Vitamins. *See also specific types*
  chemical contamination and, counteracting, 111
  in commercial pet food, 12–13
  pet, 40
  in raw foods, 13–14
  supplements, 39–40
Vomiting, 310, 312, 326

W

Warts, 327
Waste products
  chemical contamination and, 195
  diseases transmitted by, 168–69
  exercise and, cleaning out, 93
  fasts and, cleaning out, 93, 195
  sanitation and, 166–67
Water
  in ear canal, 263
  fluoride in, 111
  in liquid fasts, 209
  pollution, 111–12
Weight problems, 327–29
Wheat berries, for grazing, 34
Wheat-germ oil, as supplement, 40
Wheat grass, growing, 34
Whipworms, 331
White oxide of arsenic, in treating sick pets, 188, 203
Wild animals, rabies and, 296
Wood tick, transmission of Rocky Mountain spotted fever and, 169
Worms
  animals affected by, 330
  hookworms, 168, 330–31

identifying, 330–31
naturopathic approach to ridding pets of, 333–35
roundworms, 168, 330
tapeworms, 168, 330
treating, 331–35
whipworms, 331

X

X-rays, radiation from, 296

Y

Yeast, as food flavoring, 36, 37
Yeast sprinkle, as food flavoring, 37

Z

Zinc, in counteracting chemical contamination, 111